D0122089

CLINICAL PRACTICE MANAGEMENT

Robert J. Solomon, PhD

Graduate School of Business
The College of William and Mary
Williamsburg, Virginia

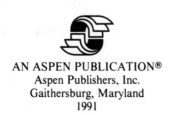

AN ASPEN PUBLICATION®
Aspen Publishers, Inc.
Gaithersburg, Maryland
1991

Library of Congress Cataloging-in-Publication Data

Solomon, Robert J., 1947—
Clinical practice management / Robert J. Solomon.
p. cm.

Includes index.
ISBN: 0-8342-0224-7
1. Medicine—Practice. 2. Medical offices—Management. I. Title
[DNLM: 1. Computer Systems. 2. Financial Management—methods.
3. Marketing of Health Services. 4. Personnel Management—methods.
5. Practice Management, Medical. W 80 S689c]
R728.S55 1991
610'.68—dc20
DNLM/DLC
for Library of Congress
91-4619
CIP

Editorial Services: Lisa Hajjar
Library of Congress Catalog Card Number: 91-4619
ISBN: 0-8342-0224-7

Printed in the United States of America

1 2 3 4 5

Dedicated
to the memory of my father, Charles W. Solomon, DDS,
to my mother, Helen B. Solomon,
and to my wife, Bernadette

Table of Contents

Acknowledgments

Many people have contributed to the completion of this book either through their remarks concerning its content or by reading and commenting upon chapter drafts. I thank the following individuals for this assistance: Fred L. Adair, PhD; Bruce P. Barnett, MD, MBA; William E. Fulmer, PhD; William T. Geary, PhD; Paul Grehl; Robert R. Johnson, PhD; Bernadette M. Jones, MSW; William Logan; Henry E. Mallue, JD, EDD; Stephen M. Mautner; Garland Tillery; William H. Warren, PhD; and Ned Waxman, JD.

Chapter 1

Introduction

In recent years increasing competition in medicine has forced many doctors to recognize the importance of the business aspects of health care for their prosperity and even survival. Some doctors have aggressively adopted formal management, marketing, and financial methods. They have observed that these methods can result in more effective delivery of services, increased profits, organizational growth, and a greater sense of personal control. Effectiveness, profit, growth, and control are objectives that medical practices share with most other businesses.

In some ways a medical practice is like any other business, and thus doctors can benefit from the methods and concepts that have proven useful in other types of business. For example, observing how long it takes to collect fees (aging of accounts) is an accepted business procedure that certainly has application in a medical practice. Similarly, utilizing marketing methods that present an appropriate organizational (practice) image as well as attract customers (patients) is as important for a medical practice as it is for a Xerox or an IBM. In short, the lessons learned by the Xeroxes and IBMs of the world should not have to be rediscovered by medical practices.

Medical practices *are* businesses. Unfortunately, the recognition of this fact by doctors and by those who train them has been a recent phenomenon. Doctors have historically been insulated from the razor of competition by the monopoly granted to them by their state licenses. When coupled with the relatively few practitioners produced by medical schools, this has ensured that doctors could set fees that would pay for operating expenses and provide a profit. It is also not surprising that the education provided by many medical schools has neglected or minimized training in the business aspects of operating a private medical practice. Medical school curricula are designed by academics, who are often unfamiliar with and uninterested in the nonmedical aspects of the health care profession.

Although medical practices are businesses, they do have their unique aspects. Providing medical services is not the same as producing bolts or selling soap.

There are qualitative considerations to operating a medical practice that would be lost in simply transferring accepted business practices to the medical world. This uniqueness is a result of several factors. The close, personal relationship that often exists between the patient and the doctor removes many of the adversarial boundaries normally defining a client's relationship to a business. If the doctor-patient relationship is not properly addressed, a conflict can arise between the humanitarian aspects of health care and the financial and ethical considerations that are necessary for organizational survival. The importance of professional services to the life of the patient, the cost of the services, and the history of accepted practices in the medical profession all must temper what otherwise might be acceptable business procedures.

How can the doctor achieve the objectives of effectiveness, profit, growth, and control? The answer is to utilize methods, procedures, and techniques that have been developed and successfully applied in other types of business but to modify them when necessary to fit the unique aspects of a private medical practice. How can the doctor identify the areas in which proficiency is necessary? A business school curriculum is a good place to start, since it is designed to educate those with no business background in all of the major aspects of operating a business. It can serve as a useful checklist of areas in which a medical practice must be able to function efficiently. All of the aspects of business discussed in this book are described below.

MANAGEMENT

Management is the glue that holds a practice together. It is the process of obtaining, organizing, and commanding all of the human resources associated with a practice. Whether you are a solo physician with a secretary, or a group practice with many associates and employees, the quality of management will determine whether personnel operate as independent dukedoms constantly fighting border disputes or act synergistically to achieve your vision of what your practice should be.

There are many aspects of managing a practice's human resources, including:

- *Employment methods:* knowing how to hire both professional and clerical employees.
- *Compensation:* determining equitable pay and benefits for employees.
- *Performance appraisal:* evaluating the job performance of employees and using this information to make personnel decisions, such as pay raises, training, termination, and so on.

- *Leadership:* guiding and inspiring professional and clerical employees to work toward the vision that you have set for your practice.
- *Motivation:* understanding what drives employees to act in specific ways when given a task to perform or a goal to achieve. By understanding what motivates employees you can structure the work/reward relationship to best achieve your objectives.
- *Organizational design:* putting the parts of the practice together so that they make sense, so that reporting relationships are logical and contribute to productivity, and so that jobs are composed of tasks that logically fit together and require an appropriate amount of work.

To be a successful doctor-manager, you must understand each aspect of management. This will enable you to develop a coherent management policy. You and your employees will consequently experience a sense of consistency and predictability in your interpersonal relationships. As a result, you will not have to be constantly looking over employees' shoulders to ensure that they are properly completing their work. In addition, employees will be able to respond to unique situations based on your vision of the goals and priorities that have been set for the organization.

MARKETING

Marketing is the process of identifying the services provided, pricing them, promoting them, and determining how they will be distributed or provided to patients. Successful service organizations are market driven. They identify what the *market* wants, and then they design or package the services to meet consumers' perceived needs.

The concept of marketing is distinctly different from that of selling. Selling is the process of persuading patients, for example, that they need a particular service. The "seller" asks the question, "Where and how can I find patients to buy the services that I currently offer?" In contrast, the "marketer" begins with patients; determines what they need, can afford, and so on; then designs, packages, prices, and provides services so that the patient has a natural affinity for it. The marketer asks, "Who are the likely consumers and what services can I offer at a profit that they will buy?"

Many doctors react to the marketing concept with skepticism. One typical response is to claim that all of the questions raised by the concept of marketing are already answered. For example, "The service that I should provide is what I was trained for in medical school" and "The patient is sick and comes to me to become healthy" are both typical statements made by doctors with a selling orientation.

Doctors with a marketing orientation understand that some of their services are in more demand or are more profitable than others. They develop and operate their practices accordingly. They also understand that treatment of medical problems may be only one part of what patients really want and only one of the services they can provide. Other things affecting the total marketability of a practice include furnishings and accoutrements (e.g., waiting room decor, professional and staff dress, etc.), courtesy, access, location, reputation, quality of facilities, and interpersonal relationships.[1] Finally, doctors with a marketing orientation understand that patients may never discover the services they can provide if they do not actively promote their practices.

Some doctors react to the marketing orientation by questioning the ethics of marketing. What you as a doctor consider ethical, given the local and national standards of the profession and the actions of competitors, is a personal matter. Certainly, what is generally considered to be ethically acceptable today is different from what was considered acceptable in the recent past. The marketing chapter of this book is designed to familiarize you with the marketing mindset and to give you the tools to implement effective marketing consistent with your personal ethical standards.

MANAGEMENT ACCOUNTING

Management accounting is the process of using accounting information to make management decisions. As a doctor you will be a *consumer* of accounting information, which will be generated for you by others, such as your business manager or accountant. Your objective is not to replace your accountant but to better utilize the available accounting information and to actively manage your practice based on this information. Management accounting addresses operational questions such as these: If I increase the size of my practice, what effect will this have on my profit? Which procedures, insurance companies, associated physicians, and so on, are responsible for my revenues? How much cash should I be able to collect in the next eight months? How much should I spend on overhead? How do I deter theft and embezzlement? What is a reasonable collections standard? What financial reports should I examine on a daily, weekly, and monthly basis in order to effectively run my business?

As a result of your management accounting knowledge, you will be able to more effectively and efficiently use consulting professionals, such as accountants, as well as the information that they can supply. You will also be able to use accounting data to plan for the future of your practice. By using techniques such as break-even analysis and budgeting, you can take active control over your practice's future and base strategic practice decisions on rational, considered thought, as opposed to speculation.

BUSINESS LAW

A medical practice constantly interacts with other entities, such as patients, insurance companies, landlords, suppliers, employees, and contractors. Many of these interactions have legal implications. Ideally, the time to address the legal implications of an arrangement is *before* it goes into effect. Documents must anticipate anything that can go wrong, provide for what you would like to have occur if something does go wrong, and be legally binding. You certainly will want to consult an attorney during this process and have him or her draft all written agreements.

There will be situations, however, in which you must make decisions without being able to contact your attorney immediately. By knowing how to recognize the legal implications of such situations, you may be able to avoid a legal blunder in the "heat of battle." The objective of the chapter on business law is to provide you with knowledge of basic business law concepts so that you will be able to respond in more appropriate ways on a daily basis, and will also know when and how to utilize your attorney.

COMPUTER SOFTWARE AND HARDWARE

Computer software and hardware can enhance your ability to manage your practice. For example, doctors are finding medical office management software (MOMS) increasingly useful. MOMS can be used to maintain patient financial records, including ledger cards, and to generate insurance bills, patient statements, and various management reports. Choosing the MOMS that best meets your specific needs is the single most important computer decision you will make. The chapter on computers will help you to determine which MOMS characteristics are most meaningful given the nature of your practice.

Computers also can be used for a number of other practice functions, including accounting, word processing, and database management. Accounting software allows you to produce many useful management reports independent of your accountant. Effective word processing software will increase the effectiveness of your clerical staff. Databases contain information about specific subjects. MOMS, for example, is a patient financial and treatment database. You may also want to construct other databases, such as a referral database, so that you can easily track where your referrals are coming from and why they chose your practice.

Software and hardware selection decisions are crucial and will affect the productivity of your practice for years to come. Mistakes can be costly. The chapter on computers is intended to (1) help you determine what your role should be in the selection and purchase process, (2) provide you with information that you will need to manage this process, and (3) familiarize you with possible roles for consultants.

STRATEGIC MANAGEMENT

Strategic management is the process of developing a plan for business success. It involves thinking about events in a larger context than today's immediate needs. Many doctors have no strategic plan. Their practices develop in response to their immediate personal goals or the transitory demands of the market place. Without a strategy, each management decision will be treated as a unique event. There will be no basis for determining whether specific decisions contribute to or work against important practice or personal objectives. As a result, many doctors who neglect to develop practice strategies find themselves disappointed or surprised with how their practices have matured over the years.

Many businesses fail or do not generate the expected level of profit for reasons that are entirely predictable. Strategic planning can help you to identify potential practice design problems and conceptualization and more profitable and satisfying practice models. The strategic management chapter discusses tools for identifying and developing a specific strategy for your practice. It will also provide several generic strategies that you can use as a basis for developing your specific strategy.

COLLECTION

Revenue is the wealth that you have generated through your clinical efforts. Your practice's collection methods must be thorough enough to convert a large proportion of this revenue into cash. Many businesses generate enough revenue to survive but nevertheless fail because they do not convert the revenue into cash efficiently. This can be a particular problem for medical practices, because they often must collect from both patients and insurance companies. This division of the debt between patients and insurance companies creates many opportunities for the collection process to fail.

The chapter on collection will teach you how to develop a collection plan for your practice that will improve your ability to collect from both patients and insurance companies. You will learn how to use management reports to identify insurance filing problems, unpaid claims, and unreliable insurance companies. You will learn how to manage the claim filing process so that problems are caught early and are prevented from growing into larger, profit-threatening or even practice-threatening issues. You will also learn why patients don't pay their medical bills, what your employees can do to increase their collection effectiveness, the strengths and weaknesses of alternative billing arrangements, and methods for preventing patient collection problems.

EXPECTATIONS

The professional relationships you have with your patients and fellow physicians will not prepare you for the relationships you will have with them in your role as entrepreneur, business associate, or employer. In each of these roles, the concepts of friendship and altruism are inappropriate. Reliance on friendship and altruism will result in disappointment and disillusionment. It may ultimately result in financial failure. A more appropriate standard for operating a medical practice is to apply the concept of equity.

Equity entails a continuous balance between what is given and received between any pair in an exchange. When equity is achieved, one party does not bear an undue burden in the hope that the inequity will be reconciled at some future date. Similarly, past arrangements are simply that—they are history. There is no unstated burden that is owed and that must be accounted for in some future arrangement. Focusing on equity may seem cold, impersonal, and in many ways inflexible. It may, in fact, be all of these things, but it is also a strategy that takes into account the reality of how people behave when money, pride, and power are at stake.

Operating a private practice requires an incredible amount of work. You will undoubtedly come to the conclusion that none of your employees have your motivation, perspective, or talent. You will have no vacations, simply time when you are unavailable to make the best decision or to head off the impending crisis. You must have a strategy for effectively responding to a job with unending and limitless demands. You cannot always be available. You cannot always *let* yourself be available.

The emotional experience of operating a private medical practice is a very real, important issue. Understanding and anticipating the emotional impact of opening and maintaining a practice is ultimately every bit as important as developing an effective marketing strategy or determining whether your cash flow will cover the next payroll. This chapter will help you to anticipate, understand, and master the personal and emotional aspects of being a doctor who operates a health care business.

HOW TO USE THIS BOOK

The following rules should help you to use this book more effectively.

Rule 1: Don't try to do everything yourself. Learn when to delegate work to subordinates and when to contract work out to consultants.

There are no magic shortcuts to operating an efficient and effective practice. Some of the methods presented in this book are complex, and they will take some time to learn and to implement. A common reaction when confronted with a complex matter is to wish that it would go away, then to dismiss it by stating, "I don't have the time to deal with this" or "It really isn't very important anyway." When you learn, for example, how to hire employees (Chapter 2), the methods may at first appear intimidating and time consuming. Your initial reaction may be to wish that there were simpler, equally effective ways of hiring employees or to pretend that hiring decisions really aren't very important. These would be dysfunctional reactions. If there were better ways of hiring, the Xeroxes and IBMs of the world would have invented them by now. Resign yourself to the fact that managing your business requires specific technical business knowledge. Acquiring the necessary skills and learning to apply them effectively will take some time. Failure to do so can be exceedingly expensive. Once acquired, however, these skills will differentiate you from many of your private practice peers and provide you with a competitive advantage.

When you don't have the time or the desire to personally deal with a complex matter, delegate it to a subordinate or contract it to a consultant. Remember, you are running a company that primarily generates revenue because you do clinical work, not because you personally hire employees or develop marketing plans. Why, then, is it necessary for you to be personally knowledgeable about the methods and techniques discussed in this book? The answer is that *you* are the chief executive officer (CEO) of your company, *you* bear the ultimate responsibility for what goes on in your company, and *you* will suffer the consequences if someone else fails to properly perform his or her duties. It is essential, therefore, for you to know how things should work in order to step in at critical times and to be capable of effectively evaluating the performance of subordinates and consultants.

Throughout this book you will find suggestions regarding which tasks you or your partners should personally perform, which tasks subordinates should probably perform, and which tasks are likely candidates for consultants. These are only suggestions. Use your judgment by balancing the time and task commitments that you and your subordinates already have against the cost of hiring a consultant.

Rule 2: Don't implement too many changes at once.

As you read this book, you may develop a panicky feeling that your practice is on the edge of chaos or that doom is just around the corner. This book probably contains many ideas and suggestions that you don't currently use. That you haven't been taking advantage of these ideas and methods does not mean that your practice is not coping with problems. Companies are in many ways like people.

They are resilient, can endure considerable injury, and generally find ways to adapt and respond to their environment.

Another possible reaction as you progress through this book is overenthusiasm. You may become like the child with a new hammer who quickly determines that everything needs hammering. Similarly, you may be motivated to simultaneously rework too many major practice policies and procedures.

Both panic and elation can be counterproductive, because they both can lead you to introduce too much change too suddenly. If you are currently operating a practice, a more realistic way to use this book is to rank by importance those things that you feel should be changed. Begin the change process by working down your list. Organizations and people can only absorb a limited amount of change at any given time. The chapter on organizational issues provides a number of ideas to consider when introducing organizational change. Rule 2 is important because careful, well-planned change will make your practice more productive, whereas ill-considered, uncoordinated change can create unintended confusion, turmoil, and damage.

> **Rule 3:** If you are just opening your practice, approximate as many of the management systems and ideas as possible rather than concentrating on one or two and totally neglecting the remainder.

The ideas discussed in this book are robust in the sense that they are still valuable even if realized in less-than-ideal form. Trying to fully comprehend and simultaneously implement all of the methods discussed could be an exhausting, distracting, and counterproductive start-up strategy. There is simply too much to learn and apply in too short a period of time. For example, you may be simultaneously trying to obtain a lease, develop a marketing plan, evaluate computer hardware and software, make certain that the money is available to open, and hire a business manager. It is impossible to concurrently do all of these things for the first time and do them well.

Rule 3 tells you, for example, to approximate as best you can under the circumstances what you know to be appropriate hiring methods. Don't reject the ideas that you have learned about selection methods just because you don't have the time to do an ideal job of evaluating business manager applicants. Delay work on those things that can be delayed, and try at a minimum to implement the *philosophy* of selection discussed in Chapter 2. If necessary, hire a consultant and postpone spending money on other, less immediate concerns. In short, don't easily give up your objectives in any area of operations. Set priorities, make compromises when necessary, always understand where your greatest exposure is at the moment, and then protect yourself against it to the extent allowed by your circumstances.

CONCLUSION

This book covers the major business subjects contained in a Master of Business Administration (MBA) curriculum as they relate to private medical practices. The object is to provide the doctor with an understanding of how the science (and art) of business administration can be applied to operating a private medical practice.

Doctors must make choices concerning the allocation of their time. This book takes the position that the private practice doctor is the CEO of a business and is ultimately responsible for the survival of that business. As such, the doctor must know enough about how a business *should* operate to be able to evaluate the performance of subordinates and consultants, step in at appropriate critical times in the management process, and determine overall practice strategy. This book is designed to provide this necessary knowledge.

NOTE

1. F. Crane and J. Lynch, "Consumer Selection of Physicians and Dentists: An Examination of Choice Criteria and Cue Usage," *Journal of Health Care Marketing* 8, no. 3 (1988): 16–19.

Chapter 2

Employment Methods

CHAPTER OBJECTIVES

This chapter will tell you how to hire employees using scientific selection methods and thus keep personnel costs due to turnover, absenteeism, poor job performance, and training to a minimum. You will learn

- how to use interviewing, testing, references, resumés, and work samples to ensure hiring the best available personnel
- how to organize the employment process so that it is as inexpensive and time efficient as possible
- your role in the employment process as well as the roles of subordinates and consultants
- how to recruit so that you can choose from a well-qualified pool of applicants

INTRODUCTION

Personnel management procedures include hiring employees, training them for their positions, evaluating their job performance, and determining their compensation levels. This chapter will focus on the employee hiring process. Using effective employment methods will help you to (1) reduce employee turnover; (2) cut training time and training costs; and (3) improve the productivity of employees and the quality of patient services.

Many doctors blame their personnel problems on their employees. Employees certainly are responsible for their own incompetent behavior. You, however, are responsible for hiring them. Whenever and wherever a mess occurs in your company, you also will have the ultimate responsibility for fixing it.

11

It is your responsibility to determine before hiring whether an applicant is capable of performing the job. A generally applicable employee selection strategy is to have applicants perform tasks that will simulate eventual job performance, and to do this in such a way that you can evaluate applicants against each other. In order to use this strategy, you must first determine which tasks are actually performed on the job. If you don't really understand what an employee does, then you will not know what to look for when you are evaluating applicants. The process of discovering what employees really do when they are working is called *job analysis*.

Next, you must choose the appropriate tools for making the hiring decision. These tools include interviews, tests, references, and resumés, to name a few. Since each tool has distinct strengths and weaknesses, you will have to learn when to use each one. Many medical practices limit their choice of employment methods to interviews or, perhaps, to a particular test routinely used for all jobs. This strategy will result in less-than-ideal employment decisions. It is analogous to having only two tools in your garage and using them for all jobs performed around the house. Try digging a ditch with a rake or cutting the lawn with a hedge trimmer. It *can* be done, but the costs in terms of time, effort, and the quality of the final product are ridiculously high.

It is also important to generate a large pool of applicants. Even if you develop a perfectly good employment procedure, it will not help you much if competent applicants do not apply for the job. The process of generating an applicant pool is called *recruiting*. It is important to know how to recruit a good applicant pool as well as how to select from it effectively.

Finally, you will need a *selection strategy* for sifting through the applicant pool. In addition to identifying the best applicant, you must be able to apply your selection tools efficiently and cost-effectively. If you don't have a workable selection strategy, you will get bogged down in a swamp of applicants and will waste valuable time evaluating candidates who should have been eliminated at the beginning of the process.

The following discussion of these topics focuses on the hiring of clerical, administrative, and supervisory personnel, such as office managers, computer operators, and secretaries. These will be referred to collectively as "front office" jobs. Most hiring conducted by medical practices is concerned with these front office positions. The strategy and tools for hiring physicians and other professionals is generally the same as for hiring front office personnel. Those considerations unique to filling professional positions will be discussed in a separate section of this chapter.

In summary, you should develop a hiring method for a job in the following manner. First, you should determine the tasks that are performed on the job. Second, you should identify appropriate selection tools. Third, you should develop a recruiting strategy. Fourth, you should construct a decision-making procedure for identifying the best applicant. Finally, you should do all of these things in a simple, timely, and inexpensive manner. After all, you are not in the business of hiring, you are in the business of practicing medicine, which is where you should devote your time.

The methods described in this chapter will be discussed as things that *you* should do. In a technical sense, you are ultimately responsible for whatever goes on in your practice. However, all of the methods discussed can be carried out by a well trained subordinate or a consultant. Because of the value of your time, you will want to involve yourself personally only at selected critical points in the process—and then only for certain jobs. Nevertheless, it is essential that you understand what should be done so that you can assign the tasks to subordinates or consultants appropriately and determine whether they have completed the work properly. At various points in this chapter, suggestions regarding who should normally perform particular tasks will be made.

JOB ANALYSIS AND SELECTION FACTORS

In order to hire the right person for a job, you must first understand the content of the job in detail. If you don't know what skills and abilities are needed to perform the job, then you cannot determine whether an applicant has the appropriate skills or abilities. Employee selection, therefore, always starts with collecting information about the job. The process of collecting this information is called *job analysis,* and the resulting document describing the job is called a *job description.* Exhibit 2-1 is a sample job description.

Job analysis can be performed in a number of different ways. If there is an employee currently performing the job, you can interview that employee. You want to know exactly what the employee does and how often he or she does it. You might ask the employee to verbally walk you through a typical workday. Also have the employee describe any tasks that are performed only weekly or monthly.

Another good way of obtaining job analysis information is to observe the employee performing the job. Keep in mind that, because of your presence, the employee may change the job content or speed up or slow down the performance of tasks. (Although an employee may tend to exaggerate the importance or frequency of some tasks, it is rare that he or she will fabricate or totally eliminate tasks. This is especially true in a small organization such as a medical practice, where the employee might well expect that you generally know the content of the job.)

Finally, sometimes you can obtain important information about a job by briefly performing the job yourself. This technique will familiarize you with the small points that might easily be missed in an interview. For example, I recently did a job analysis of a computer operator/secretary position. By doing the job myself for a few minutes, I discovered that it is not unusual for a patient to be at the window

Exhibit 2-1 Job Description for the Position of Computer Operator/Secretary

---

Primary Duties

The Computer Operator/Secretary is the primary expert in the operation of the computer system. Duties include the operation of all computer hardware and software, troubleshooting problems with hardware and software, learning how to use new hardware and software, training new employees in the operation of hardware and software, making recommendations for the acquisition of new hardware and software, and developing procedures and taking the responsibility for ensuring that all databases are backed up on a regular basis.

In addition, it is the responsibility of the Computer Operator/Secretary to identify methods and procedures for the operation of the office in the event that the computer system becomes temporarily inoperative and to train appropriate personnel regarding these methods and procedures.

The Computer Operator/Secretary must be proficient in the operation of MediMac, word processing (Word 4.0), database (Filemaker II), and spreadsheet (Excel) programs.

Secretarial duties include patient interaction, answering telephones, scheduling appointments, collecting fees, word processing, and other duties and responsibilities as assigned by the supervisor.

Major Job Performance Factors

- Operating and troubleshooting computer hardware and software
- Proficiency in various programs, including MediMac, Word 4.0, Excel, Filemaker II
- Patient interaction—personal and telephone
- Office activities—word processing, filing, scheduling appointments
- Collecting fees

Supervision

The Computer Operator/Secretary reports to the business manager.

---

paying for a session and scheduling a new appointment while the telephone is ringing and someone else is grabbing the appointment book. Performing the work conveyed an intensity that was not readily apparent from interviewing or observing the job incumbent.

Any job analysis method can lead to judgments that may be altered when the information is checked using an alternative method. A good example of this was a job analysis I conducted for a bus company. After interviewing several bus drivers, I was very impressed with the complexity of the job—to such a degree that I was inclined to rate the job as only slightly less demanding than that of astronaut or polar explorer. To check my observations, I bought a ticket and rode the buses for a few hours. This put things back into perspective. The tasks were performed exactly as the drivers had described to me in the interviews. The circumstances under which they were performed, however, were very different. The drivers had not tried to deceive me. Quite the contrary, they were very aware of what they did on a daily basis and had accurately conveyed this to me. But all of us probably feel that our jobs are a little more difficult or a little more important than an independent observer might report.

Once you have a good sense of what the job entails, write a job description. The job description in Exhibit 2-1 is typical. Job descriptions should be written in concise, clear language. There is no point to using excessive, flowery, or imprecise language. The object is to identify the major job performance issues. It is not necessary for the job description to describe the position down to the last detail. Don't be worried, therefore, if your job description is a "little rough." The next step involves reducing the job description down to a handful of major performance issues. As long as you don't miss a major job responsibility, the remaining steps will not be jeopardized.

The whole job analysis and description process should not take much time. You should be able to interview a typical clerical incumbent in about 30 minutes. Perhaps observation of any critical or confusing parts of the job will take another 20 minutes. Writing the job description should take no more than 30 minutes. In a little over an hour you can construct a document that will help to ensure you will hire the best applicant. The cost associated with this process is minimal when you consider how many hours it might take to fix the problems that would result from hiring the wrong person. In addition, the job description only needs to be changed if the job changes. It is quite possible, therefore, to use the same job description for many years and for the selection of several job holders.

You should construct job descriptions before you need them. When employees give notice or are fired, you must move as quickly as possible. In addition, terminated employees and employees who resign because they are unhappy tend not to be cooperative. It is best, therefore, to write the descriptions in advance so that they will be available in an emergency. You will also use job descriptions in most other personnel management procedures, including performance evaluation and training. Thus, having job descriptions on hand will expedite these procedures.

If you are starting a new medical practice, you obviously can't interview the job incumbent. There are, however, a number of ways to obtain the information you need. Start by mentally visualizing all of the tasks that must be performed in the practice, then separate them into logical clusters. These logical clusters will be jobs. As you will see in a later chapter, the practice of visualizing a logical cluster of tasks is an important method for creating the structure of an efficient organization. If you couple this "what if" analysis with a healthy dose of adaptability and flexibility, your initial job descriptions will be adequate. Another way of acquiring job analysis information is to obtain access to a colleague's practice and unobtrusively observe and interview the personnel there.

Once you have constructed a job description for a position you want to fill, you must now distill it down to the major employment issues, which are called *selection factors*. The typical selection factors for a clerical position include typing, filing, telephone skills, verbal skills, assertiveness, and clerical speed. Applicants will be evaluated with respect to these factors. There are three reasons for this reduction process:

1. It would take too much time to evaluate applicants on their ability to perform *all* tasks that make up the job. You must concentrate, therefore, on the most important job performance issues.
2. Not all tasks are important. If they are not important, then you don't want to waste time basing your selection on them.
3. Many tasks cluster together because they require the same fundamental skills or knowledge. For example, it is not necessary to assess whether an applicant can type letters as opposed to memos or address labels. There is an underlying factor here: *typing ability*. If the applicant possesses the basic skill of typing, it is reasonable to assume that this skill can be applied to a number of circumstances that only differ superficially.

Table 2-1 contains the selection factors for a computer operator/secretary position. By comparing Exhibit 2-1 and Table 2-1, you can see the logical connection between the job description and the selection factors. Generally, you can adequately describe a job using between four and seven selection factors. If you draft more than eight selection factors, look at them carefully to see if you can combine a few. If you can't, then you should consider whether the job is too broad for any one person to perform adequately. It may be that a broad job can be performed when you first open your practice, because the workload is relatively light. As your practice grows and the workload increases, however, the employee may become overburdened.

The selection factors will now form the basis of your selection procedure. Remember, the object of this procedure is to determine *in advance of hiring* whether

---

Table 2-1 Selection Factors for the Job of Computer Operator/Secretary

Factor	Description
Software and hardware skills	Ability to learn and use Word 4.0, Filemaker II, Excel, MediMac, or similar types of programs
Typing skills	Ability to type correctly and speedily
Interpersonal skills	Ability to communicate in socially appropriate ways with others
Anticipatory skills	Ability to anticipate the effects of actions on patients and peers
Language skills	Ability to speak and write in grammatically correct ways

the applicants are capable of performing the job. The general strategy of selection, therefore, is to have applicants perform tasks that will indicate their eventual job performance and to do this in such a way that you can compare applicants against each other.

Who Should Conduct Job Analyses and Write Job Descriptions?

The most appropriate persons to perform these tasks are the supervisors of the positions. You should only consider becoming personally involved for positions that report directly to you, such as the position of nurse or business manager. If you decide that you don't want to be personally involved in the job analysis of a position that reports to you, then an employee whose position is at the same level or another supervisor would be an appropriate choice. For example, an office manager could analyze a business manager position and vice versa. Business managers and office managers should analyze positions that are directly subordinate to them.

Assuming that you will delegate these tasks to someone, you should examine the final list of selection factors and compare them to the job description. You should be able to discern a logical relationship between the two documents. Personally performing this check will serve as a control, providing some assurance that the analysis was properly performed.

All of this work could easily be contracted out to a consultant. If you choose to use a consultant, it is a good idea to have the consultant simultaneously train one of your employees in job analysis methods, since these skills are easily learned. By doing this, you will reduce the likelihood of having to pay future consulting fees. A management consultant should be able to do a job analysis in one to two hours, and write the job description and identify selection factors in another one to two hours. These time estimates are longer than those for medical practice personnel, because consultants will be less familiar with the content of the jobs and will produce more polished documents, thus requiring additional time.

SELECTION TOOLS

The Interview

The interview is the most commonly used selection tool. Unfortunately, given the way that it is normally used, it is also one of the least effective.[1] Management research, beginning as early as 1915, has consistently indicated that interviews tend to have low reliability. This means that if you were to interview the same person on two different occasions, your conclusions might not agree. Similarly, if two interviewers interviewed the same applicant, they also might not reach the same conclusions. Research also indicates that the interview has low validity.[2] This means that interviewer predictions of eventual employee job performance tend to be inaccurate. If this is the case, why is the interview the most commonly used selection tool and why has its use persisted over the years?

The answers to these questions tell us a lot about employers and a lot about the misuse of the interview. Many employers view the hiring process as a test of their own personal intuition. They don't view the interview as a distinct tool. Instead, they believe that their personal intuition is the tool and that the interview simply provides a time, a place, and an excuse to utilize their intuition. If in fact the interview is really nothing more than an opportunity to apply intuition and perspicacity, then it requires no prior preparation. In addition, most employers don't want to take the time to prepare a proper interview. As a result, the interview is typically a morass of questions that are either "pets" (posed to all applicants irrespective of the job) or created on the spot with little or no thought regarding what is being measured or how to evaluate the applicant's response.

Irrespective of the research evidence, interviewers are usually convinced that they make good employment decisions.[3] Two factors usually operate to create this fallacious belief in success. First, we all tend to remember the past selectively. Good employment decisions tend to be remembered and bad ones tend to be forgotten or explained away. Second, there will always be a natural incidence of success in choosing from any pool of applicants. Even if you make selections by tossing coins, some of those chosen will be successful employees. If a job is minimally demanding or if your recruiting is effective, many of the applicants might well have the appropriate skills. As a consequence, even poor interviewing will result in some hiring success, and the interviewer will be led to overestimate his or her contribution to this success. The interviewer will then continue to use the interview in ways that contribute little or nothing to obtaining better employees. The danger of this unfounded assumption of competence is that the interviewer will use the same poor interview techniques for difficult and demanding jobs and will obtain unsatisfactory results.

Fortunately, all of this does not mean that the interview is useless; rather, it is a testimonial to its routine misuse. In general, the best selection methods require applicants to perform as they would on the job. Consider what you are asking applicants to do during an interview: to communicate and interact in a social situation. Therefore, there *is* a strategy for successfully using the interview. Going back to the idea of selection factors, you should only use the interview for selection factors involving communication and interpersonal skills.

You would probably unconsciously abide by this rule in certain extreme cases. Few employers, for example, would ask an applicant if he or she is a good typist. Obviously, a simple typing test is a superior way to assess typing competence. Once we go beyond these obvious examples, however, employers are inclined to misuse the interview in other absurd, if less obvious, ways. For example, if you use the interview to assess technical skills, reliability, learning ability, intelligence, or work attitudes, you are misusing this tool. These factors can be more accurately and easily assessed using other methods.

When using the interview to assess communication and interpersonal skills, construct a *structured* interview. To do this, write your questions ahead of time. Each question should directly relate to a specific selection factor. By writing the questions ahead of time, you will be certain to

1. ask questions that relate directly to employment factors
2. pose the same questions to all applicants
3. avoid asking questions for which it is difficult or impossible to determine what constitute good answers

Think about the *characteristics* of good and poor responses to your questions. I stress the word characteristics because you will never be able to anticipate all of the answers that applicants will give to a question. You can develop a concept, however, of what would be typical of a better answer. You can then use this to evaluate applicant responses. In larger organizations, it is often useful to define and label specific scoring categories. It is usually sufficient to anticipate three levels of response to a question, such as "outstanding," "acceptable," and "not acceptable." Sample structured questions and response categories are found in Exhibit 2-2. The number of evaluation categories is arbitrary and should depend on what you find to be useful. Some questions could generate five easily separated categories, whereas other questions could be evaluated with only two categories.

Whether or not you formally generate and write down scoring categories, it is important to think about the characteristics of good and bad responses so that (1) you don't allow your experiences with applicants to influence the criteria that you develop, and (2) you don't waste time asking questions that don't give you the information you need or for which you aren't certain what constitute better answers.

When you are conducting the interview, you should concentrate on what the applicant is saying and take notes for later evaluation. After the interview, you can rewrite your notes into a more complete narrative evaluation so that you can more easily recall the applicant's responses. You can also then classify the responses into scoring categories. If the applicant says something that you want to pursue, feel free to pursue it. Be certain, however, to come back to the point of departure and proceed from there.

It is very important to understand that your evaluation criteria express a value system. For example, look at Question 3 in Exhibit 2-2. Some doctors would favor the last ("poor") answer and would evaluate applicants who suggest discussing the personal and business implications of a personal problem as having poor supervi-

Exhibit 2-2 Structured Interview Questions and Response Categories for Supervisor Skills

---

Supervisory Skills: Exhibiting patience and tactfulness when dealing with fellow employees, remaining open to new ideas and suggestions, and listening to and understanding employee needs.

1. How would you handle a situation in which there is a deterioration in a subordinate's performance?
   a. Good: answer refers to attempts to determine the cause and to institute corrective actions.
   b. Fair: answer refers to confrontation with and warning of subordinate.
   c. Poor: answer refers to dismissal of subordinate with no attempt at corrective action or to corrective actions that do not directly address the performance problem.
2. Lori is a secretary who collects patient fees and does typing and other clerical tasks. She comes to you with an idea for improving the negotiation of patient fees. Negotiation of patient fees is your job, not hers. How would you respond?
   a. Good: answer refers to sincere evaluation of the subordinate's suggestion and to attempt to understand the reasons why it was suggested.
   b. Poor: answer refers to superficial acceptance without evaluation, or to outright rejection of the idea of a subordinate making such a suggestion.
3. An employee comes to you to discuss a personal problem. How would you respond to this situation?
   a. Good: answer characterized by setting aside time to examine with the employee the problem's possible job-related consequences as well as the personal consequences.
   b. Fair: answer characterized by a discussion of the job-related consequences.
   c. Poor: answer characterized by a discussion of the personal consequences.
   d. Very Poor: answer characterized by refusal to discuss the problem and telling the employee, implicitly or explicitly, to leave personal problems at home.

---

sory skills. The scoring categories should reflect *your* preferences. There is nothing wrong with this as long as you understand your preferences and consciously build them into the applicant evaluation process. Problems arise when you select employees on one basis but then ask them to perform in a contrary manner. If you feel that the best strategy for running an office is to refuse to discuss personal problems, then don't hire applicants whose natural inclination, as reflected by their answers, is to deal with such problems.

In order to achieve consistency between your preferences and employee characteristics, you may have to engage in some serious introspection. For example, discussing personal problems with someone is socially acceptable. It sounds like the nice, appropriate thing to do. But after some reflection, you may conclude that this type of response should not characterize your practice. Once you determine your real preferences, be certain to build them into your evaluation criteria.

Keep in mind that the interview will best assess applicants' abilities when they are using their skills as they would use them on the job. For example, if you are trying to assess medical terminology skills, then develop questions around discussions with previous job incumbents that required the understanding and correct utilization of medical language. On the other hand, if you are trying to assess general language skills, including the ability to use good grammar, get the applicant to talk on any familiar topic, such as hobbies, career goals, or previous jobs. Concentrate on *how* they communicate as opposed to the *content* of their communication.

If you are familiar with the job and have developed a clear list of selection factors, it should take you no longer than an hour to develop questions and evaluation criteria for all the factors. Keep in mind that the questions and evaluation criteria for each factor may be used for any other job that requires that same factor. If you have several clerical jobs that require good verbal skills, you can use the same questions and criteria for that factor.

Who Should Do the Interviewing?

Interviewing is a task within the capacity of most business managers and office managers. In general, it should not be contracted out to a consultant unless none of your staff has the time available. The personal involvement of your staff in selecting their associates will more than compensate for their initial lack of structured interviewing experience. Generally, an employee will be more knowledgeable than a consultant about the position. Finally, using employees to conduct structured interviews will develop their interview skills, thereby giving you the flexibility to respond to unexpected employment needs and keep your consulting costs down.

Whether you get personally involved should depend on the position. If you will be working closely with whoever is selected, you will probably want some involvement. Obviously, you will only want to use your time to interview the best applicants—those who have already cleared several other selection hurdles. Positions more removed from the focus of your activities might not require your personal attention. This is, however, a matter of personal preference. Some doctors insist on personally interviewing all of their employees.

Testing

Testing is one of the most effective ways to assess an applicant's ability. Unfortunately, many employers who could greatly benefit from it do not utilize testing. There seem to be three general reasons for this. First, it never occurs to some doctors that they could use testing. Second, some feel uncomfortable using an unfamiliar technology. Third, some believe that federal equal employment opportunity (EEO) laws have made testing difficult to use, if not illegal.

Should these reasons prevent you from utilizing testing? As to the first, obviously not. You are now informed: Testing is an available alternative that is cost-

effective and applicable to jobs found in medical practices. As to the second, although you may currently be unfamiliar with how to use testing, you can develop
the competence to test in an effective, professional manner or hire those who have
it. As to the third, there is nothing in the 1964 Civil Rights Act, the Equal Employment Opportunity Commission's *Uniform Guidelines*,[4] or any other piece of federal civil rights legislation that precludes you from using employment tests. The
Uniform Guidelines do raise some issues with which you should be familiar, but
these relate to *any* employment method, including unstructured and structured
interviewing. (These issues are discussed in Chapter 9.) It is sufficient at this point
to understand that the *Uniform Guidelines* do not cover most medical practices,
and they also do not require employers to do anything that they shouldn't do
anyway.

When considering testing, it is important to think in terms of the job-related
factors you are trying to assess. Some factors, such as typing, filing, and other
clerical skills, verbal skills, writing skills, and so on, are directly used and can be
observed on the job. Other factors, such as intelligence, work ethic, sense of responsibility, motivation, supervisory capacity, and so on, *support* the behaviors
that are manifested on the job but are less directly observable. These factors form
part of the *context* within which the work is performed, and can also be evaluated
through testing.

Performance and Ability Testing

Performance and ability (PA) tests assess skills that are directly manifested on
the job, such as typing, filing, and other clerical skills, verbal skills, numerical
skills, writing skills, and computer skills. There are many published PA tests. Exhibit 2-3 contains an example of a commonly used test for assessing clerical speed.

In PA testing, you can either use published tests or construct your own tests,
which are called *work samples*. The latter alternative is not as difficult as it may
appear. However, let's first examine how to use published PA tests.

The first thing that you must do is find out what tests are available. There are a
number of published reference books that can provide you with descriptions of
tests and information on how to obtain them. One of the best is *Tests: A Comprehensive Reference for Assessment in Psychology, Education, and Business*.[5] An
alternative, more academic in its orientation, is *The Tenth Mental Measurements
Yearbook*.[6] In addition, test review books are generally available in college libraries. An example of a test review is found in Exhibit 2-4. Test reviews can provide
much useful information, including what the test measures, how long it takes to
administer, appropriate uses, scoring, cost, and where to obtain the test.

By using references such as *Tests*, you can get a good idea of what tests may
assess the selection factors you have identified as important for a job. Once you
find a test that seems appropriate in terms of factor coverage, testing time, and
cost, call the publisher. Most of the big publishing houses have toll-free telephone

Exhibit 2-3 Number Perception Test

Hay Aptitude Test Battery

NUMBER PERCEPTION TEST

Form A

Name: _____   Date: _____

DIRECTIONS

Compare each pair of numbers. If the two numbers are exactly the same, place a check mark (√) in the space provided in the column marked "Same." If the two numbers are different, leave the space blank.

SAMPLE PROBLEMS

				Same
1.	7384	---	7384	√
2.	25961	---	25967	

The two numbers in Example 1 are exactly the same. Therefore, a check mark has been placed in the space provided in the column marked "Same." Since the numbers in Example 2 are different, the space has been left blank.

Below are 15 pairs of numbers for you to complete as a practice exercise. Work as fast as you can without making mistakes. Work down the column. <u>Do not skip</u>. REMEMBER : Check the pairs of numbers that are the same. Go ahead.

			Same
6984	---	6984	
92058	---	92058	
7623	---	7613	
819	---	891	
1359	---	1359	

			Same
28496	---	28496	
196	---	197	
50471	---	54071	
387051	---	387051	
4607	---	4607	

			Same
5438	---	5438	
63925	---	63952	
97555	---	97556	
47613	---	47613	
2516	---	2616	

Do the problems on the next two pages in the same way. If you make a mistake, cross it out. It is quicker than trying to erase. Work <u>QUICKLY</u> and <u>CAREFULLY</u>.

Source: Reprinted with permission of E.F. Wonderlic Personnel Test, Inc., Northfield, IL, © 1990.

numbers. Describe the job that you will be using the test for and discuss the appropriateness of the test for your application. If there is enough time, have the publisher mail you literature on the test or order a specimen set. A specimen set usu-

Exhibit 2-4 Sample Test Review

HAY APTITUDE TEST BATTERY: NUMBER PERCEPTION
Edward N. Hay

Purpose: Measures ability to check pairs of numbers and indentify those that are the same. Used for selection of office and clerical personnel.

Description: 200 item paper-pencil measuring speed and accuracy of numerical checking. Each test item consists of a pair of numbers that the applicant must decide are either the same or different. Test items designed to include most common clerical errors. May be administered and timed via optional cassette tape. Examiner required. Suitable for group use. Available in French.

Timed: 4 minutes
Range: Adult
Scoring: Hand key
Cost: 25 forms $17.00
Publisher: E.F. Wonderlic & Associates, Inc.

Source: Reprinted from *Tests: A Comprehensive Reference for Assessment in Psychology, Education, and Business* by R.C. Sweetland and D.J. Keyser, p. 767, with permission of PRO-ED, Inc., © 1983.

ally includes one copy of the test, the test manual, and other literature describing the test's appropriate application.

Whenever you obtain a test, pay particular attention to its manual. A good test manual should contain easily understood administration and scoring instructions. It should also contain information on the appropriate use of the test and the test's reliability and validity. Reliability is the ability of a test to give consistent results. With a reliable test, applicants would get similar test scores if tested on two separate occasions. Validity concerns the question of whether a test really does measure what it is intended to measure. If a test is called "The XYZ Test of Verbal

Skills," it possesses validity if it really does measure verbal skills. Test manuals often provide a reference list of published papers and books. Many of these publications discuss using the test for specific jobs. By consulting some of these publications, reviewing information in the test manual, and carefully looking through the test yourself, you should be able to gain a sense of the test's appropriateness for your application.

Work Samples

In a work sample, you use a portion of the actual job to assess job applicants. A work sample provides a very effective way to evaluate applicants, because it gives each applicant the opportunity to actually perform part of the job. *A work sample is only appropriate when you do not intend to train whoever is selected in the particular skill.* For example, typing ability is a good work sample candidate, because you certainly wouldn't intend to train a new employee to type.

Here is how to construct a typing skills work sample. (The same basic procedures can be used to assess any other skill.) Select a document from your current files. It should be typical of the kind of typing normally performed in your practice (e.g., a letter, report, speech, etc.). Generally, it is best to make the work sample long enough so that even the very best applicants won't be able to finish. This will ensure that you get plenty of "range" in the scores.

It is very important to standardize the work sample testing conditions so that everyone is tested under similar conditions. In addition, the testing conditions should simulate normal working conditions. If, for example, typing is performed in a rather noisy front office, with people talking and telephones ringing, then the test should occur under like circumstances. If typing is normally performed in a quiet back room, then this is where to conduct the test. To some degree, using realistic working conditions may reduce standardization, since different applicants will encounter somewhat different conditions. Telephones will ring a different number of times, employees may be more or less vocal in the background, and so on. As long as the testing conditions are not extreme, the knowledge gained by testing skills under realistic conditions is probably worth the reduced standardization. Naturally, extreme circumstances, such as a patient interrupting the applicant during testing, will require retesting.

Give the applicants plenty of time to learn the "feel" of your typing equipment. If the typing will be done on a complex word processor or computer, you may want to tell applicants not to reproduce the format of the original document, but to concentrate instead on speed and accuracy. The test should provide enough time for the applicants to fully exhibit their typing speed and accuracy. A five-minute test is usually adequate, but, depending on the type of document and the typing demands of the job, you may choose to use a somewhat longer test to better simulate working conditions. After a test is completed, it is a good idea to ask whether the applicant felt it was a good test. If the applicant wants a retest, provide a new document to type.

Use your common sense to develop reasonable scoring criteria. An obvious scoring criterion is the average number of words per minute typed in the test. Another obvious scoring criterion is the number of typing errors. If you want to combine the two criteria, you could subtract the number of errors from the average number of words per minute. The particular scoring criteria that you adopt are not as crucial as the consistency with which you apply them. As long as the rules are generally reasonable and consistently applied, the resulting rank ordering of applicants should reflect their skill levels.

There are many other opportunities to develop work samples. For example, you can assess telephone skills by staging a work sample during an interview. Play the role of a caller and have the applicant turn away from you so as not to react to your facial expressions or body language. Then develop a conversation to assess the applicant's abilities to use language, respond appropriately to questions, and so on. Keep the evaluation criteria simple. This will increase reliability. Develop two or three evaluation criteria, such as these:

- Adequate: handled all questions and situations using appropriate language or tact.
- Minimal: had some problems with appropriate language or tact.
- Inadequate: had substantial problems with appropriate language or tact.

In addition, keep your notes to support your conclusions. Later, you may want to review your evaluation of an applicant, and your original notes will allow you to reevaluate and weight the test conclusions.

Other factors amenable to work sample assessment include writing, filing, checkbook balancing, interacting with patients (using a simulated patient), negotiating patient payment plans or fees (using a simulated patient), and completing insurance forms.

It is important not to confuse style preferences with skill. For example, if there is a particular way you like the telephone answered, it is not appropriate to expect your preference to be anticipated by applicants. Instead, you should be looking for fundamental telephone answering skills, such as use of tact and appropriate language.

Psychological Testing

PA testing can be used for many important job-related factors, but there are other factors that are less directly observable yet nevertheless very important. These factors can usually be assessed by using psychological testing. Psychological testing assesses traits such as intelligence, introversion, work ethic, sense of responsibility, motivation, and supervisory capacity. You might want some of these traits to be possessed by all of your employees. If so, you might want to do some psychological testing for all jobs.

Another way to use psychological testing is as a substitute for *some* PA testing. For example, suppose that a job requires the use of the word processing program Word 4.0. You could select applicants based on current ability to use this program. You might discover, however, that there are relatively few applicants who actually have experience with Word 4.0, and as a result you find yourself rejecting many otherwise desirable applicants. As an alternative strategy, you could evaluate applicants based on their likelihood of successfully learning the program. For example, you could base selection on intelligence, since people with higher intelligence learn complex skills more thoroughly and more quickly than those with lower intelligence. You could also base selection on the PA factor of clerical speed, since speed is necessary in order to effectively use any word processing program. Applicants who score high on both of these measures stand a good chance of being able to quickly learn and effectively use the word processing program.

As with PA tests, you can use reference books such as *Tests* to identify potentially useful psychological tests. Distribution of some psychological tests is restricted to those with appropriate qualifications. If you fail to meet the publisher's qualifications, don't try to circumvent these restrictions, since such a failure indicates that you need a more sophisticated understanding of testing theory or specific training in the test in order to use it effectively. Remember, if you use a test improperly, you may deceive yourself regarding the quality of applicants whom you hire. Continue looking for another test that assesses the same factor. There are thousands of tests available, and usually any given factor can be assessed using literally dozens of published tests. The difference between restricted and unrestricted tests is often analogous to the difference between some prescription and nonprescription strengths of a drug. The "nonprescription" test may be more than adequate for your purpose.

If you can't find an unrestricted alternative, or you wish to use a test you aren't qualified to administer, hire a consultant. Generally, a cost-effective way of finding a knowledgeable consultant is to contact the business, psychology, or education department at a local college. If the test is appropriate, the consultant will train you or your staff to administer it correctly and will arrange for you to obtain the testing materials. Remember, once you find a test that satisfactorily measures job-related factors, you will be able to use it for any other job that requires those same performance factors. Once again, your initial investment of time may well pay long-term dividends.

Many published tests are supported by scoring services. A scoring service will provide you with an interpretive report at a reasonable cost, with turnaround in a week or less. Some services provide scoring over the telephone, thereby providing an immediate evaluation. The quality and quantity of data provided in these reports is generally very high. The cost varies from about ten to twenty-five dollars. A scoring service should be used, therefore, only for finalists for important positions.

Other Types of Testing

Polygraphs, which are also called *lie detectors,* are used for assessing deceptiveness. Most of us have been conditioned to react physiologically when we are dishonest, and the polygraph attempts to measure these reactions. Unfortunately, research evidence strongly indicates that the polygraph is not a useful employment method.[7] Many states have outlawed its use, and federal legislation that went into effect in September 1988 has greatly restricted the situations in private employment where polygraph assessment is legal. In summary, don't use polygraph testing.

Some employers use "honesty" tests as an alternative to polygraph testing. Honesty tests ask applicants questions that supposedly are correlated with stealing or deceitful behavior. As of this writing, research findings are too meager to demonstrate conclusively whether honesty tests are valid and whether they are sufficiently predictive of future behavior to be useful when making employment decisions. Although a number of validity studies report evidence that these tests work, the studies I have read are methodologically unsound. For example, some studies use the polygraph as the standard to determine deception. If you decide to use an honesty test, be certain to examine the evidence for validity presented by the publisher. You may also want to contact a consultant to obtain a professional opinion regarding the test and the publisher's data.

White-collar crime is certainly a major problem in the United States. However, no matter what a test is named, if it doesn't do what it purports to do, you are only deceiving yourself by basing decisions on it. Organizations, including medical practices, can control some of the problems supposedly addressed by polygraph and honesty testing by implementing well-designed and consistently applied financial controls and employee performance reviews. This may be analogous to closing the door after the wolf has entered the chicken coop, but if you close the door fast enough and the chickens scream loudly enough, you may prevent the most serious damage.

Drug testing of applicants may be appropriate under certain circumstances. Because drug testing is a relatively expensive procedure, you should give careful consideration to when and how you use it. There are a number of different drug tests. The least expensive, at a cost of about ten to fifteen dollars, is thin layer chromatography (TLC). It is also the most subjective. Enzyme immunoassay (EIA) and radioimmunoassay (RIA) are slightly more expensive but provide more definitive results. These tests can detect the eight major abused drugs or drug classes: amphetamines, barbiturates, benzodiazepine, cannabinoids, cocaine, methaqualone, opiates, and phencyclidine. EIA and RIA are the most commonly used employment drug tests and cost between fifteen and twenty dollars. Finally, gas chromatography and mass spectroscopy offer much greater sensitivity than EIA, RIA, and TLC. Since their price is currently over fifty dollars per test, they must be reserved for situations in which extreme accuracy is essential.

All of the tests discussed are susceptible to various degrees of cross-reaction. A cross-reaction is when a licit substance, such as poppy seeds, falsely indicates the presence of an illicit substance, such as heroin. With these facts in mind, you may want to consider testing an applicant in the following instances:

1. The applicant, once hired, would have ready access to prescription drugs or large sums of cash.
2. You have obtained information that leads you to believe the applicant may have a history of illicit drug abuse.
3. The drug screen is the final employment hurdle.

In such situations, employers will generally use an EIA or RIA test. If a positive finding is returned, the possibility of a false positive is evaluated using either gas chromatography or mass spectroscopy. Obviously, it is essential that the company doing your drug testing retains all samples so that retesting is feasible.

Who Should Design and Conduct Your Testing?

Testing is truly a double-edged sword. It gives you considerable power, but considerable knowledge is required if this power is not to be abused. In order to use testing effectively, you must distinguish between (1) selecting published psychological and performance tests; (2) constructing work samples; and (3) scoring and evaluating performance. As was pointed out above, you can do your own test selection. Most doctors, however, will find it to be more cost-effective to hire a consultant to develop the selection procedures, including test procedures. If the job content remains fairly constant, you can reuse these procedures if the job becomes open again. As you have seen, the tests used should match the skill requirements of the job. Keep this in mind when you evaluate a consultant's recommendations. Some consultants have their "pets." Irrespective of the job, they use the same employment tests. The consultant should be able to make a very convincing argument for using each employment test, including demonstrating that each one measures some important aspect of job performance.

Ideally, the employment tests a consultant recommends should be scorable by your staff or a scoring service. Even if you decide to have the consultant evaluate the current applicants' test scores, it would be desirable for staff to have the ability to evaluate performance. Become suspicious if a consultant recommends tests—

other than work samples—that are "self-developed" or only scorable by the consultant. To lock yourself into this kind of arrangement may limit your future flexibility as well as result in inflated consulting fees. There are simply too many good, inexpensive PA and psychological tests that will meet your needs on the market.

Your staff should be able to do a creditable job of constructing work samples. Your role in this process is to review the content of work samples to make certain they are fair and representative. If you have neither the time nor the desire to do this, then contact a consultant. It should require very little consultation time to review a work sample, evaluate its appropriateness, and make recommendations for any necessary modifications.

Test administration, scoring, and evaluation generally are within the capability of you and your office staff. Once again, you may choose to use a consultant to perform these tasks. The trade-off will be between the convenience of using a consultant and the timeliness and cost savings achieved by doing the work in-house.

THE RESUMÉ

Resumés are valuable sources of information for two reasons. First, resumés are samples of applicants' behavior. They are statements that applicants prepare themselves at their own pace, stating what they feel is important about themselves, and what qualifies them for the job. Look first, therefore, at a resumé as a sample of behavior. Second, each resumé is a statement of what the applicant has been doing with his or her life.

When examining a resumé as a behavior sample, consider the orderliness, neatness, and organization. How clearly and concisely does it convey information? If the applicant takes two pages to express what could be presented in one page, this is an indication that the applicant will not be able to construct concise documents or arguments or "get to the point" on the job. Does it appear that some thought has gone toward organizing information in a logical manner? If the resumé is confusing or illogically organized, this is an indication that the applicant may not be able to present information in a logical, understandable manner to you, your employees, and your patients. Are the spelling, punctuation, and grammar correct? If you find mistakes, it means that the applicant (1) does not have basic language skills; (2) is a lazy or sloppy worker; or (3) tends to be rushed and make mistakes.

After you have evaluated the resumé as a sample product, you should then evaluate its content. First, examine the applicant's previous experience and education to determine whether he or she has skills required for the job. This doesn't mean that the applicant must have performed a job with the same job title or worked in your branch of medicine. For example, bookkeeping in a medical practice is little different from bookkeeping in any other type of professional or service organization. An applicant who has worked for an accounting firm, a lawyer, or an architect should have little difficulty making the transition to a medical practice.

Examine how frequently the applicant has changed jobs. Eliminate applicants who have a history of frequent job changes. They are job hoppers who will be dissatisfied in any situation, and their dissatisfaction will cause disruption and dissension in your practice. Look for a logical order or progression in the job changes. Good applicants will show a history of increased skills and responsibilities. An applicant who has gone from being a bookkeeper to a secretary to a business manager may be futilely searching for a kind of satisfaction probably never to be achieved. If you see this type of searching behavior, carefully explore the issue with the applicant during the interview. If there is no legitimate explanation, don't let this applicant's personal problem become your problem.

Examine the resumé for unexplained gaps in employment. If you find any, the applicant must account for them. An employment gap sometimes indicates failure at some job, failure that may or may not have been the applicant's fault. Discuss any gaps with the applicant during the interview. You will have to make a judgment concerning the reasonableness of the applicant's explanation.

On many jobs, education and experience are to some degree interchangeable. An applicant for a bookkeeping position who has had no previous experience but has received appropriate, documented education might well be able to perform the job. Jobs requiring skills that normally aren't obtained through formal education are best performed by people who have had previous experience. This of course creates a problem for the inexperienced applicant: how to obtain experience if the only people who are hired are people with experience. This is a problem, but it is not *your* problem.

Don't personally screen all applicant resumés, unless the job reports directly to you. However, don't delegate this task to subordinates if the job does report to you. Your ability to judge whom you can work with can only be matched, never exceeded, by the judgment of others.

REFERENCES AND RECOMMENDATIONS

References and recommendations are very difficult tools to use, because you can never be certain what motivates those who provide them. (For an examination of the issues involved in giving references, see the discussion of the tort of defamation in Chapter 9.) Employers can have many reasons for giving former employees a good reference, including keeping their own unemployment insurance rates down and fear of legal action on the part of the former employee. It is important to determine the reference's ability to evaluate the applicant and the extent of his or her knowledge of the applicant's job performance. Finally, remember that everyone can find someone who will provide a good reference. Joseph Goebbels would certainly have received a good reference if you had happened to talk to Adolph Hitler.

Consider references only from people who had an employment relationship with the applicant. A personal reference is generally worthless, because the motivation of the person giving the reference is totally unknown. You may be talking to the applicant's brother-in-law. (You may be doing this even with an employer reference. It is wise to ask whether the employee is related to the person providing the reference.)

The best way to use a reference is as a means to verify or validate information that you have obtained elsewhere in the employment process. Personally, I find it is best to talk on the telephone with whoever is giving a reference. You can often obtain more information than the person is willing to commit to writing, and on occasion the person will inadvertently reveal some unintended information by voice inflection, pauses, and so on.

If you are using the reference for verification, then you should construct a list of questions to ask. For example, if psychological testing indicates that an applicant should have outstanding interpersonal abilities, attempt to verify this by asking, "Could you describe some of John's most outstanding qualities?" Hopefully, the person will mention the applicant's interpersonal abilities. If not, you might then say, "Give me an example of an incident that is typical of John's ability to work with others." Similarly, if an applicant has indicated that a significant part of her job involved insurance collection, you could ask the reference, "What were some of the major duties that Sally had?" The answer should verify whether insurance billing was a primary or secondary responsibility.

Asking good questions and designing a strategy to use the reference to confirm or disconfirm hypotheses generated in previous employment steps will take time and effort on your part. As a result, obtaining references should be the final step in the selection process. Ideally, it should only be used for the top one or two applicants, as determined by your other employment methods.

Who Should Evaluate References and Recommendations?

Once again, you should only become personally involved in the case of jobs that report directly to you. If you don't feel that your staff is capable of performing the evaluation, and you are personally uninterested or don't have the time, contract it out to a consultant.

THE APPLICATION FORM

Generally, the initial screening of applicants will be based on resumés, followed by short telephone interviews. Survivors will then be invited in for additional interviewing, testing, and so on. It is desirable at this point to have all applicants complete an application form. This will make it easier to compare applicants on education, previous experience, and so on. The alternative is to dig this information out of the resumés, which is a frustrating, time-consuming job. Another important reason for using an application form is that it can provide justification for immediate dismissal of an employee who lied about qualifications, credentials, previous experience, and so on. The application form should state that supplying false information may result in the denial or termination of employment.[8]

Application forms should only request job-relevant information. Do not ask applicants about their race, religion, sex, national origin, or age, since these are not relevant to job performance. You may preclude a legal challenge to your employment decision by not collecting this information. Exhibit 2-5 is a sample application form. State laws vary considerably regarding what questions are permissible, and you should contact your attorney before using any application form. For example, federal law allows the use of *Ms., Mrs., Miss,* and *Mr.* on application forms, whereas some states, such as New York and Michigan, forbid this practice.[9] (Refer to Chapter 9 for a more complete discussion of equal employment opportunity and how to utilize your attorney.)

Finally, if the employee is to work without a written contract, the application form should contain a strong "at-will" employment statement. At-will employment will give you flexibility to terminate an unsatisfactory employee. (Refer to Chapter 9 for a discussion of at-will and written contract employment arrangements.)

RECRUITING

Recruiting is the process of getting applicants to apply for a job. The object is to attract those applicants who (1) are likely to have the required skills, and (2) will find the job attractive and will want to work for you.

The most commonly used recruiting tools for front office positions are "word of mouth" and newspaper advertisements. Word-of-mouth recruiting has the advantage of quickly conveying information to people who have indicated to you or your employees that they are in the job market. If your current employees are high performers, word-of-mouth recruiting will help screen out unsuitable applicants. Usually, competent employees will not recommend people they *know* are incompetent, because they will not want to work with them. Word-of-mouth recruiting can also result in your employees' persuading friends or associates to *enter* the job market and become applicants. Many people are not dissatisfied enough with their current job to take the risk of searching for a new job. Others may not be willing to expend the effort required to search for a new position. If opportunity knocks, however, they may respond. The danger of word-of-mouth recruiting is that the

Exhibit 2-5 Sample Employment Application Form

APPLICATION FOR EMPLOYMENT WITH GREENWICH MEDICAL ASSOCIATES, P.C.

Last Name		First Name			Middle Name			

Present Address (Street, City, State, Zip Code)		Telephone Number		Social Security Number	

Position Applying For	Date Available

Names & Addresses Of Schools Attended	Dates From	To	Degree	Major or Subject Area	Major G.P.A.	Overall

Licenses or Certificates	Granting Agency	Expiration Date

Honor Societies, Professional Societies, Etc.:

List All Previous Work Experience. Begin With Most Recent Position Held. Use Additional application forms if necessary.

Employer's Name & Address	Supervisor's Name & Title	Job Title & Work Description	Salary	Employed From	To

Work or Educational References.

Name of Reference	Name of Organization	This Reference Was Your:

I acknowledge that I am seeking employment with Greenwich Medical Associates, P.C. I further state that all of the information which I have provided is true. By signing this application form I acknowledge that employment may be denied or terminated if I have supplied false or misleading information. I also understand that the position that I am applying for is an at will position, and that if I am hired my employment can be terminated at the sole discretion of the employer.

Job Applicant's Signature: _____   Date: _____

Source: Courtesy of Greenwich Psychological Associates, P.C., Virginia Beach, VA.

employee who learns of a position from a friend may feel an allegiance to the friend that competes with the allegiance to the employer.

Classified newspaper advertising is another excellent way of generating an applicant pool for front office positions. The advertisement should clearly state the major duties of the job, the compensation level, and the work hours so that applicants can self-select based on these considerations. Newspaper ads generate a low proportion of useful resumés (between 50 and 75 percent of the applicants will be eliminated in the resumé-screening process). These ads compensate for this by generating large numbers of applicants.

Generally, employment agencies are not a desirable recruiting source. If you hire one of their applicants, you will usually have to pay some form of fee. In addition, their screening methods are often ineffective. Unless you are willing to delegate the whole selection process to the employment agency, you will still have to use some or all of your own selection procedures. Employment agencies *can* be useful for supplying temporary replacements, thus allowing enough time to find well-qualified applicants.

Other potential recruiting sources include local colleges and technical schools. In general, these sources are best used for jobs that require little or no previous experience. But for such jobs, schools have several distinct advantages:

1. A school placement office can send you a large number of applicants with little effort on your part.
2. Applicants with little or no experience will generally work for lower wages than experienced applicants. If the job doesn't require experience, why pay for it?
3. A school may do some preliminary screening so that you only get the better applicants. One way to increase the chances of this happening is to tell the placement office that you will evaluate a few of their applicants and will discontinue recruiting there if the quality of applicants is low.

Who Should Do Your Recruiting?

You should become personally involved in strategic-level recruiting decisions, such as determining recruiting media and the recruiting budget. All of the actual recruiting tasks, including writing ad copy, contacting recruiting sources, and so on, may be performed by your staff.

SELECTION STRATEGY

After reviewing all of the selection tools that are available, you may feel that doing a good job of hiring employees is a time-consuming and complicated process. It doesn't have to be. The key to hiring good employees and doing it in a timely, cost-effective manner is understanding how to organize your employee search procedures. You must have an efficient and effective selection strategy.

The first step in implementing a successful selection strategy is to create a large applicant pool as quickly as possible. The applicant pool is the set of applicants who apply for the job. It is a waste of time and effort to sequentially identify and evaluate a few applicants, then repeat the whole process. First, there is always a time delay between recruiting efforts and the receipt of resumés. Obviously, if you have to repeat the whole process even once, you will waste considerable time simply waiting for the arrival of resumés.

A second and perhaps more important consideration is that a sequential recruiting process may not identify the most qualified applicant. For example, suppose you only use a limited recruiting method—such as word of mouth—that generates a selection pool of two or three applicants. One of these applicants may appear to be an adequate although not outstanding prospect. As a result you find yourself in the difficult position of having to decide between offering this applicant the job or resuming your recruiting efforts. There will be a strong temptation to hire the "bird in hand," since this will relieve your anxiety and allow you to move on to other more pressing matters—such as practicing medicine. It may be, however, that a far more qualified applicant is out there and that a broader initial search, using a newspaper ad, for example, would have identified this applicant. The effort required to evaluate the superior applicant would have been no greater than that expended on the mediocre applicant.

Also requisite for developing a successful selection strategy is to understand how to sequence the events and how to process all of the applicant information. The best way of sequencing is to use "multiple hurdles." This means that you order the selection process into sequential stages so that subsequent employment methods are only applied to the survivors from previous stages. An effective sequencing uses the least expensive and least time-consuming procedures early in the employment process and reserves the more expensive and more time-consuming procedures for those applicants who have survived the initial hurdles. For example, a reasonable order of events for a clerical position might be as follows:

1. resumé review
2. telephone interview of applicants
3. testing and face-to-face interview of applicants
4. telephone reference check

Ideally, you would only conduct the telephone reference check for your top candidate.

An example of a selection sequence for processing 26 applicants is illustrated in Table 2-2. In Step 1, the 26 resumés are classified as "good" or "bad." Only the 14 "good" applicants are interviewed by telephone. Of these survivors, seven pass the telephone interview and are invited in for testing and initial face-to-face interviewing. After testing and interviewing, two applicants, D and A, stand out. These two are invited back for a second interview. The object of this interview is to resolve any questions raised by the first interview and testing, and to provide a realistic preview of the work so that any uninterested applicant will self-select out. Applicant D is evaluated as superior and expresses interest in the job, so her ref-

Table 2-2 Sequence of Employment Steps

Step	Time	Initial Evaluation		Subsequent Evaluation			Rank (in order)	Offer Recipient
		Good	Bad	Superior	Adequate	Inadequate		
1. Resumé Review	4 hrs.	A,B,C,D,E,F, G,H,I,L,M,P, Q,W	J,K,N,O,R,S, T,U,V,X,Y,Z					
2. Telephone Interview	3.25 hrs.	A,D,E,H,L,M, Q	B,C,F,G,I,P,W					
3. Test	1 hr.*			A,D,E	H,M	L,Q		
Interview	3 hrs.			A,D,H,Q	E,M,L			
4. Second Interview	1.5 hrs.						D,A	
5. Reference Check	.25 hrs.							D

*Directions only.

erences are checked. The references' comments are consistent with the previous testing and interviewing, so she is offered the position. If she declines the job, A's references will be checked, and A might be offered the job. If A were to decline, then you would have to decide whether to interview E and H a second time or obtain a new applicant pool.

Sometimes there is a temptation during the selection process to be overly quantitative and to try to combine the information from several selection procedures into one or a few grand numbers. Avoid this temptation. Unless you are very familiar with statistics, you may easily create a useless index and deceive yourself regarding the meaningfulness and accuracy of your decisions. For example, don't combine numbers from a structured interview with those from a typing or psychological test to create one index. You will do better to examine narrative reports and testing outcomes and to categorize applicants subjectively into two or three broad groups (Great, Okay, Bad).

You will also benefit from providing applicants with detailed realistic information about the job (a so-called realistic job preview) early in the selection process. This will enable uninterested applicants to drop out of the process, saving you the trouble of evaluating their qualifications. For example, always indicate the salary range for the position in the newspaper ad and discuss it in the telephone interview. Similarly, you should describe the job in some detail in the telephone interview so that uninterested applicants can drop out at that point. During the first face-to-face interview, give the applicant a written job description and, if possible, show the applicant where he or she would work. Fill in any gaps left by the job description, and provide a fair statement of the work, warts and all. Applicants who have unrealistic job expectations and would be likely to quit after a short time on the job tend to self-select out of the applicant pool if told the honest truth.

Table 2-2 indicates that 26 applicants could be evaluated and a job offer realistically made with the expenditure of about 13 hours of someone's time. It is also possible to reduce the time expended if you are willing to risk lengthening the employment process. For example, suppose that A and D greatly impressed you during their telephone interviews. You could delay testing and interviewing E, H, L, M, and Q until after you tested and interviewed A and D. If you then conclude that either A or D is about as good as an applicant can get, you could further delay evaluating the others until you reach a final decision on A and D. If you eventually hire A or D, you will save at least 5 hours. The danger here is that one of the other applicants might be superior.

Finally, an effective selection strategy is one that is put into practice with *patience*. It is disruptive and perhaps frightening to have an important position vacant. It is far worse, however, to fill the position with the wrong person. Your employment methods may give you answers you don't like. They may indicate that many applicants who initially appeared to be well qualified are not good employment risks. Be persistent and don't easily take a less-than-adequate applicant just to fill the position and move on to other issues.

Employee selection is analogous to betting. The interviews, tests, work samples, and other selection tools and procedures change the odds, but they do not guarantee that you will hire an adequate employee. If you are using valid, job-related employment methods, applicants who perform better on the selection procedures will have higher probabilities of succeeding on the job. From your perspective as an employer, there are two types of selection mistakes which you can make: (1) You can fail to hire an applicant who would have been successful; or (2) you can hire an applicant who will fail. The first is called a *false-negative error* and the second a *false-positive error*. From your perspective as an employer, a false-positive error is far more expensive and dangerous than a false-negative error. It is better not to hire someone who would succeed than to hire someone who would fail. Therefore, you want to bias your decision making so that you minimize the probability of making a false-positive error, even though that may increase the chance of making several false-negative errors and continuing the employment process.

Following is an explanation of the relationship between false-positives, false-negatives, and successful employment decisions. Figure 2-1 illustrates the relationship. The horizontal axis of each graph represents applicant performance on the selection procedure. The vertical axis represents the job performance that would occur if all the applicants were actually hired.[10] Each dot in the scatterplot represents how a particular applicant scored on both the selection procedure and on job performance.[11] The line encircling the scatterplot provides a visual summary of the selection procedure–job performance relationship. Notice that as selection procedure performance increases, job performance *generally* increases, although this does not happen in every instance. Nevertheless, higher selection procedure performance is strongly correlated with higher job performance. An applicant who performs well on the selection procedure is more likely to perform well on the job than an applicant who performs poorly on the selection procedure.

The vertical axis of Graph A in Figure 2-1 has been bisected to distinguish acceptable and unacceptable job performance. The effect of hiring at any given level of selection procedure performance can be observed by drawing a vertical line through the scatterplot. The scatterplot is now divided into four areas: the false-positive area, the false-negative area, the true-positive area, and the true-negative area.

True-negatives occur when the selection procedure predicts that the applicant will fail and the applicant does in fact fail. True-positives occur when the selection procedure predicts that the applicant will succeed and the applicant does in fact succeed. Notice the size of the true-positive area relative to the size of the false-positive area. The ratio of these two areas is an index of the employment method's effectiveness.

Now examine Graph B in Figure 2-1. The only difference between this graph and Graph A is that the Hire–Don't Hire line has been moved to the right. This means that the employer is demanding higher selection procedure performance

Graph A

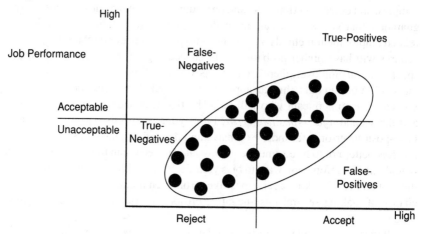

Graph B

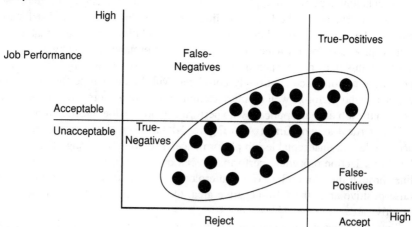

Figure 2-1 False Positives and Negatives, and True Positives and Negatives

before selecting an applicant. Notice the effect this has on the selection procedure's effectiveness. The ratio of the true-positive area to the false-positive area has increased. Notice also that the ratio of the true-positive area to the false-negative area has decreased. *By demanding higher applicant scores, you will increase the probability that those whom you hire will succeed, but at the cost of rejecting more applicants who would have been successful.*

It should be apparent that theoretically an employer could demand a selection procedure performance score so high that the probability of applicant success would be 100 percent. The limiting factor, however, is that the employer has to fill the position, and it may take a very long time to find an applicant who scores high enough for that degree of certainty. More to the point, this illustration demonstrates that you should not jump at the first applicant whose selection procedure performance scores are acceptable. Be patient enough to bring in sufficient applicants to give yourself a good chance of finding high-scoring applicants. This will increase the probability of success.

The implications of this illustration are as follows:

1. Employment methods that are far less than perfect can, nevertheless, be very effective if you can demand high enough applicant scores.
2. High applicant scores are more likely to occur if you recruit effectively. Your advertising, working conditions, pay rates, and so on, must help attract many qualified applicants.
3. The value of finding high-scoring applicants must be balanced against the cost and time involved in evaluating larger numbers of applicants.

Who Should Design Your Selection Strategy?

The selection strategy used for a job is critical to filling the position successfully and economically. It is very important, therefore, that you devote your best thinking to the design of the selection strategy for all jobs in your practice. If the strategy is to be developed in the practice, then your personal involvement is critical. If you don't feel fully confident in your ability to develop a selection strategy or don't have the time to do a good job, then retain a consultant. Once a selection strategy has been designed for a job, it can be used again for that job. Over time, therefore, your practice will acquire selection strategies for all jobs. These strategies need not change unless the content of jobs change or you become dissatisfied with the quality of your employees.

A PERSONAL CASE

In retrospect, one of the biggest employment mistakes I made occurred when an applicant pool wore me down. Due to bad luck, poor applicants, ineffective recruiting, whatever, applicant after applicant failed to survive some critical part of the employment process. One particular problem was that many applicants were scoring at high levels on the Fake Good scale of the California Psychological Inventory. A high Fake Good score may mean that the applicant is trying to present a false impression on the test. It would be reasonable to assume that such an applicant might well have problems with honesty and sincerity on the job. Unfortunately, the high Fake Good applicants generally performed better than others in the interview and on the various ability tests. In effect, the Fake Good scale was the only thing keeping the medical practice from hiring a business manager. The physician was growing more anxious as applicant after applicant was rejected. I explained the problem to the physician, and we jointly chose to conclude that the Fake Good scale wasn't working properly. With the Fake Good scale no longer an impediment, I recommended an applicant who, although well into the questionable range on that scale, had excellent performances otherwise.

Needless to say, the employee's subsequent job performance was marked by covering-up problems, deception, manipulation of employees, and outright mendacity. The personal and financial costs of searching for a few more days or weeks would have been far less burdensome than the problems caused by hiring this applicant. This experience proved to me that there are times when one must "tough it out." Hire a temporary employee, use a contractor to continue billing, or whatever is necessary, but don't easily compromise your hiring standards.

A CASE APPLICATION

The purpose of this case description is to provide you with an example of how selection methods and strategy can be applied in a real employment situation. It illustrates how you can use the general guidelines presented above in a realistic and practical manner. The case also illustrates how you can adjust your employment procedures to take advantage of the changing reality of the selection process.

A family practice employing six physicians was seeking a new business manager. The current business manager had fallen behind in collection and did not have the organizational skills, efficiency, or motivation to fix the problem. The job description for the position (Exhibit 2-6) was organized into five technical skill factors, two interpersonal skill factors, and one personal trait, which were to be evaluated using resumés, interviews, work samples, psychological tests, and reference checks (Table 2-3). The sequence of selection methods was as follows:

1. resumé review
2. telephone interview
3. face-to-face interview and psychological test
4. second face-to-face interview and work samples
5. reference check

Exhibit 2-6 Business Manager Job Description

---

1. *Revenue Collection.* Responsible for the collection of all revenue. This includes using current office procedures and developing new ones to ensure the collection of all copayments and the collection of insurance. This will involve working with the other front office staff to develop these procedures and make them work. Responsible for making certain that all accounts are paid within a reasonable time, which is normally not to exceed 90 days past current.
2. *Insurance Billing.* Generating accurate insurance bills and mailing them on a regular basis (the schedule to be determined by the director).
3. *Payroll.* Maintaining and generating accurate payroll records (including a collection record for each physician), determining monthly income based on collection, and calculating appropriate deductions. Preparing appropriate paperwork and transmitting it to the office manager, who maintains the checkbook and generates checks.
4. *Taxes.* Creating and maintaining all paperwork and databases necessary for paying payroll taxes efficiently and for providing tax authorities with documents showing the accuracy and timeliness of tax payments. Paying all payroll and corporate taxes in a timely manner.
5. *Posting and Accounting for All Payments.* Posting all payments made into the MediMac system. Reconciling all payments made the previous day with cash, checks, insurance remits, credit card receipts, and so on, thus ensuring accuracy and accountability.
6. *Fee Negotiation and Collection.* Negotiating patient fees. Following accounts that are delinquent and ensuring the timely collection of fees. Notifying physicians when their patients' payments are delinquent.
7. *Management Reports.* Generating or causing to be generated the management reports that are necessary for daily operations and for providing accountability and problem identification. These reports include, but are not limited to, Aging Analyses, Earned Receipts by Producer, and Daily Receipts.
8. *Problem Identification and Resolution.* Identifying problems in any area of the practice, bringing them to the attention of the director, and proposing and implementing solutions.
9. *Teamwork.* Working with the computer operator, office manager, and physicians to
   • ensure continuous communication
   • identify problems regardless of their source or cause
   • keep the managing physician informed
   • assist the managing physician with problem solving
   • create a positive atmosphere in the office
   • work effectively with coworkers, subordinates, and patients
10. *Additional.* Additional duties and responsibilities as they are determined to be appropriate by the managing physician.

Recruiting methods included word of mouth and two newspaper advertisements spaced one week apart. These generated 18 resumés. Exhibit 2-7 contains the resumé of the applicant who was eventually selected for that position. This resumé shows competence on most, if not all, of the selection factors.

Ann's resumé was well organized and contained appropriate language, with correct spelling and grammar. The information was presented in a neat, well-

Table 2-3 Business Manager Job Description Factors, Selection Factors, and Selection Procedures

Job Description Factor	Selection Factor	Selection Procedure
Revenue collection	Technical skill	Resumé Work sample Interview
Insurance billing	Technical skill	Resumé Work sample
Payroll	Technical skill	Interview Work sample
Taxes	Technical skill	Interview Work sample
Fee negotiation	Interpersonal skill	Work sample
Management reports	Technical skill	Work sample
Problem identification	Trait	Psychological test
Teamwork	Interpersonal skill	Psychological test

organized, logical, and concise manner. Her resumé made an acceptable *initial* impression. It indicated that the following things were important to her: (1) revenue collection, (2) developing systems to deal with business problems, (3) efficiency, and (4) interpersonal relations on the job. Their importance to her, however, does not guarantee she does these things well. Her resumé indicated previous experience with revenue collection, insurance billing, payroll, management reports, and problem identification. The time break between the last two jobs was accounted for in the initial telephone contact.

Next, Ann was interviewed on the telephone by Dr. Frederick, the managing physician. His objectives were to acquire more detailed information about her previous work experience, assess her verbal skills, familiarize her with the job description to clarify whether the job interested her, and determine whether the salary range for the job was acceptable. The telephone interview was organized so that the most fundamental qualification issues were discussed first. It also could thus be quickly ended if the applicant was not appropriate for the job.

The telephone interview began by verifying that Ann was still in the job market. Next, the job was described to her in considerable detail. She was encouraged to ask questions at any point during the interview. After the job description had been reviewed, she was once again asked if she was still interested in the position. Benefits were then discussed, including the salary range, vacation time, sick leave, the retirement plan, and medical insurance. Once again, she was asked if she was still interested in the position. Finally, she was told that the next step would in-

Exhibit 2-7 Resumé of Business Manager Applicant

Ann Johnson
342 Main Street
Virginia Beach, Virginia 23456
(804) 555-1212

Experience

Andrew Carey, M.D., Surgeon
1867 Oats Road
Eastville, Connecticut 06387
Position: Business Manager (November 1984 to August 1988)

My objective, as an effective business manager, was to ensure a consistent income for the practice by utilizing proven, effective means of collection. With this end in mind, I initiated a turnover system so that within 12 hours after a patient's visit the insurance had been processed. By thoroughly understanding the mechanisms of different insurers, we were able to achieve a 98 percent collection rate month after month. By streamlining different tasks and implementing time management principles, much of the loose paperwork was eliminated and fewer errors were made. Consistent with this objective was my desire to create a satisfying environment for the employees. All employees had their own spheres of importance and expertise, which afforded them some control over their work and resulted in higher productivity.

John Blanchard, M.D.
Professor and Chairperson
New England Medical School
Westville, Connecticut 06774
Position: Practice Manager–Executive Secretary (March 1982 to July 1983)

The position encompassed two areas: (1) private practice manager and (2) secretary to the chairperson of OB-GYN. As practice manager, I was responsible for patient records, transcription, coding, charges, and patient scheduling. As secretary to the chairperson, I was involved with the residency program for obstetrics and gynecology.

Nutmeg Roofing
87 Westover Street
Westville, Connecticut 06774
Position: Office Manager (September 1978 to June 1980)

I ordered supplies and maintained inventory, payroll, accounts receivable and payable and did the preliminary figures for the quarterly taxes.

Education

New England Business College, Eastville, Connecticut, 1986. Principles of Accounting, Business Management, English, Principles of Information Processing.

Connecticut Community College, Eastville, Connecticut, 1985. Biology, English, English Literature, American Literature.

Smith Business School, Westville, Connecticut, 1981. Medical Terminology I, II; Physiology I, II; Medical Transcription, I, II; Insurance I, II; Psychology; English; Typing I, II; Shorthand I, II.

clude a face-to-face interview and testing. She was informed that testing was included in the next step so that she could drop out if that was a problem for her. An evaluation of her performance in the telephone interview is included in Exhibit 2-8. Dr. Frederick decided that Ann was a very promising candidate, so he scheduled her for an interview. His reasons for immediately scheduling interviews with promising candidates were as follows:

> When I conclude during the telephone interview that the applicant is a *very* good candidate, I schedule the next step in the employment process before I end the call, so that I don't waste time recontacting the applicant. This can be advantageous for three reasons. First, I can easily waste a day or two trying to recontact and schedule an applicant who is in demand. Second, the selection process works two ways. The applicant is also making decisions. I am in competition with other employers, and if the applicant is tied down tomorrow morning interviewing with me, then she *can't* be interviewing with my competition. Finally, scheduling the next step will shake out the serious from the non-serious applicants. The danger in scheduling the applicant at the end of the telephone interview is that she may not be as good as the next two or three

Exhibit 2-8 Structured Telephone Interview Format and Evaluation

---

Interview

1. Identify yourself.
2. Ask whether still in job market.
3. Describe the position to applicant and tell applicant to ask questions at any point during this interview.
4. Ask what applicant is looking for.
   a. Position with responsibility. Enjoys getting the money in. Place where she fits in. Long-term relationship.
5. Ask applicant to describe previous work experience.
   a. Handled accounts to $650,000 by herself without computer. Stressed her ability to organize, look for efficient ways of working. Has done insurance billing, posting, collections. No experience with local CHAMPUS, some with state BC/BS.
6. Discuss salary and benefits.
   a. No problem.
7. Next step is interview and testing.

Evaluation of Skills

Language was always appropriate. No observable mistakes in grammar or syntax. Asked relevant questions at several points—possibly indicates good problem-solving ability. Technical skills appear to be appropriate. Overall, she appears to be intelligent, qualified, and interested.

---

that I will assess on the telephone, but I can always call back and cancel. . . . In reality, deciding whether to immediately offer the second step or postponing that decision is usually not difficult. Those applicants who are really good stand out.[12]

The next step in the selection procedure consisted of a structured interview and administering the California Psychological Inventory (CPI). The interview focused on technical questions related to insurance billing and collections. The object was to explore the depth of the applicant's knowledge and assess her ability to make the shift into another medical field. Exhibit 2-9 contains the interview questions and the interviewer's notes regarding her responses. The first five questions were used with all applicants. The sixth question was specific to this applicant, because her last job had been in another state and her previous experience had been in another medical field.

The most important consideration on this job was collections, so the interview questions focused on this factor. Obviously, it was impossible for Dr. Frederick to assess every facet of her knowledge of collections, so he identified particularly important areas that would give an indication of the depth and degree of her knowledge. In addition, he used the structured questions as points of departure. If the applicant said something that raised another question or made a comment that didn't seem quite right, Dr. Frederick followed up until he felt confident he had satisfactorily resolved any uncertainties.

The CPI is a 462-item questionnaire that assesses 24 traits related to psychological adjustment, work attitudes, and interpersonal skills. It takes about an hour to complete, and it is self-administered, so it doesn't consume any personnel time during administration. Computer scoring is available, or the CPI can be interpreted using the test manual and other reference resources. Exhibit 2-10 lists the CPI traits that were scored on applicants for this job. Dr. Frederick forwarded Ann's completed CPI to a consultant for scoring and interpretation. Examination of Ann's profile indicated that she had many traits that would contribute to success on the job. Exhibit 2-11 contains Ann's CPI interpretive report.

The interview took 45 minutes to complete, and the CPI took 65 minutes. Dr. Frederick, however, was only present during the interview. As a result of Ann's superior performance in the interview, her CPI results, and her stated interest in the position, it was decided to suspend assessment of other applicants until a decision could be made on her. It made sense, therefore, to change the ordering of assessment procedures and to immediately proceed with the telephone reference checks since these would consume less time than the second interview. The comments of her references are reported in Exhibit 2-12. On the basis of all this information, Ann was asked back for a second interview and work sample testing.

The work sample testing was designed to end any remaining doubts regarding Ann's knowledge of revenue collections and insurance. The applicant was pre-

Exhibit 2-9 Structured Interview Questions and Responses

---

1. What is the procedure you use when a patient has more than one insurance carrier? Answer indicated that she would identify the primary, hold billing on the secondary until the primary had paid. Addressed some of the difficulties of identifying the primary. Overall, an informed answer, quickly given.

2. How do you handle a delinquent account? (Follow with role-playing.) Initial answers pointed to the necessity to act quickly but with reason. If patient is in office, meet face to face. First, ask if there are any personal circumstances to account for not paying. Depending on the situation, use humor, sternness, etc., to achieve the goal. Obtain a partial payment or credit card if necessary. If patient is not present, use telephone call first, then short series of letters. Applicant indicated that she did not like to use form letters. This was then role-played. I stated, "Okay, I'm the patient. Talk to me." She was direct, courteous, and asked me to make behavioral commitments. Overall, appropriate answers given quickly. Answers stressed reason, control, logic, need to be systematic, etc.

3. How do you handle a delinquent insurance company? Responded with humor. Stated that she really "liked to go after them." When pushed on how to identify outstanding claims, she stated that she assumed that there would be some reports available. When asked what reports she needed, she responded by stating aging analysis and aged insurance. Both are appropriate. Also indicated that she has simply looked through patient files. When pressed on how she would identify slow payers, she indicated that the key was systematic review of accounts, ideally on a weekly basis. When asked how she would review 800 accounts in a week, she stated that she would separate out the bad ones based on aging and would review those regularly. Overall, her answers were adequate. She seemed somewhat hampered or frustrated by not knowing our procedures.

4. What do you consider to be an acceptable standard for accounts receivable? Previously indicated a standard of two times current as the upper end of what would be acceptable, implying that this was marginally not acceptable. Body language and verbalizations indicated that she thought our accounts were out of control.

5. How would you go about reducing this practice's accounts receivable? Didn't have a particular strategy and seemed somewhat confused or surprised by the question. Her first response was that it would take long hard work. She then asked if there was anyone else in the practice who could assist. This indicated to me the standard strategy of looking for available tools that could be utilized on a project. She then asked how long she would have to get the "AR plug" fixed. I indicated that it should all be gone, as well as current accounts properly handled, in six months. She stated and/or indicated through expressions that this was a reasonable if not generous time period.

6. Your background is in working in a surgical practice in Connecticut. What problems do you anticipate in doing billing in a family practice in Virginia? Indicated that there were differences between fields but they were not major—related to knowing what codes to use, what diagnoses would be paid for, etc. In regard to the insurance companies, she stated that it was just a matter of getting on the phone and asking a lot of questions. She didn't minimize the difficulty of shifting across medical fields or having to deal with new insurers, but she clearly was not intimidated by it, nor did she express overconfidence. A very appropriate and reasonable answer.

Exhibit 2-10 California Psychological Inventory Factors

Dominance (Do): Self-confidence and assertiveness
Capacity for Status (Cs): Need for success, ambition, and independence
Sociability (Sy): Friendliness, enjoyment of people
Social Presence (Sp): Self-assurance, spontaneity
Self-Acceptance (Sa): Opinion of self
Independence (In): Self-sufficiency, resourcefulness, self-confidence
Empathy (Em): Understanding the feelings of others
Socialization (So): Ability to conform, acceptance of rules, etc.
Self-Control (Sc): Control of emotions, self-discipline
Good Impression (Gi): Trying to do what will please others
Communality (Cm): Ability to "fit in" with others
Well-Being (Wb): Optimism about the future
Tolerance (To): Tolerance for others' beliefs and values
Achievement via Conformity (Ac): Drive to do well, ability to work in situations where there
are rules and standards
Achievement via Independence (Ai): Drive to do well, ability to work in unstructured work
settings
Intellectual Efficiency (Ie): Efficient use of intellectual abilities
Psychological Mindedness (Py): Interest in the reasons why people act the way that they do
Flexibility (Fx): Liking change and variety
Femininity/Masculinity (F/M): Sensitivity to criticism, emotional vulnerability, action orientation
Work Orientation (Wo): Sense of dedication to work, strength of work ethic
Management Potential (Mp): Talent and desire for management role
Leadership Potential (Lpi): Foresight and decision-making ability
Fake Good Scale: Designed to identify protocols that were faked to look overly favorable.

Sources: Adapted from *California Psychological Inventory Administrator's Guide* by H.G. Gough, pp. 6–7, Consulting Psychological Press, 1987, and from *A Practical Guide to CPI Interpretation* by L.W. McAllister, Consulting Psychological Press, 1988.

sented with a real account that had a large outstanding balance. She was told to analyze the account and identify any problems with it. She analyzed the account by identifying copayments, insurance payments, and write-offs for each procedure, and she then assembled personal and insurance balances. When asked what she would do regarding the personal balance, she stated, "I'd call the patient on the telephone, because the balance is large and long overdue." Since that type of conversation had already been role-played in the first interview (Question 2, Exhibit 2-9), there was no need to role-play it again. Her ability to successfully bill insurance companies was assessed by presenting her with several insurance forms containing errors, such as a missing diagnosis code. She responded by correctly noting the additional pieces of information that needed to be entered on the insurance forms.

The second interview focused on specifying the needs of the practice's director, Dr. Frederick, and providing Ann with a realistic preview of the job and the per-

Exhibit 2-11 Interpretation of California Psychological Inventory

CPI Overall Conclusions

A dominant theme is the applicant's strong sense of obligation and strong need to meet the expectations of others. She wants to fit in and meet the needs of those whom she values. There is a strong need to be needed, but there is also evidence of assertiveness and perhaps aloofness and detachment. She is perceptive of others' needs and abilities, likes to be with other people and work with them, and is competent in interpersonal situations, but ultimately her trust in her own ability to get things done is greater than her willingness to delegate to others.

She is serious, proper, stable, competent, rational, able to accept constructive criticism, disciplined, and concerned about her performance. There is a desire for structure and predictability and sticking to plans, which probably results in an aversion to risk taking.

Her behaviors are always appropriate, she strives for competence, and she adheres to the Protestant work ethic. She works hard, intelligently, and efficiently, and her efforts are characterized by planning, setting of priorities, and anticipation of consequences. Overall, her personality and work are characterized by optimism and a positive attitude. Her behavior pattern is opposite to the passive-aggressive behavior pattern.

Response Set Evaluation

The Fake Good scale was within normal limits. There is no indication of an attempt to fake good.

Class Evaluation

The high degree of consistency within classes indicated that class interpretation was appropriate. Class I scales indicate a self-confident person who is outgoing, competent in interpersonal situations, and person-oriented. The *relatively* low Self-Acceptance score may indicate that she tries to put her evaluation of her own capabilities into a reasonable perspective, if not to minimize them consciously, so as not to appear as self-aggrandizing.

Class II scales suggest a person who has a sense of duty, behavioral control, and a dislike of taking risks.

Class III scales indicate that she is achievement-oriented and uses intellectual strategies as opposed to a brute force to deal with problems.

Class IV scales are mixed and cannot be interpreted as a set.

Structure Evaluation

Structural scale characteristics indicate that she is a weak Alpha, an ambitious, action-oriented, productive type of person, a doer who does socially acceptable things and feels comfortable in interpersonal relationships. At their worst, Alphas can be self-centered, opportunistic, and manipulative. She has an exceedingly high v.3 score. This indicates that the positive aspects of the type are highly developed in her. This in turn indicates a high degree of self-reflection and optimism regarding the future.

Selected Individual Scale Interpretations

She has a responsible level of dominance (Do), indicating that she is not overbearing but can be assertive when necessary.

The capacity for status (Cs) scale indicates that she aspires upward, should be sensitive to management's perspective, and can handle stress and pressure.

continues

Exhibit 2-11 continued

The sociability (Sy) scale indicates she has the ability to relate to people in an appropriate manner, enjoys interpersonal relationships, but is not a "backslapper" or inappropriately boisterous. Her sociability level is associated with sincerity, honesty, and compliance with social norms.

The social presence (Sp) scale indicates enthusiasm and ties in well with her sociability level, indicating a comfort with social situations.

The self-acceptance (Sa) scale is inconsistent with the previous two scales. This may indicate a conscious attempt to keep her own self-impression under control and to be modest and socially appropriate regarding her own skills.

Her independence (In) is at a level indicating appropriate goal-oriented behavior and an appropriate degree of assertiveness.

The empathy (Em) scale indicates insight into her interpersonal behavior. As a result, her behaviors are viewed as reasonable by others.

Her responsibility level suggests a sense of responsibility and a desire to follow through on obligations.

The self-control (Sc) scale indicates a preoccupation with detail, a tendency toward compulsiveness, and a reliance on facts instead of intuition. She plans ahead and is good at developing systems and procedures for getting things done. She thinks before she acts but may also repress feelings and occasionally explode.

Her tolerance (To) level indicates a nonjudgmental, tolerant appreciation for differences and a trust of others.

The achievement scales suggest that she is comfortable working in organized structured situations, but at the same time she can act independently and only needs a minimum of supervision.

The intellectual efficiency (Ie) scale indicates that planning, anticipation of events, and establishing priorities are very important to her. She does not act impulsively.

Her level of psychological mindedness (Py) suggests that she is more comfortable in dealing with concepts and abstractions than delegating responsibility. She is perceptive of others' needs and empathic. She would rather do a task herself than delegate it.

Her flexibility (Fx) level indicates deliberateness and determination. She is not afraid of change but probably is realistically cautious and skeptical regarding it.

Her femininity/masculinity (F/M) level indicates a balance between being tough-minded and sensitive to the needs of others.

Special Scales

Her work orientation (Wo) level is very high. This suggests she is reliable, disciplined, and dependable. Similarly, her management potential (Mp) is well above average. This indicates she creates a good impression; is confident, socially effective, emotionally stable, mature, realistic, optimistic, and well organized; shows foresight; and gets things done.

sonnel with whom she would work. Salary and benefits were discussed in detail, and a job offer was made. This second interview and the work sample testing took two hours. The telephone reference checks took 15 minutes.

The time expended by practice personnel for Ann's selection was as follows:

Resumé Review	.10 Hrs.
Telephone Interview	.50 Hrs.
Interview and Testing	.75 Hrs.

Reference Check	.25 Hrs.
Second Interview and Work Sample	2.00 Hrs.
Total	**3.60 Hrs.**

In this instance, the entire selection process was conducted by Dr. Frederick, the practice's director. Dr. Frederick described his job as 80 percent clinical work and 20 percent administration. He felt that the business manager position was so important that he should personally assume the responsibility for filling it.

This case illustrates how a medical practice can fill a critical position in a timely, cost-effective manner, while at the same time obtaining an employee with an excellent chance of success. It also illustrates how procedures can be streamlined in ways that would be difficult or impossible for larger organizations.

SELECTING PROFESSIONAL EMPLOYEES

The strategy and methods for filling front office positions are also appropriate for filling professional positions. It is likewise essential to understand the type of work that will be performed and to evaluate the applicants' ability to perform this work. The major difference is that the applicants for some professional positions will not consider psychological testing or any other paper-and-pencil testing to be acceptable. Since hiring is a two-way process in which applicants also evaluate the employer's suitability, using selection methods that are not considered acceptable is risky.

In reality, this is not a major problem. Testing a doctor's skills is most appropriately handled by using work samples, references, and the resumé. For example,

Exhibit 2-12 Reference Questions and Evaluations

Questions
1. What were the duties and responsibilities of the job that she performed for you?
2. Describe her style of working with others.
3. How did she respond to evaluation of her performance?
4. Describe her attitude towards work and life.

Evaluations

Dr. Blanchard had minimum recollection of her. He checked with his nurse and stated that "the nurse remembers her very favorably."

Dr. Smith was very pleased with her performance. He hired her for a secretarial position, which she found out about through a newspaper ad. She quickly exhibited a multitude of skills, and as the practice grew she took on additional responsibilities. She was "tactful" and "wise." She did a lot of insurance billing, and he perceived her as very capable in that capacity. Her attitude was very positive, she worked well with others, and her actions indicated that she kept the "practice's interest in mind."

---

the last stage in the selection of a physician could involve the finalists' working at the medical practice for a morning. On a work sample day, the practice physician would inform each patient that "Dr. X is helping us out today, and we will be working together with you this morning." The practice physician would retain the ultimate responsibility for and control over the situation. She would observe Dr. X's skills and progressively allow him more latitude in the examination and treatment of patients. During this process, she would evaluate his diagnostic ability, communication with staff, rapport with patients, prescribing, and so on.

Work sampling is also appropriate for nursing positions. Once again, allowing applicants at the last stage of selection to exhibit their skills under close supervision is an appropriate and effective employment method.

An applicant's acceptance of psychological testing is generally related to the difference in status between your position and the position to be filled. A physician who requires nurse applicants to complete a CPI will probably not get much resistance. On the other hand, a physician who requires this of a fellow physician should expect to generate hostility.

Newspaper ads and word of mouth are appropriate for professional recruiting. Other recruiting sources include medical journals and newsletters as well as professional conferences. Perhaps the best strategy for recruiting doctors is to be active in the local medical community. If you are well known and have a good reputation, other doctors will seek you out when they are exploring employment alternatives. Attending local medical society meetings, networking with peers, joining the country club, and affiliating with a nearby university that trains doctors are all subtle, long-term, and effective recruiting strategies.

EQUAL EMPLOYMENT OPPORTUNITY

You should use all of your selection methods without regard to the race, religion, sex, national origin, or age of applicants. Specific guidelines to ensure that your methods comply with the content and spirit of legal requirements are discussed in Chapter 9.

CONCLUSION

You should now understand that there are many tools, procedures, and methods for selecting and hiring employees. By using the strategy presented above, you will be able to develop a selection method that will assess job-related skills in a timely, cost-effective manner. Such a method will greatly increase your chance of hiring employees who will perform satisfactorily. You should also understand your own role in the selection process, as well as the roles of staff and consultants.

NOTES

1. W. Cascio, *Applied Psychology in Personnel Management,* 3d ed. (Englewood Cliffs, N.J.: Prentice-Hall, 1987), 264.

2. J. Hunter and R. Hunter, "Validity and Utility of Alternative Predictors of Job Performance," *Psychological Bulletin* 96 (1984): 72–98.

3. R. Arvey and J. Campion, "The Employment Interview: A Summary and Review of Recent Research," *Personnel Psychology* 35 (1982): 281–322.

4. "Uniform Guidelines on Employee Selection Procedures," *Federal Register,* 1978, vol. 43, 38290–315.

5. R. Sweetland and D. Keyser, *Tests: A Comprehensive Reference for Assessment in Psychology, Education, and Business* (Austin, Tex.: PRO-ED, Inc., 1983).

6. J. Conoley and J. Kramer, *The Tenth Mental Measurements Yearbook* (Lincoln, Neb.: University of Nebraska, 1989).

7. L. Saxe, D. Dougherty, and T. Cross, "The Validity of Polygraph Testing," *American Psychologist* 40 (1985): 355–66.

8. Courts have held that inadvertent or minor misstatements may not be reason for termination. For example, misspelling an address or transposing a telephone number would be very questionable reasons for dismissal.

9. S. Kahn, B. Brown, and B. Zepke, *Personnel Director's Legal Guide: 1988 Cumulative Supplement* (Boston: Warren, Gorham, and Lamont, 1988), s2-19-s2-20.

10. Some large companies will hire applicants at random to test new employment methods. As a result, they will be able to observe how applicants whom the selection procedure predicted would fail actually perform on the job. This strategy for evaluating the predictiveness of a selection procedure is called *predictive validation.*

11. Few medical practices would hire the number of applicants represented in Figure 2-1. The same phenomenon could be observed, however, by plotting the performance of applicants hired over a very long period of time. Even though a practice may only be filling one position, the same forces illustrated by this example will be at work.

12. Personal correspondence. Name withheld by request.

Chapter 3

Evaluating, Disciplining, and Terminating Employees

CHAPTER OBJECTIVES

In this chapter you will learn how to evaluate the job performance of your employees so that you can improve their effectiveness and, as a result, the effectiveness of your practice. In addition, you will learn how to discipline employees in ways to (1) improve their job performance, and (2) provide documentation to prevent or combat any legal challenge to an eventual termination. Finally, you will learn how and when to terminate an employee. Terminating an employee in the correct way can prevent a number of legal, financial, and employee morale consequences.

INTRODUCTION

Not all employees will do what you want them to do. The reasons might include:

- limitations in ability that prevent an employee from properly performing the job
- personality characteristics that limit an employee's willingness to follow directions
- the widespread view that institutions and organizations, such as medical practices, exist to serve the needs of the employees as opposed to the employers
- giving an employee ambiguous or contradictory directions

Inadequate employee job performance has the potential to lower the quality of health care provided by your practice, to reduce its profits, and even to jeopardize its existence. It is essential, therefore, that you be able to evaluate job performance swiftly and effectively, change employee performance when it is inadequate, and terminate employees who will not or cannot improve their performance.

The process of determining how well an employee is performing on the job is called a *performance appraisal,* and the document that results from this process is called a *performance evaluation.* An employee's performance evaluations will form the basis for subsequent personnel actions, including pay raises, training, promotion, discipline, and termination. The performance appraisal process includes

- evaluating the quality and quantity of work performed
- constructing a performance evaluation document to record the conclusions reached as a result of the performance appraisal
- informing the employee of your observations
- using this information to improve job performance by providing, for example, training, coaching, additional equipment, incentives, and so on

All medical practice supervisors must become accomplished in performance appraisal methods. If clerical personnel are supervised by a business manager, then the business manager must be proficient in these skills. The doctor should only personally conduct performance appraisals on direct subordinates, such as the business manager, surgical assistant, nurse, and office manager. The doctor, however, may be a source of performance appraisal information about any employee. For example, the doctor may provide the business manager with observations regarding a receptionist's job performance, which the business manager will then take into consideration when writing the receptionist's performance evaluation.

Performance appraisals serve a number of functions essential to the success of a practice. For example, performance appraisals tell employees that management is aware of their performance, that it matters, and that the practice has standards distinguishing acceptable from unacceptable work. If employees believe that nobody cares or that nobody will notice whether job performance is adequate, they may perform in ways to meet their own needs instead of the needs of the practice. The feedback that supervisors give to employees is also an important motivational tool. All of us like to have our accomplishments acknowledged by others. Performance appraisals provide a psychological boost to employees who do well and a "kick in the pants" to those with performance problems.

Performance appraisals also provide employees with direct guidance regarding how you wish them to perform their jobs. If your business manager is devoting too much time to producing unused financial reports and not enough time to working old accounts, then comment on it *now.* In the absence of your comments, the business manager may assume that you approve of the current apportionment of work. By documenting your dissatisfaction and then evaluating and rewarding the business manager's future apportionment, you will tie behavior to rewards, thereby motivating the employee to perform in the interest of the practice.

Performance appraisals can also tell you what additional training, supervision, and task changes might be needed by your employees. For example, if you find that your accounting data are not being kept in a timely enough manner, this may indicate that the employee who is responsible needs more direction regarding when you expect the data to be available. It also may indicate that the employee needs some additional training in the use of your accounting software or that the employee's workload is too heavy and some accounting tasks should be transferred to another employee or to your accountant.

Finally, performance appraisals are essential for making good compensation, promotion, disciplinary, and termination decisions. Since compensation, promotion, discipline, and termination should be based on job performance, the adequacy of your decisions in these areas will be limited by the quality of your performance evaluations.

Performance appraisals constitute a cornerstone of successful management. As a result, you and any other practice supervisors must be skilled in the use of performance appraisal methods. Immediate feedback and formal, periodic performance reviews are components of a good performance appraisal system. Immediate feedback controls and motivates behavior on a daily basis and provides data for periodic reviews. Periodic performance reviews, which might occur quarterly, semiannually, or annually, provide context and structure for the daily observations and guidance for the future.

CONDUCTING EMPLOYEE PERFORMANCE REVIEWS

Immediate Feedback

The single most effective performance appraisal procedure is to observe and comment on employee performance *as it occurs*. Immediate feedback has a number of benefits. If job performance is good, your comments will provide motivation and encouragement. If job performance is poor, you will immediately begin to modify the substandard behavior. If an employee's performance is inadequate and you don't comment on it, you have implicitly told the employee that the performance is acceptable. For example, if a deadline for completing a letter is missed by a day and you don't remark on this, then you have indicated that deadlines are not really that important. Delaying your comments until a periodic annual or semiannual performance review may result in many missed deadlines. In addition, if you do not comment on inadequate performance as it occurs, some employees may conclude that you are afraid of a confrontation. Employees who perceive that their supervisor is afraid of distasteful or confrontational situations may use this knowledge to achieve their objectives at the expense of the practice.

Many doctors have difficulty providing immediate feedback, particularly when it is critical. It can be difficult to sit across a table from an employee and say, "John, I have a problem with how you are. . . ." It is much easier to be critical of an employee to your spouse or to your golfing partner, because they are likely to nod in agreement. All this does, however, is provide a safe outlet and temporarily relieve your frustration. It does not achieve the most important objective: changing the employee's behavior. On the other hand, some doctors are only too happy to be critical of an employee, while being slow to provide deserved compliments. This is a quick way to generate employee turnover. Effectively using immediate feedback is a difficult skill to master. It takes both experience and good judgment to distinguish between the occasional inconsequential error or achievement and a failure or triumph of real significance.

An important tool to use in conjunction with feedback is a *critical incident file* (see Exhibit 3-1). A critical incident file contains brief comments regarding noteworthy events in the working life of an employee. The word *critical* in this instance means out of the ordinary *and* important. A critical incident file should include comments about praiseworthy as well as blameworthy incidents. The comments should be very brief. If they are not, then the time involved in documenting incidents will become burdensome and the file will not be maintained.

The critical incident file will be particularly useful at the time of an employee's periodic review. It will provide the supervisor with behavioral examples from the entire year, thus allowing a more balanced and accurate evaluation. Without a critical incident file, the supervisor's memory may become selective. He or she may tend to remember only more recent events or may disproportionately recall positive (or negative) incidents. Since the critical incident file should be maintained by the employee's supervisor, you should maintain critical incident files only for direct subordinates. Keep them handy so that it will be convenient to add comments.

Exhibit 3-1 Critical Incident File Excerpts

2/11/90	VISA bill not paid on time. $36.62 finance charge.
4/29/90	941 tax form not prepared until the last day. Preparation done only after I reminded her.
7/17/90	Ran long computer reports during day instead of overnight, tying up computer during day. When asked, she had no reason for doing this. Poor time management.
11/3/90	Went out of her way to make Frank feel welcome on his first day by taking him to lunch.
12/9/90	Got us a $6,000 advance from CHAMPUS against claims that they are slow paying on.

Each employee should be able to review the contents of his or her own critical incident file. Remember, the object is to improve job performance. You can't do that by keeping your comments, either positive or negative, secret. Correspondingly, any incident worthy to be entered into an employee's critical incident file is important enough to be discussed with the employee near the time of the occurrence. By commenting on performance as it occurs and then documenting important deviations from the norm in a critical incident file, you will make the assessment of performance an integral part of your management technique. Other practice managers should do the same.

Periodic performance appraisal interviews should be conducted regularly. Typically, these interviews are done annually, although new employees should receive a periodic review after two or three months on the job. By telling new employees at the time of employment that they will be formally evaluated in two or three months, you achieve two objectives. First, you give the new employee an extra incentive to learn the new job and to excel. Second, you emphasize that you are very concerned about job performance and will recognize when the employee's performance is inadequate or outstanding or in between. In effect, this initial periodic review provides an opportunity to shape the development of a new employee.

Periodic reviews of a continuing employee provide an opportunity to evaluate the employee's record and establish a coherent plan for improvement. Without the periodic reviews, the feedback provided by daily supervision can amount to a series of unconnected comments. The reviews help to place these comments into a larger perspective and allow plans for improvement to be based on the employee's current strengths, weaknesses, and personal goals.

Evaluation Errors

There are a number of errors that supervisors can make when evaluating job performance. Leniency errors occur when supervisors consistently rate employees either too high or too low. Some supervisors tend to consistently evaluate subordinates too favorably (positive leniency bias) because they think that a more accurate evaluation would have an adverse impact on morale. Some give high evaluations because they have not been paying close enough attention to subordinate performance, and no one ever objected to a high evaluation. Other supervisors feel that a less-than-outstanding evaluation reflects poorly on their own leadership ability. Finally, some supervisors lack assertiveness, and they become overly dependent on acceptance and approval from their subordinates. Giving an accurate appraisal may threaten this approval.

Similarly, there are a number of reasons why some supervisors consistently downgrade subordinate performance. Some supervisors project their own failings onto their subordinates. If it is always a subordinate's fault, they do not have to accept personal responsibility. Other supervisors have unreasonably high standards. It is important to remember that a medical practice owner will generally have a far greater degree of commitment to the practice than an employee. Therefore, an owner must try hard to be realistic about the degree of commitment and performance that can be expected from employees. Consistently giving low evaluations and demanding performance that employees perceive as unreasonable will only result in employee dissatisfaction and turnover.

Another common evaluation mistake is called a *halo error*. A halo error occurs when a supervisor allows an employee's performance on one job factor to influence the evaluation of another factor. For example, if Sarah is outstanding at word processing, the supervisor should not allow this to influence the evaluation of her performance on communications with patients. These are separate issues and should be treated as such in the performance appraisal process. A particularly insidious type of halo error occurs when the supervisor allows a factor that is *not* job relevant, such as physical attractiveness, to influence some or all of the evaluations of job-relevant factors. Sometimes this halo process can be very subtle, and it may be occurring at an unconscious or semiconscious level.

Performance Standards

Performance standards (Exhibit 3-2) are statements describing what an employee in a particular job must do or achieve in order to perform adequately. Performance standards relate to the *job*. Irrespective of who occupies the position, the incumbent will be expected to meet the performance standards for that job.

Performance standards should not be confused with employee goals. A goal is a personal objective that may equal or exceed a particular performance standard. For example, a performance standard for the position of business manager may be to keep total accounts receivable below 2 times current billings. Any business manager who does this is doing at least an adequate job on this factor. A specific goal for Jane, however, may be to reduce accounts receivable this year from 1.9 to 1.75 times current billings.

Many large organizations like to have written performance standards for virtually all factors on most jobs. This is a waste of time. It is difficult to write meaningful performance standards for some factors, and others are so obvious that it makes no sense to ponder the issues. For example, the following might be a performance standard for patient relations: "Employee is always courteous and attentive to patient needs." This statement is so bland that it is virtually meaningless. It states the obvious and provides no guidance to the employee. Don't waste your time or your employees' time writing or trying to apply meaningless performance standards. On the other hand, if you have a clear standard of acceptable behavior and the job performance issue is important, then it will be helpful to your employees if you share the standard with them. Performance standards should always be dis-

Exhibit 3-2 Performance Standards

Checkbook

- Checkbook is reconciled with the bank statement no later than five days after the statement is received.
- Monthly income should always balance against the monthly collection for physicians plus other income.

Accounts Receivable

- Total accounts receivable (AR) should never exceed two times current AR.
- AR report should be run each week.
- Cash box should be balanced against receipts printout each day.

Word Processing

- Documents should contain no typing, spelling, or grammatical errors.
- Documents should be completed no later than three days after they are submitted for typing.

Database Maintenance

- Referral database should be revised at least weekly.
- MediMac should be revised daily.
- All other databases should be revised at least weekly.
- All databases should be backed up daily.

Referrals

- Twenty-five percent of a physician's referrals should be self-generated.
- Thank you letters should be written on at least a weekly basis.
- Two public information seminars should be presented each year.

---

cussed with employees at the time of employment. They should also be communicated to employees in written form, either as part of the job description or in a separate document.

Rating Forms

Many supervisors consider completing a rating form (Exhibit 3-3) to be equivalent to doing a performance appraisal. Completing a rating form should instead be viewed simply as a way of recording the evaluation information and conclusions. Rating forms can be useful if you have to make comparisons between many employees. For example, when a large company is evaluating current employees for promotion, it would be very time consuming, if not impossible, to evaluate 100 narrative performance appraisal reports to determine who is most worthy of the promotion. A rating form such as the one in Exhibit 3-3 provides a means to de-

Exhibit 3-3 Typical Performance Appraisal Rating Scales

1. When unsure about a problem, discusses it with supervisor.						
Almost Always	1	2	3	4	5	Almost Never
2. Has mastered the information provided in technical manuals for the office equipment and software used on the job.						
Almost Always	1	2	3	4	5	Almost Never
3. Has a sense of humor even with difficult patients.						
Almost Always	1	2	3	4	5	Almost Never
4. Accepts and adapts to change.						
Almost Always	1	2	3	4	5	Almost Never
5. Adequately delegates work.						
Almost Always	1	2	3	4	5	Almost Never
6. Gets written reports completed on time.						
Almost Always	1	2	3	4	5	Almost Never
7. Gets all appropriate paperwork signed by patients.						
Almost Always	1	2	3	4	5	Almost Never
8. Communicates appropriately with patients.						
Almost Always	1	2	3	4	5	Almost Never

termine efficiently who has the highest performance evaluation. Evaluation forms of this type have their own special problems: (1) They take time and effort to construct; (2) unless long and complex, they make it difficult for a supervisor to describe all aspects of a subordinate's performance; and (3) they are particularly subject to the rating errors discussed above.

Since medical practices rarely need to make comparisons between large numbers of employees, rating forms such as the one in Exhibit 3-3 are not necessary. Usually, performance appraisals in medical practices are aimed at assessing a few employees in great depth. The object is to compare the employee against the demands of the job instead of with other employees. A narrative evaluation constructed around the job description factors for the position is the most appropriate type of evaluation form for achieving this. Excerpts from a narrative evaluation report are found in Exhibit 3-4. This type of evaluation is useful for making compensation, termination, and training decisions as well as comparing performance levels from past years with current levels.

Evaluation Data

The data that you will use to evaluate an employee can be classified as either objective or subjective. Objective data are produced in the normal course of work

Exhibit 3-4 Excerpts from a Narrative Performance Appraisal

Position: Computer Operator/Secretary
February 13, 1991

Computer Operations

Your performance with MediMac has been outstanding. You understand the program better than anyone else in the office, and you use it very effectively. You have successfully installed the new updates and deleted cases, and you have become more assertive in getting help from HealthCare Communications. There has been a noticeable improvement in the quality of data entry into MediMac. This is partly due to a personnel change, but it is also a result of your making this a priority for you and those who report to you. This factor is a very critical part of your job, and you have provided confidence in the quality of the data and reports as a result of your good work habits and consistency.

You need additional training with Filemaker II. Your databases don't have consistent variable categories, so it is difficult to sort and search on a variable category. In addition, you occasionally get behind on entering cases, so that the databases are sometimes more than a week out of date, which constitutes a failure to meet the performance standard. Developing your ability to use this program is a high priority.

Relations with Patients

You continue to do an outstanding job of working with patients. You always perform your duties in a professional manner, even with the most difficult patients. As you indicated, your judgment in crisis situations has been excellent. You and the other front office people have done an outstanding job of handling new referrals. This has produced an initial visit "show rate" of 93 percent, which is outstanding.

Setting Priorities

Previously, this had been a problem area. You have improved in this area because you are more willing to be assertive with those who place inappropriate demands on you. You are also more willing to communicate with others, allowing you to set reasonable priorities.

Communications and Problem Solving

Your improving assertiveness skills have helped you to communicate more effectively with physicians and with HealthCare Communications about its software, and these skills are now adequate. You now also do a good job of providing consistent feedback on whether tasks have been completed. Previously, this had been a problem. In order to improve still further and turn this into a real strength, consider taking an assertiveness course.

---

activities. Examples include "typing error rate," "percent of insurance dollars collected within 90 days," "number of patients treated per week," "number of referrals generated per month," and so on. You must be very careful when using objective data. Unless you fully understand the numbers, they can be misleading. For example, suppose that you are evaluating a physician based on the number of referrals that he has generated over the past year. Can you separate referrals generated by the practice, such as those caused by a Yellow Pages ad that mentions your colleague's name, from referrals generated directly by the physician? Similarly, suppose that you are evaluating your business manager's performance collecting revenues. An increase in the accounts receivable may indicate a performance problem or that your practice is growing. If the practice is growing, you may have to adjust the accounts receivable numbers to obtain a valid picture of the business manager's performance. You could, for example, take the accounts receivable money that is 90 days old as a percentage of the current accounts receivable, thereby adjusting for practice growth. Objective data can be very useful for evaluating an employee's performance if the data truly reflect the performance.

Subjective data include your personal interpretation of events, such as your judgment of an employee's ability to work with patients, diagnostic skills, supervisory skills, and knowledge of software. Subjective data are generally susceptible to the rating errors mentioned above. Most of the data available for evaluating medical practice employees are subjective. Even those practices that maintain databases on productivity and finances find that in the final analysis performance appraisals are fundamentally subjective, since the objective data usually are relevant to only a part of each job. Eventually, someone must weight and integrate the subjective and objective appraisal information.

When jobs contain evaluation issues that are both objective and subjective in nature, be especially vigilant for halo errors. It is very easy to let subjective data bask in the halo of objective data. For example, you have good hard evidence that Fred is doing a great job generating referrals for the practice. You may tend to unconsciously or semiconsciously allow this fact to bias your evaluations of other less measurable issues, such as his bedside manner, diagnostic skills, and treatment of staff. Similarly, Frances does a great job of collecting revenue, but she tends to look the other way when subordinates complete assignments late. Once again, you may be inclined to overrate her supervisory ability out of gratitude for her ability to keep the money flowing. It is important for supervisors to evaluate factors separately, thereby providing the employee with the opportunity to improve in those areas that need development.

Conducting the Periodic Appraisal

The first step in the periodic appraisal process is to schedule a date for the review. Provide enough notice so that you and the employee will have time to prepare. Ask the employee to write a self-evaluation. The employee's remarks should be organized around the major job performance issues noted in the job description. Tell the employee to get the written remarks to you at least a week before the day of the periodic review. The process of writing a self-evaluation causes the employee to think about his or her job performance, to examine it as a supervisor might, and to begin thinking about what needs to be done in the future. The self-evaluation also tells you how the employee has interpreted your feedback and gives you an indication of what to expect in the appraisal interview. (Exhibit 3-5 contains a self-evaluation written by an incumbent in a computer operator/secretary job. Exhibit 2-1 contains the position's job description.) Schedule the periodic review at a time during normal work hours and explain to the employee that the purpose of the meeting is to review past performance and to begin planning for the next year.

The appraisal information that you will be discussing in the meeting should contain no surprises. If you are doing an adequate job of keeping the employee appraised of his performance on a daily basis, the periodic review will simply be a reiteration of what has been said over the year. At some point, it will be useful to review the employee's critical incident file. Classify incidents according to the factors noted on the job description. In addition, collect any other pieces of pertinent information, such as objective measures of job performance and comments from peers and other doctors.

It also is appropriate for you to examine your own performance relative to the subordinate. Are you contributing to any of the employee's performance problems? For example, Jane has not been able to fully utilize the capabilities of the word processing software. Has the practice provided her with proper training? Has she been given time to read the manuals and ask questions? If you are contributing

Exhibit 3-5 Computer Operator/Secretary Incumbent Self-Evaluation

In the past year and a half, I have grown both personally and professionally. I have established a good rapport with both patients and professionals. I feel that I have good instincts when it comes to dealing with patient "emergencies." The appointment book is running smoothly. I think I have gotten a handle on everyone's schedule and I am making fewer errors. I rarely if ever miss my deadlines. Although I probably shouldn't, I always make sure that documents that are literally given to me at the last minute go out on time. On a personal level, I think that I have learned to tolerate things that I cannot change, and I am not letting things get to me like I used to.

MediMac is running smoothly now, and I have been able to handle several occasions when we had a software problem. I have been better at calling HealthCare Communications when we have had a problem that I couldn't solve.

Right now I feel that my major weakness is that I don't know very much about Dr. Sample's schedule or about what he expects from Angela. I also need to be more assertive, but I think that I have made giant leaps in that department over the last year.

I want to learn how to do the checkbook and use the accounting software. I want to get away from all the word processing and take on more administrative responsibilities. I would like to work on accounts occasionally, but I don't want to do it exclusively.

I think that the office is running smoothly, and overall I think that I am doing a very good job.

to the problem, then you should take this into account when developing a realistic way of improving her performance.

You are now ready to write the employee's performance evaluation report. Your evaluation should always be put in writing. A written report provides documentation that will be useful for tracking an employee's progress over the years. Written documentation also can be useful in defending against legal challenges to personnel decisions (see Chapter 9).

Exhibit 3-4 contains excerpts from an employee's annual evaluation. When writing an evaluation, it is important to use clear, concise language. This will save you time and will provide the subordinate with an unambiguous statement regarding strengths and weaknesses. Initially, you may find it difficult to be direct, especially if there are performance problems. It is important to remember, however, that careers can be ruined by supervisors who are kind and softhearted. *Avoiding the difficult issues until performance is so inadequate that you must discipline or fire the employee is not doing anyone a favor.* It is important that your comments remain related to job performance and are not condescending or personally derogatory. In summary, stick to the facts and work with the employee to develop reasonable solutions.

Begin the performance appraisal interview by giving the employee a copy of your written analysis. Then review the sources of data that you used in developing your evaluation. This tells the employee that your evaluation is based on a thorough analysis of facts, not conjecture, and that the appraisal is important enough for you to have taken time to assemble a written document. (The facts, of course, may include the opinions of others and the observations recorded in the critical incident file.) Use the interview time to elaborate on your written appraisal and to plan for the future. Solicit employee comments, and explore any areas in which the employee has suggestions for how job performance might be improved. Although weaknesses and areas needing improvement should certainly be discussed, don't dwell on them. Most employees have strengths, and it is important to discuss these and build upon them.

Before beginning the interview, you should have a clear idea of what you wish to accomplish and any changes you wish to implement. Discuss desired changes with the subordinate to ensure that they are really feasible. Once you determine that your strategy for improvement is feasible, devise an implementation schedule. This increases the probability that the plan will be carried out.

Improving Job Performance

Job performance can be improved by selectively using four techniques:

1. training
2. incentives

3. discipline

4. job restructuring

The choice of which method or methods to use depends on the employee's current circumstances. The performance appraisal process will help you to determine the best strategy. Training is appropriate for increasing an employee's skills. If an employee's low performance is due to limited ability *and you believe that he or she has both the capacity and motivation to improve,* then training is a reasonable choice. It is also beneficial in the case of an outstanding employee who still has some room to grow.

Incentives will be more fully discussed in Chapters 4 and 5. At this point, it is sufficient to say that providing an incentive, such as a pay raise or a bonus based on production, will only change behavior when the employee sees the incentive as valuable and related to job performance. The same holds true for discipline. Threats and the removal of rewards only change performance when the rewards are desired and are perceived as tied to achievement. If the employee really doesn't want the job or the rewards, then discipline will have no effect.

Job restructuring involves changing a job to compensate for an employee's strengths and weaknesses. For example, suppose an otherwise valuable secretary has difficulty collecting fees from patients at the time of service. You try to improve performance by giving her guidelines and having her enter an assertiveness training program, read articles on self-esteem, practice collection methods using role-playing with other employees, and so on. Her performance, however, does not improve. At this point you may choose between firing the employee or examining the tasks performed on this job and the other front office jobs. If it is possible to restructure some of the jobs so that this employee will spend little if any time collecting fees, you will have solved the performance problem. Obviously, you must use this method carefully. If other employees perceive that they must bear an extra burden because of a coworker's incompetence or reluctance, you will simply be trading one kind of problem for another.

Performance Appraisal Summary

The assessment of performance should be a continuous process involving both supervisors and employees. Formal appraisals provide an opportunity for you to review an employee's progress, solicit personal goals, and plan for the future. Performance appraisals furnish you with a measure of your practice's performance, help you to motivate your employees, and provide you with critical information for making management decisions, including training, job-restructuring, compensation, and termination decisions.

You should personally conduct all performance appraisals of your direct subordinates. It is also desirable for you to observe the appraisal interviews conducted by your supervisors of their subordinates. At a minimum, you should read the evaluations and review them with your supervisors. This will help prevent supervisors from using the performance appraisal process to satisfy their own needs for power and control at the expense of their subordinates. Reading evaluations will also provide you with an efficient way of learning more about your employees and the strengths and weaknesses of your practice.

DISCIPLINE

Discipline is the act of forcefully reacting to your employees when they fail to meet your expectations. The object of discipline is to change an employee's behavior. *The object is not to degrade, embarrass, or harass the employee or force the employee to resign.* Discipline is a logical and appropriate course of action, when you determine that an employee is willfully ignoring your expectations or disregarding your orders. It is appropriate for any number of infractions, including absenteeism, tardiness, abusive or obscene language, alcohol or drug abuse, carelessness, negligence, inappropriate dress or grooming, insubordination, inadequate job performance, dishonesty, theft, and falsification of documents. In addition to changing the behavior of the affected employee, good disciplinary procedures provide standards and expectations for all other employees and thus help prevent new problems from arising.

In industrial settings where unions are involved, discipline can be an overly complex process in which the company and the employee become entangled in a complex web of hearings and procedural steps. This degree of formality and restrictiveness is not characteristic of medical practices. Nevertheless, there are some generally accepted rules that apply to cases in which disciplinary actions are used.

Discipline generally should be progressive. This means that initial disciplinary actions should be less severe than later actions. The concept of progressive discipline is consistent with the concept of due process, since the employee receives warning or notice as well as an opportunity to comply. Usually, termination should be a last resort and should take place only after preceding disciplinary steps.

Progressive discipline would be appropriate for many of the infractions noted above. Some infractions, however, are so severe that they merit immediate dismissal. Such infractions may include theft, gross insubordination, falsification of records, and so on. When discussing disciplinary procedures with your employees, it is important to make a distinction between offenses that will result in immediate dismissal and those for which progressive discipline will be instituted.

It is important to develop disciplinary procedures firm enough that employees understand that unacceptable behavior will result in undesirable consequences. It is also important, however, to make the procedures flexible enough so that you can respond to events with some discretion and be able to take into account differences between employees as well as extenuating circumstances.

Progressively applying discipline gives employees an opportunity to improve. Generally, a summary discharge for a first offense will be perceived by employees as arbitrary and unjustified. Ultimately, you do yourself an injustice if you dismiss an employee who would have succeeded if given a second chance. As you will see in Chapter 9, employment at will—the power of an employer to terminate an employee for good reason, bad reason, or no reason at all—is under attack or has been limited in many jurisdictions. In many states, summary termination for anything but the most serious offenses, such as theft or drug use on the job, can be successfully challenged in the courts. Progressively disciplining an employee provides you with a defense to an allegation of wrongful discharge, since you will be able to show that the employee was made aware of the consequences but failed to respond to warnings.

Employers can choose from a number of progressive disciplinary actions. The object should be to devise disciplinary procedures that vary in their degree of progressiveness depending on the seriousness of the infraction. Procedures for infractions of a less serious nature may progress through more steps, whereas those for infractions of a more serious nature may only have one or two. The disciplinary choices generally include

- verbal warnings (one or several)
- written reprimands (one or several)
- suspension
- termination

When a verbal warning is given, the employee should be called into the supervisor's office. This will convey the seriousness of the matter to the employee as well as preserve the employee's privacy. When giving a verbal warning, be certain to clearly state

1. the nature of the infraction
2. what you want the employee to do
3. the time period in which the employee is to react, if appropriate (e.g., if an apology is to be given, state that it must be given before a specific date)
4. the consequences if the behavior recurs

The following is an example of a verbal warning given by a physician to a business manager:

John, your actions have been insubordinate. When I tell you that I want an aging analysis for Dr. Johnson, you either do it or give me a reason why it should be a lower priority, and then let me decide. You don't fail to do it and then not inform me. If there are choices to be made, I will make them. You present me with the information that you feel is relevant, and I will then decide how you should devote your time.

My expectation is that this will never happen again. You've been a good employee, and this behavior is out of character for you. If it does happen again, however, I will have to consider further disciplinary action, which may include immediate dismissal. Do you have any questions?

The tone and content of the warning should convey your concern but should also indicate you are optimistic the employee will be able to improve. Even if you are not optimistic, indicating that you expect compliance may motivate the employee to obey. In addition, you should place the infraction in the context of the employee's normal job performance. Doing this is particularly important for an employee whose performance has generally been acceptable. This will tell the employee that many months or years of good performance are not being suddenly nullified by one event.

When discussing the consequences if the behavior is repeated, you may want to begin to build the necessary framework for a termination. This is a judgment call that you have to make based on the severity of the infraction, the likelihood that you will have to terminate the employee, the employee's previous job performance, and the employee's anticipated response. If you decide that there is the potential for eventual termination, then you may want to say, "If this behavior continues to occur, it *may* result in your eventual dismissal." At this point in the process, you don't want to encumber yourself with too many commitments regarding what you will or will not do. It is important to document each verbal warning by writing a summary of the precipitating incident and the content of the warning.

You may want to provide more than one verbal warning for infractions that in isolation are not critical to the functioning of the practice. Also, if a second infraction is dissimilar to the first or there are extenuating circumstances, then you may want to give a second verbal warning before moving on to a written warning. Once again, the object is to get the employee's attention, to impress upon the employee the serious nature of the offense, and to correct the behavior. If, given your knowledge of the employee, you feel that this can be accomplished by another verbal warning, then another verbal warning is appropriate. This second warning will also convey the message that a written warning is extremely serious and that the employee's job will be in jeopardy if one is issued.

A written reprimand should also be presented and discussed in the privacy of the supervisor's office. When discussing the reprimand with the employee, it is important to "reach back" to any preceding verbal warnings. Reaching back justifies more severe discipline, since it establishes that two or more incidents are linked and that you see them as part of a pattern of disobedience, nonperformance, and so on. Often an employee's second infraction will differ from the first. If you perceive that two or more infractions are linked, then you should treat them as linked and proceed to the next disciplinary step. On the other hand, if there has been a significant lapse of time between the two infractions, the slate should be wiped clean.

You will probably determine that some transgressions will necessitate a written reprimand as the first disciplinary step. The policy of starting with a written reprimand should be reserved for very serious infractions, infractions that would result in immediate dismissal if repeated even once. Examples might include falsification of records, blatant insubordination, and abusive language. If an employee commits an offense that requires a written reprimand as the first step, you may be dealing with someone who has a character flaw. Employees with character flaws rarely change; they simply learn to hide their transgressions. Thus, you may want to begin preparing for the eventual replacement of the offending employee.

The written reprimand should be shown to the employee. Ideally the employee should sign it, thereby indicating that he or she has reviewed the document— although not necessarily agreeing with its content. The act of signing the reprimand will also make it seem more significant, once again impressing on the employee the serious nature of the offense. Since written warnings should be reserved for very serious matters, it is important to build the framework for a termination by giving the employee clear notice that any future infraction may result in immediate dismissal with no additional warning.

Be certain to choose your words carefully so that you will have some discretion in the matter. For example, suppose that an employee has had an attendance problem. You provide a written warning and state, "If you miss another day for any reason, you will be fired." The employee then has excellent attendance for the next four months but fails to report on a day when the roads are covered with snow. You and other employees manage to get to work. The employee's work has been good, and it would be very inconvenient to replace her at this time. What do you do? It's a tough call. You certainly don't need the added consideration that you will appear to be inconsistent if you don't fire her. In addition, you don't want to give her the incorrect message that her value is so great that you won't ever fire her. Leaving yourself a little room to maneuver when giving warnings will allow you the latitude to make a decision that is best for you given the circumstances at the moment. In this case the wording "may be disciplined up to and including immediate dismissal," would have been appropriate.

Providing a second written notice is not recommended. Generally, an employee who does not respond to a verbal reprimand and a written reprimand for the same type of offense is not salvageable. Giving an endless string of written warnings only serves to undermine your authority in the eyes of your other employees, dilute the significance of a written reprimand, and postpone the inevitable.

Suspension is usually not a feasible alternative for a medical practice. The relatively small office size, coupled with the thin staffing typical of medical practices, usually means that a suspension will be more of an inconvenience to the doctor than a penalty for the employee. *If this is the case in your practice, be certain that you don't threaten employees with suspension.* This could create the misperception that a suspension will precede termination. If you make this statement either verbally or in writing, it could be construed by a court to be part of the contract between the practice and the employees (see Chapter 9). Termination of an employee without a preceding suspension might then be interpreted as a wrongful discharge. The underlying principle here is that if you make any sort of verbal or written commitment to employees, you may well have to live up to that commitment. Don't promise or threaten anything in the disciplinary process unless you are fully aware of the consequences and willing to follow through.

In order for a disciplinary procedure to be effective, it must provide employees with due process. This means that a number of generally held employee expectations must be met. For example, employees expect

- comprehensive information about job performance expectations as well as the consequences of failing to meet those expectations
- treatment that is consistent and predictable
- discipline based on facts as opposed to conjecture
- the opportunity to present a defense to a management willing to listen
- discipline that is progressive and in proportion to the infraction or pattern of infractions
- disciplinary decisions that take into account extenuating circumstances

Due process requires that employees know what is expected of them. This applies to their jobs and to the disciplinary process. Job descriptions, frequent discussions between supervisors and subordinates, and clearly stated or written disciplinary procedures ensure that employees know what is acceptable, what is not acceptable, and what will occur if employer expectations are not met.

It is also important to clearly state the disciplinary consequences. If you really intend to terminate an employee on the basis of the next infraction, then you need to say that clearly and directly. Some employers cringe at the thought of being this direct with employees; it makes them feel uncomfortable. Others believe that they will overly antagonize employees. Unfortunately, this burden goes with the responsibility of being a supervisor. It is far worse to "sandbag" employees by concealing your expectations and then surprise them with unexpected discipline. Sandbagging is inconsistent with due process, and it makes you appear to be unpredictable in the eyes of your other employees.

Consistency is a hallmark of an effective progressive discipline plan. If an employee fails to call in when ill and other employees were previously given verbal reprimands under similar circumstances, then the same standard should be applied to this employee. Similarly, if a verbal warning and two written warnings preceded previous terminations for below-standard job performance, the same three-step process should be applied consistently to all other employees. Any change in the process should be fully discussed with employees and put in writing.

Basing discipline on factual findings is essential. Employees are quick to perceive or imagine ulterior motives.[1] These perceptions can destroy the effectiveness of discipline as well as your overall credibility as a manager. When determining the facts, you must create a written record. If you are disciplining an employee for absenteeism or tardiness, then the written record (e.g., employee time cards) should clearly support the allegation. If an employee was insubordinate to you, then write down exactly what happened. If there were others present, have them also describe the incident. If records were falsified, include copes of them in the documentation.

A clear factual record can be used as support for a termination and as a defense should the employee claim to be wrongfully discharged. Defamation suits have been filed against employers by former employees who maintained that they were harmed when employers fired them without documented factual evidence.[2] Although it is not likely that an employee will pursue this course, it is always safest to have your personnel actions grounded in well-documented fact, since this will provide a legal defense as well as let you sleep at night.

Another requirement of due process is that an employee be given an opportunity to present his or her side of the case. If the employee has an explanation or can bring forth extenuating circumstances, what is the harm in listening? It does you no good to discipline an employee who in fact acted in a responsible manner or to overdiscipline an employee when there were extenuating circumstances. Employees who are treated in an arbitrary manner will feel that they have been wronged even if your reason for disciplining them is fully justified. They will then focus on their feeling that they were wronged by the process, as opposed to recognizing the significance of their own transgression. In addition, a disciplinary process that does not allow the employee to present a defense may cause other employees to question your overall commitment to fairness. This may have consequences in other areas, such as when you ask an employee to do something out of the ordinary or temporarily change work hours.

Finally, a progressive discipline plan should provide for individual differences among employees. This rule may appear to be inconsistent with the objective of providing consistent discipline. Remember, the goal of discipline is to change behavior. If a particular employee's background or previous work history indicates that differential treatment is most likely to correct the problem, then it may be justified. For example, an employee who has been with you for ten years fails to order important medical supplies and covers up the fact. Other cover-ups have consistently been addressed by issuing written reprimands. Given the employee's seniority and previous work record, it might be appropriate to issue a verbal warning instead. Discipline that provides differential treatment based on appropriate provable considerations is consistent with the notion of due process and will facilitate employee acceptance of your standards. It is important, therefore, to strike a balance between the need for applying discipline with consistency and the need to tailor discipline to the particular circumstances of each case. There is no magic answer. Your awareness of the need to balance these competing demands is essential to successfully managing this aspect of discipline.

In summary, progressive disciplinary procedures will help ensure that your employees are treated fairly, that they have sufficient opportunities to improve performance, and that you have sufficient cause and documentation to justify termination. By varying the number and type of steps for various classes of infractions, you will treat your employees fairly while retaining discretion to deal expeditiously with serious infractions. Some offenses might call for a three-step process comprising a verbal warning, a written reprimand, and termination. Other offenses might call for a written warning followed by termination. Finally, a few offenses might require immediate termination. An example of a progressive disciplinary plan is found in the discipline section of the sample employee handbook (Appendix 3A).

TERMINATION

It is important to terminate employees in such a way that you minimize legal exposure and disruption to the practice. The infraction that precipitates the termination should be documented in detail. If there are witnesses other than yourself, have them provide a written record as well. Be certain to retain any physical evidence, such as falsified records, financial data, or poorly typed documents.

Your attorney should be involved in this process at least twice. At the first point in the disciplinary process that you feel the employee *may* have to be discharged, review with your attorney your state's standards for discharge. This will help you to properly document subsequent infractions. You should also contact your attorney prior to the termination meeting. Review the evidence supporting the discharge and have your attorney suggest specific language and comment on any written documents you will give to the employee or ask the employee to sign.

Before you conduct the termination meeting, try to obtain from the employee any information that is important for practice operations, such as the location of important charts and records and the status of important accounts. You must balance the value of the information that may be obtained against the risk that the employee will determine something is amiss and use the occasion as an opportunity for sabotage.

When you conduct the termination interview, it is desirable to have another person present to witness your actions. Using direct, clear language, cite any preceding disciplinary actions. Also cite any warnings that you provided regarding the possibility of termination. Then describe the recent infraction and ask the employee if there were any extenuating circumstances. If the employee provides an explanation for his or her actions, you may choose either to proceed (if the explanation is obviously without merit) or to verify the explanation. Although it is usually better to take the time to investigate an employee's explanation, you should understand that you run the risk of sabotage.

Once you have determined that termination is justified, tell the employee the specific reason for the termination. If you have progressively disciplined the employee or if the infraction was outrageous, reminding the employee of your evidence may deter future legal action. Any severance benefits should then be clarified with the employee. At this point, you may choose to offer the employee the option of resigning. In some states, an employee who resigns cannot collect unemployment compensation. Other states merely delay eligibility for benefits when an employee resigns. A resignation, therefore, may be advantageous to you, since your unemployment insurance rate will usually increase when an employee collects compensation benefits. The employee may also benefit when looking for a new job—as a result of being able to state that he or she left voluntarily. If the employee chooses to resign, be certain that the employee signs a document stating that he or she has voluntarily resigned. This will protect you against any subsequent wrongful discharge claims.

Conduct the meeting in a calm, orderly manner. This is not the time to degrade or otherwise attack the employee. Once you have obtained a resignation or fired the employee, have the employee turn over keys and any other practice property. The employee should then *immediately* leave the practice under escort. Be certain to change security codes on any office alarms as well as computer access codes.

In some cases, contract employees may have to be given notice before termination. If this is the case, resist the temptation to have the employee provide training to a replacement or continue working after notice has been given. The relationship between the new employee and the practice will be vulnerable to poisoning by the terminated employee. In addition, the terminated employee is likely to devote as much time to sabotage as to training or working. If an employee must be given notice, you are better off paying the salary that is owed and dismissing the employee then and there. Tell the employee that you expect him or her to answer any specific questions by telephone and that receipt of the final paycheck or severance pay is contingent upon this cooperation.

Finally, you may want to consider timing the termination so that it meets your needs. Although notification of termination should take place within a reasonable time after the infraction, that does not mean that you must terminate the employee on the same day as the infraction. You may want to buy some time to begin the recruiting process. For example, tell the employee that you want to meet tomorrow or two days hence and schedule the meeting for the end of that day. If the employee raises any defense to the termination, say that you need some time to consider the arguments. This could buy you another two days. There are risks to this strategy. If the employee believes that he or she will be fired anyway, sabotage becomes a possibility. In addition, if the discharge is merited, do you really want the employee working for you even for another two or three days? These are choices that only you can make, but they should be choices to which you give careful consideration.

You may conclude that the discipline and termination process must take a lot of time. The following two cases illustrate that this is not necessarily so.

Lucy was hired to fill a secretarial position on January 12. The position involved typing, answering phones, scheduling appointments, collecting fees, and so on. Her test and interview performance was adequate, although not outstanding. The previous job incumbent had been fired, and there was considerable pressure to fill the job. The job market was tight, so Dr. Smith's business manager determined that "adequate" was good enough. Lucy received on-the-job training for four days, and her coach worked in the adjacent room.

Lucy seemed to be always behind. Little of her assigned typing was completed on time. Patients were left on hold for long periods of time, and she appeared to move slowly in a very busy office. On her sixth day of work, Dr. Smith happened to observe Lucy taking a new referral over the telephone. She was exceedingly slow. It took her over 15 minutes to obtain all of the information and schedule the patient. On the following day, the business manager noted that a new referral hung up on Lucy during the middle of the referral process. Once again, the observation was that she was painfully slow. The typing never seemed to quite get finished, and the front office staff was beginning to have trouble finding some patient charts. Apparently they had been misfiled.

Eight days after Lucy had been hired, the business manager met with her and reviewed her performance inadequacies. He then gave her guidance regarding needed improvements. He also told her that if her performance did not improve, she *might* lose her job. Two days after the verbal warning, the business manager met with her again and told her that he knew that she was trying hard but that her performance had not improved. If there was no change, she would have to be terminated. The business manager summarized the conversation, told Lucy that the practice could not wait much longer for her to become proficient, and said that he would enter his notes in her personnel folder as a written warning. The next day, January 25, there were three double bookings in Lucy's appointment book.

The business manager called her into his office at 4:00 P.M. He told her he knew that she had done her best and that the extra pressure of knowing she was being watched may have made it more difficult for her. Her job performance, however, had not improved. He then terminated her for inadequate job performance. Dr. Smith had been consulted on the impending termination, and he agreed to provide one week of severance pay, which, along with her back pay, was given to her at the end of the termination interview.

JoAnne was hired to fill a billing position. She performed well on her employment tests and in her interviews. She dressed nicely and appeared to be a confident, verbal, and skilled applicant. Three days after she was hired, she left a message for Dr. Franklin in which she stated, "I just wanted to remind you that I will need to take next week off to go to an out-of-town wedding." Dr. Franklin was shocked. He didn't remember being told during the employment interview about the wedding, and he certainly hadn't agreed to the leave. In addition, he recalled stressing the importance of reliability in both the telephone interview and the personal interview.

Dr. Franklin telephoned JoAnne and confronted her with the discrepancy. JoAnne told Dr. Franklin that she had to attend the wedding and that she couldn't believe she had neglected to tell him. Dr. Franklin was convinced that JoAnne was attempting to manipulate him. Dr. Franklin told her that she had acted dishonestly by taking the job without informing her future employer of this significant commitment. Dr. Franklin then told JoAnne that he was firing her for dishonesty and for purposely misleading him in order to get the job.

THE EMPLOYEE HANDBOOK

An employee handbook can be an effective means of conveying the kind of information discussed in this chapter to employees. The purpose of the handbook is to provide a reference describing your personnel policies and practices and how they affect employees. All too often, doctors attempt to treat their employees as though they are "friends." Although it is important to treat employees fairly, it is a mistake to assume that employees are your friends. To some extent the employer-employee relationship is adversarial, since your needs may be inconsistent with an employee's personal desires. Maintaining an arm's-length relationship with your employees is important to ensure that they meet your expectations. An employee handbook is one way of saying, "This is a business, we have standards and expectations that we intend to enforce, and we are all here to meet my needs and my patients' needs first."

Exhibit 3-6 contains some topics that you may want to include in an employee handbook. Since some of the policies will be different for professional and non-professional employees, it is best to have different handbooks for each class of employee. Appendix 3A contains a sample employee handbook for salaried, non-professional employees.

Exhibit 3-6 Possible Employee Handbook Topics

Job Performance Expectations	Pay Practices
Working Hours	Paydays
Notification of Absence	Overtime Pay
Bad Weather Policy	Travel Expenses
Confidentiality	Benefits
Personal Use of Practice Property	Employee Evaluation
Time	Employee Evaluation Plan
Vacation Policy	Probation
Holidays	Annual Performance Appraisal
Sick Leave Policy	Performance Standards
Time Off for Personal Business	Employee Problems
Leaves of Absence	Discipline Procedures

Medical practices are not required to have employee handbooks. The information they typically contain, however, does need to be communicated to employees. Some doctors, especially those with only one or two employees, may feel that an employee handbook is an overly bureaucratic way of presenting information that could be communicated in ten minutes of face-to-face discussion. Recognize, however, that memories can be selective and that misunderstandings can escalate into disagreements, which can sour the employer-employee relationship. If practice policies and expectations are in writing, there is less chance for misunderstandings to occur. Choose the medium you feel most comfortable with. If you choose to convey the necessary information verbally, a good time to do this is during the employee's orientation period. If you choose to write an employee handbook, you may want to consider the following advice:

1. Put a disclaimer at the beginning of the handbook stating that the handbook is not part of the employee's contract. This will give you maximum flexibility in dealing with your employees. The main object is to avoid inadvertently modifying an employee's written or unwritten employment contract. (See also "Employment Issues" in Chapter 9.)

2. You will never be able to anticipate all of the situations that will arise. Use wording, therefore, that provides you with the flexibility to act with discretion and in the practice's best interest. This is particularly important when defining causes for termination. Although you want to provide due process, you do not want to unduly restrict your prerogative to terminate an employee when you determine that this is necessary.

3. Recall previous employee disputes. These can give you some idea of the specific policies you want to set as well as the potential problem areas you need to address.

CONCLUSION

This chapter discussed some of the most important employee management skills. After reading it, you should be able to use performance appraisal as an employee development tool to increase the productivity of your employees and thereby improve your practice's ability to deliver effective health care services.

Discipline may be necessary when employees do not meet your performance expectations. You should understand how to create a progressive disciplinary process that provides employees with assurances that they will be treated fairly and with respect. At the same time you should have gained an appreciation for why you need flexibility in administering discipline. The discussion in this chapter should help you to balance these two competing needs when you develop discipline procedures for your own practice.

Termination is the outcome of unsuccessful performance appraisal and discipline. If you practice medicine long enough, you will eventually have to terminate an employee. You should now be able to terminate an employee in such a way that the termination is minimally disruptive to the practice and can be defended if challenged.

Finally, guidelines were presented for developing an employee handbook. By issuing an employee handbook, you can contribute to due process by informing employees of the consequences of adequate and inadequate job performance. An employee handbook can also clarify your expectations of employees and prevent problems that could result from a misunderstanding of your expectations.

NOTES

1. J.R. Redeker, *Employee Discipline Policies and Practices* (Washington, D.C.: Bureau of National Affairs, 1989).

2. Ibid., 103.

Appendix 3A

Sample Employee Handbook

This handbook is designed to acquaint you with information that you will find useful as an employee of this practice. It is not part of your contract with the practice, nor does it in any way change your at-will employment status with the practice. It will tell you, however, about general practice policies and how they affect you. If you ever have questions about the issues discussed in this handbook, please talk to me or to the business manager.

Frederick Wilson, M.D.
Director

JOB PERFORMANCE EXPECTATIONS

We provide an important service to our patients. We expect that you will act courteously, promptly, and effectively to meet our patients' needs. As a small company, our success and your job security depend on your ability and willingness to learn your job and do it well. In addition, you should be aware that you will occasionally have to work with patients undergoing a medical emergency. Knowing your job thoroughly and doing your job effectively may save a patient's life.

Among other things, we expect the following:

- You will work to the best of your ability.
- You will be honest.
- You will immediately discuss with the business manager or the practice director any events that affect your ability to do your work or that could harm another employee, our patients, or the practice in any way.

In return, you can expect that the practice will

- consider your suggestions
- treat you with respect and courtesy
- compensate you in a manner consistent with your job performance and the success of the practice
- manage its affairs in an ethical manner
- not discriminate on the basis of race, religion, sex, national origin, or age

A. Supervision

Figure 3A-1 shows the reporting relationships in the practice. You report directly to the business manager. Part of the business manager's job is to help you to set priorities and to ensure that you have the training and resources necessary to do your job. It is important for you to develop a close working relationship with the business manager. You should go to the business manager whenever you need help. The business manager, for example, can help you by

- setting priorities
- determining what to do when there is too much work and not enough time

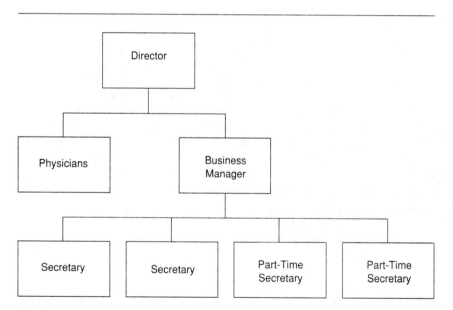

Figure 3A-1 Practice Reporting Relationships

- providing additional training
- resolving problems you are having with a physician or fellow employee
- providing direction whenever you are uncertain about what to do or you don't understand the reason for an office policy or procedure

In addition, if you have any ideas for improving the operation of the office, discuss them with the business manager.

Whenever you are given an assignment, it is expected that it will be properly completed on time. We depend on everyone doing his or her work as instructed. If you see that you cannot meet a deadline, it is essential that you immediately inform the business manager. This will allow the business manager to make *choices* regarding priorities and work assignments.

If you ever have a problem with a practice policy or one of your work assignments, it is essential that you discuss the problem *immediately and directly* with the business manager. Problems might arise, for example, in any of the following areas:

- working hours
- vacation time
- work assignments
- supervisor decisions
- collection methods
- job description changes

If you feel that the problem is still not resolved, then you should discuss this with the director. It would be destructive to the practice to take the problems to other employees or to the physicians. They cannot solve your problem.

It is very important for all employees to be treated with courtesy and respect. If you feel that a physician or another employee does not treat you with proper courtesy or respect, it is important for you to address this directly with the physician or employee. If you cannot get the problem solved, then discuss the problem with the business manager. If the business manager cannot solve the problem, then you should inform the director.

B. Working Hours

Since all of our jobs are interrelated, it is important for you to be ready to work by 8:00 A.M. The normal workday ends at 5:00 P.M. You are responsible for transportation arrangements to ensure you regularly arrive on time and are able to provide a full day of work. The business manager is responsible for coordinating lunch breaks, which are one hour, to ensure adequate waiting room and telephone coverage. Everyone should return from lunch no later than 1:30 p.m.

C. Notification of Absence

If you find that you will be absent because of illness or a true emergency, call either the business manager or the director. If you know the night before, call one of them at home. If you are calling in the morning before the phones are taken off of answering, call through on the third line (555-2275). Don't leave a message on answering unless you cannot contact either the business manager or the director.

D. Bad Weather Policy

Normally, the office will not close during bad weather. In the rare instance that it is necessary to close the office, you will be called and advised that the office will be closed for the day. If you find that you cannot get to work, immediately call the business manager or the director.

E. Personal Use of Practice Property

Please clear the personal use of practice facilities or equipment through the director in advance. For example, if you want to stay after hours to do some personal typing, copying, or computing, the director must be fully aware of your intentions and give approval. If significant amounts of supplies will be consumed, you will be expected to pay for them.

TIME OFF

A. Vacations and Sick Leave

You accrue a full day of personal time for each full calendar month that you work. This time may be used as sick leave or vacation time. You may accrue up to 15 days, at which point you must either use the time or receive payment for it.

Vacation leave must always be approved by the business manager. Although vacation leave will not be unreasonably denied, the request must be consistent with the business needs of the practice and the needs of our patients.

B. Time Off for Personal Business

Most personal matters should be taken care of on weekends or outside of normal working hours. In unusual circumstances, the business manager may allow you to shift your hours to accommodate a personal need. Any request must be approved ahead of time by the business manager and must be consistent with the business needs of the practice and the needs of our patients.

C. Leaves of Absence

Generally, leaves of absence will not be granted. We are a small practice, and unless you have accrued the leave time, we cannot give you unearned time off.

COMPENSATION

A. Paydays

Paydays are on the 1st and the 16th of each calendar month. If a normal payday falls on a weekend or a holiday, the actual payday will be the last business day before the normal payday. Each employee must complete and sign a time card and give it to the business manager the day before payday.

B. Overtime

All overtime must be approved in advance by the business manager or the director. All employees who are not exempt from the wage and hour laws will be paid overtime at 1.5 times the normal hourly pay rate. All overtime work must be reported on your time sheet.

C. Travel Expenses

If the business manager or the director asks you to travel for the practice, you will be paid $0.255 per mile and reimbursed for any incidental expenses, such as tolls.

PERFORMANCE APPRAISAL

Adequate job performance is essential to providing our patients with the best possible care. It is important for you to know how you are doing in order for you to provide the best possible service to our patients and satisfy your own personal growth and career goals. As a result, performance appraisals are a regular part of working at this practice. Normally, all new employees undergo a formal appraisal after 90 days of employment. In addition, all employees are evaluated after each year of employment.

The performance appraisal process is very important, so we have developed specific procedures for conducting an appraisal. As the time for the appraisal approaches, you will evaluate your own job performance. You will then meet with the business manager and/or the director in order to discuss your performance, set goals for the future, and consider any suggestions you have regarding how you can work more effectively.

DISCIPLINE PROCEDURES

On occasion it is necessary to discipline an employee. The practice reserves the right to determine the appropriate disciplinary action—up to and including termination—based on its sole and unrestricted interpretation of the events. Generally, less serious infractions, such as failing to call in when sick or taking overly long lunch hours, will result in progressive discipline:

First offense	Verbal warning
Second offense	Written warning
Third offense	Disciplinary action up to and including immediate termination

If more than six months has transpired between two infractions of the same nature, the practice may at its discretion consider the second infraction to be a first offense. Inadequate job performance may also result in progressive disciplinary action. Examples of inadequate job performance include

- incomplete work
- inadequate quality of work
- work completed late
- failure to apply practice policies and procedures
- hiding information from the business manager or director

The strategy for dealing with such performance deficiencies will be based on the degree of seriousness. Generally, the object will be to provide feedback, training, and an opportunity for the employee to improve. *Progressive discipline, however, will only be applied to job performance problems to the extent that it does not jeopardize the well-being of our patients or the practice.*

Offenses of a very serious nature, such as theft, insubordination, falsification of practice records, misappropriation of company property, and lying, will be dealt with by disciplinary actions up to and including immediate termination.

Based on the circumstances of the case, the business manager and/or the director will meet with the employee and determine if discipline is necessary. The employee will be given an opportunity to present information, including information about mitigating circumstances. All disciplinary decisions are ultimately made at the sole and unrestricted discretion of the practice. The director will review and approve all termination decisions.

Chapter 4

Compensating Employees

CHAPTER OBJECTIVES

An effective compensation plan will help you to hire, retain, and motivate good employees while at the same time keeping your payroll costs under control. The object of this chapter is to provide you with a strategy and procedures for determining how much to pay each of your employees. Although compensation is largely dispensed in the form of direct wages, you also will be providing some benefits, including perhaps life insurance, health insurance, a retirement plan, vacation time, sick leave, educational benefits, and profit sharing. Benefits will be discussed as a means of fine-tuning your compensation plan to best meet your needs and those of your employees.

INTRODUCTION

Compensation plans can be constructed by you or by a consultant. Most smaller practices will find that they can determine salary rates for front office personnel without the use of a consultant. The methods described in this chapter are helpful for quickly determining fair rates for practice jobs. You may conclude, however, that use of these methods is "overkill" for determining salaries for two or three front office jobs. If that is the case, you can improve the results obtained from an intuitive approach to compensation by applying the *theory of compensation* discussed below. If you understand *what* compensation should be based on, you will be able to make better intuitive judgments and arrive at more equitable salaries.

Larger practices will find that basing a compensation plan solely on intuitive judgments of the appropriate salaries for positions will tend to create personnel and compensation problems. In particular, employees might become dissatisfied with their pay, which can manifest itself in such symptoms as absenteeism, tardiness, and low quality or quantity of production. Alternatively, the size of your payroll might become excessive. If you notice either of these conditions, you should have a closer look at your compensation plan. The information contained in this chapter will help you to perform that examination. If you contract the work out to a consultant, then this chapter will help you to understand how the consultant will examine the problem and to place the consultant's recommendations in a theoretical and an applied context.

EQUITY: A THEORY AND STRATEGY FOR DETERMINING COMPENSATION

The goal of any compensation plan is to achieve equity in the minds of employees. Equity is a judgment made by the employee regarding the fairness of compensation. Equity judgments are not absolute, but they are instead comparative. An employee judges the equity of compensation by making a comparison of his or her rewards to the rewards and work inputs of others. Equity is therefore a cognitive *ratio* of rewards to performance for the employee, which he then compares to the ratio of rewards to performance for significant others. Three equity conditions can be expressed conceptually as formulae:

$$\frac{R_e}{I_e} = \frac{R_o}{I_o} \quad \text{Equity}$$

$$\frac{R_e}{I_e} < \frac{R_o}{I_o} \quad \text{Inequity due to underreward}$$

$$\frac{R_e}{I_e} > \frac{R_o}{I_o} \quad \text{Inequity due to overreward}$$

Where:

R_e is the total of all rewards received by the employee
I_e is the employee's input
R_o is the total of all rewards received by another employee
I_o is the other employee's input

The reward component in the equations includes all rewards associated with the job. In addition to salary, this would include any other nonmonetary benefits such as friendships, status, working conditions, etc. The work inputs, similarly, would include all items that the employee perceives him- or herself as contributing, including items that may not be mentioned in the job description. An important point to remember throughout this discussion is that equity is ultimately judged by the *employee,* and the employee's judgment regarding what is equitable may differ substantially from the conclusions of an independent, unbiased observer. This is significant, because the equity of your compensation plan ultimately will be judged through your employees' eyes, not yours.

Employees do not consciously calculate mathematical equity ratios for themselves and others. Although some equity judgments may result from conscious comparisons, most equity judgments are based on semiconscious or unconscious evaluations. In addition, many of the data that the employee uses to form an equity judgment are "messy." For example, although your business manager has good data regarding the rewards you provide, he may somewhat distort his input by overevaluating the importance of his job. Also, suppose he compares his rewards and input to those of a business manager at another practice. His data regarding this other manager's rewards might be very problematic. They might include the clothes the other manager wears, the car she drives, the neighborhood she lives in, "hints" she has dropped indicating satisfaction with her compensation, and so on. The data regarding the other business manager's input might also be questionable. These might include self-promotional remarks made by the other business manager, a halo effect based on the reputation of the other practice, comments made by a Blue Cross claims representative regarding the ease or difficulty of working with the other business manager, and so on. Your business manager then combines all of these data at a semiconscious or unconscious level to form an impression of the equity of his compensation.

Given these circumstances, there is a real possibility that what you perceive to be fair, just, and equitable may not be similarly perceived by your employees. The degree to which your employees will perceive their compensation as equitable will be affected by a number of issues besides salary, including

- the general climate of employee relations in your practice
- the quality of your performance appraisal feedback
- the "reasonableness" of employees in choosing peers for comparison
- other characteristics of your compensation plan

The employee relations climate will have a pervasive impact on many aspects of your practice. If there is disharmony and unpleasantness, employees will add them to the I_e component. For example, suppose that in your "heart of hearts" you know that you can be an overbearing beast with your nurse. When the nurse calculates her equity ratio, she adds "working with an overbearing beast" to the I_e component. To some degree, this will offset the value that you will be adding to the R_e component with your compensation package. The offset will be even greater if your nurse has a friend whom she uses to make her equity comparison and the friend works for a doctor who is always calm and reasonable. On the other hand, if you have very good employee relations with your nurse, and this is prized by the nurse, this can add value to the R_e component.

The quality and truthfulness of your performance appraisals will also have a profound impact on your employees' perceptions of fairness. Suppose that you have a nurse with some serious performance problems, which you choose not to address in the performance review. Given the lack of criticism, the nurse will assume that his performance is at least adequate. If you then give him a pay raise based on your recognition of his inadequate performance, he will perceive this reward as inequitable. Similarly, providing a glowing appraisal for an employee who is competent but certainly not outstanding will result in an average pay raise being viewed as inequitable. Performance appraisal feedback sets the stage for your employees' equity judgments.

Since the perception of equity is partly based on comparisons with peers, which peers are chosen will certainly have an impact on the evaluation of your compensation plan. Unfortunately, this matter is largely out of your control. If you have an employee who makes unreasonable comparisons, there is little that you can do. Generally, employees do not discuss these comparisons with their employer, and, as you have seen, they may only be vaguely aware of the comparison process.

This brings us to something over which you have considerable control: your compensation plan. By using the methods discussed in this chapter, you will be able to determine equitable compensation rates in your market and develop a compensation plan that creates equitable compensation differences corresponding to the various jobs and employees in your practice. You can also increase the fairness of the plan by talking with your employees in order to understand better the types of compensation that they desire. Sometimes practices can provide, in lieu of direct wages, benefits that are of great value to employees and of little or no additional cost to the practice. For example, suppose that you pay 100 percent of each employee's health insurance premium, but the employee must pay the additional premium for family coverage. By having the practice pay the whole premium and reducing the employee's salary by an equivalent amount, you effectively allow the employee to pay for the health insurance in pre-tax dollars at no additional cost to the practice. (The practice will actually save money, since the employer's FICA contribution does not have to be paid on benefits such as health insurance premiums.) Other options might include paying for child day-care services or education, once again in lieu of salary. Using information about desired benefits to determine the characteristics of your compensation plan will increase the probability that the plan will be perceived as equitable.

USING EQUITY TO CONSTRUCT A COMPENSATION PLAN

In order to effectively use equity concepts, it is important to make a distinction between compensating jobs and compensating employees. Jobs have value to your practice irrespective of the job incumbent. For example, no matter how well a secretary performs, the value of the job has an upper limit. This is why secretaries are not paid $40,000 per year. No matter how well the incumbent performs, regardless of the employee's years of service, dedication, and commitment, *the work itself* simply does not merit this level of compensation. Similarly, the value of each job has a lower limit. Assuming that the incumbent is competent enough to retain in the position, the duties dictate that the incumbent be paid at least a certain amount. There is a pay range, therefore, that exists for each *job* irrespective of the characteristics or performance level of the incumbent.

In order to establish an effective compensation plan, you must think of the pay for each job as being composed of an equitable pay range that is associated with the position independent of the job incumbent. You then determine the employee's pay level—from within this range—based on job performance, seniority, possibility of turnover, and so on. For example, the pay range for a business manager position might be $16,000 to $20,500. Based on the experience of a particular applicant and immediate market factors, you would arrive at some salary within this range.

Determining a reasonable salary for an employee requires consideration of three distinct types of equity. *Internal equity comparisons* are comparisons between jobs within the practice. Your business manager, for example, might compare the input and rewards associated with her job with the input and rewards associated with the positions of nurse, secretary, and medical technician—and perhaps even your position. Once again, the data regarding the contributions and rewards of each of these positions may vary in accuracy and will certainly be subjective. Nevertheless, each employee will make internal equity comparisons. Your compensation plan, therefore, should have some internal consistency. Jobs that are generally recognized as having lower value, being less demanding, or requiring less training should, all other things being equal, be paid less. *Internal equity dictates that you maintain a salary structure within your practice that reflects the differences between the demands, duties, and responsibilities of the various jobs.* Your compensation plan, therefore, should have a means of achieving internal equity.

External equity comparisons are made between the jobs in your practice and similar jobs in other practices. External equity is the perception of the so-called going rate or market rate for a job. The positions being compared can be medical or nonmedical. This is especially true for jobs not directly concerned with medicine, such as clerical and other nonmedical positions. Equitable rates for nonmedical positions are to some extent determined by banks, law firms, construction companies, and so on. If your compensation plan does not have external equity, you will not be able to attract or retain good employees.

Both internal and external equity comparisons are comparisons between *jobs*. *Individual equity comparisons* are comparisons between employees. In its simplest form, individual equity relates to the differences in pay received by different incumbents in the same job. For example, if you employ two nurses, then any difference in pay will be subject to individual equity judgments. Once again, either one or both nurses may be operating on the basis of poor or inaccurate information. Nevertheless, they will make inferences and take actions based on their assessments.

Often, employees will make individual equity comparisons across jobs. For example, nurses might compare themselves with secretaries by discounting job and performance differences. If employees can "account" for all of the perceived salary differences as due to job and performance differences, then they will conclude that their pay is equitable. If there is a discrepancy, they will perceive themselves as either under- or overpaid.

Employees combine their internal, external, and individual equity data to form conclusions about the fairness of their compensation. For example, a secretary might go through the following cognitive exercise (not necessarily consciously):

> I'm making $13,500 per year. I think that is pretty good. I saw an ad in the newspaper last month that offered $12,500 for a medical secretary over at Dr. Bowen's practice. The job sounded like it was less demanding. I know that Dr. Bowen doesn't have word processing equipment, so you don't have to know all of the programs that I have mastered. On the other hand, that probably means that his secretaries have to work harder to do the same amount of work. I prefer to work in a word processing office anyway.
>
> Susie, our business manager, is probably paid about seven or eight thousand more than me. I've been here almost two years. She just bought a new Ford Taurus with all of the options—those cars cost about $17,000! Her being single and all, why she must be making $21,000 or $22,000. Also, she always dresses very well. Not real expensive, but stylish and up-to-date. Yeah, she's probably making about $21,000 or $22,000. She's responsible for collecting all of the money, making certain that all of the bills are paid, and supervising the rest of us. She's made a number of mistakes lately—forgot to pay the 941 taxes on time and issued six incorrect W-2s a few months ago. Also, insurance collections have been slow, and I know that Dr. Simpson is not happy about that. He also knows that sometimes she has problems getting along with some of the rest of us.
>
> Dr. Simpson always tells me that I am doing a super job. In my last performance review, he gave me the highest evaluations in four of the five evaluation factors. My super performance should make up for some of the difference in the importance of our jobs. It would be fair if Susie made four or five thousand dollars more than me, but not six or seven thousand. She does have a more important job, but I am better at what I do that she is at what she does.
>
> I really think that she is being paid at least $21,000. That's not really fair. If she gets that much, then I should be making another one or two thousand. She just isn't worth that much more than me.

I know that secretaries at some of the local offices of big companies like TRW and DuPont have salaries in the mid to upper teens. Alice works for DuPont and she as much as told me that.

Maybe I really put too much into this job. When I switched schedules to cover when Francis was sick, I didn't get anything for it other than a thanks from Dr. Simpson. If he really wanted to thank me, he would pay me more. He obviously has the money—look at what he is paying Susie! I guess I should stop putting myself out. I should do a good, competent job but not do anything extra.

This case illustrates how an employee can integrate several sources of information and combine external, internal, and individual equity data to reach an overall judgment regarding the fairness of compensation. It also illustrates one other very important point: Employees *always* achieve equity *one way or another!* When employees feel that their rewards are inequitably low, they will achieve equity by reducing input. When employees cannot reduce inputs enough to achieve equity, then they will take more extreme measures, including open disobedience, passive-aggressive noncompliance, sabotage, and ultimately resignation.

Employees who perceive that they are overpaid will also achieve equity. They will increase the quality or quantity of their work or will psychologically adjust their perceptions of their input or the rewards they receive. Some doctors may be tempted to increase the compensation of valued employees to inequitably high levels to "freeze" them and deter turnover. This strategy is dangerous, because it creates internal inequity relative to other employees, thereby causing dissatisfaction and motivating other employees to act out or leave. Of course, the compensation of all employees could be raised to inequitably high levels, but this would inflate the size of your payroll to unnecessary levels.

Generally, employees are less concerned about external equity than about internal and individual equity. This is because it is relatively easy to rationalize working for somewhat lower pay than an employee in another practice. For example, "The work atmosphere is nicer here," "Parking is easier," "This practice has a great future," "Dr. Jones is a pleasure to work for," and so on, are all justifications for working for somewhat lower pay. If, however, the pay is less than that of another employee in the same practice, it is much more difficult to produce convincing rationalizations, since the comparison is with someone working under the same circumstances.

Because of these internal and individual equity considerations, it is not sufficient to simply pay the going rate to each employee. Using the average rates for jobs in your local labor market will not necessarily produce a pay plan that is internally equitable. The market rate for a job is based on an amalgam of below-average, average, and above-average performers in organizations with varying mixes of job types. Adopting this average will in no way take into account real performance differences between your employees or the mix of jobs and tasks as they exist in your practice. As a result, you need ways to build external, internal, and individual equity into your compensation plan based on the mix of jobs and performance levels in your practice.

TOOLS FOR BUILDING EQUITY

Companies use specific tools to achieve external, internal, and individual equity. External equity is achieved by finding the going rate for jobs in your market. Often, this is accomplished by using wage and salary surveys. As the name implies, a wage and salary survey involves obtaining data from a sample of employers. Internal equity is achieved by using job evaluation methods. Job evaluation methods determine the relative worth of jobs based on their content and then use external equity information to assign pay rates to jobs. Individual equity is achieved through the use of performance appraisals and seniority rules. By making employee compensation decisions based on performance evaluations, you will ensure that employee compensation differences among employees with the same job are associated with employee input (job performance). To the extent that employees accept seniority as a basis for compensation, they will also perceive salary differences resulting from longevity differences as equitable.

External Equity

The standard way of obtaining external equity information is with a wage and salary survey. Table 4-1 is from a wage and salary survey published by the U.S. Bureau of Labor Statistics. Wage and salary surveys can be obtained in three ways. First, you can conduct a survey yourself. Many large companies conduct their own surveys. Large companies can afford to employ technical personnel with the required specialized skills. They also have a need for accurate data on large numbers of jobs. This is not a viable, cost-effective alternative, however, for a private medical practice that only needs infrequent data on a few jobs.

A second alternative is to commission a consultant to conduct a wage and salary survey. This will provide you with accurate, current data for jobs that are comparable to the ones in your practice. The disadvantage of this approach is the relatively high cost of conducting a private study. Once again, larger organizations that are constantly filling many positions and have a continuous need for current data may find this to be a cost-effective alternative. This is not the case, however, for the private medical practice.

A variation on this approach is to encourage your local medical association to conduct a wage and salary survey as a service for all its members. Typically, the association would hire a consultant. Each practice that wanted a copy of the survey

Table 4-1 Hourly Earnings of Selected Occupations in Norfolk–Virginia Beach–Newport News, Virginia, June 1989

Occupation	Number of workers	Hourly earnings (in dollars) Mean	Median	Middle range
Secretaries	589	9.99	9.28	8.13–11.54
Secretaries I	65	7.98	8.01	7.21– 8.35
Secretaries II	45	8.57	7.73	6.84– 9.55
Secretaries III	222	9.39	8.98	8.12–10.45
Secretaries IV	160	10.66	10.25	9.55–11.54
Secretaries V	78	12.74	11.98	10.58–14.42
Stenographers	11	13.74	13.38	—
Stenographers I	11	13.74	13.38	—
Typists	140	6.23	6.01	5.74– 6.76
Typists I	138	6.22	6.01	5.74– 6.76
Word processors	99	6.77	7.02	5.72– 7.60
Word processors I	48	5.96	5.72	5.20– 7.10
Word processors II	51	7.53	7.16	6.75– 8.20
Key entry operators	237	6.44	6.16	5.61– 7.35
Key entry operators I	202	6.18	6.00	5.58– 6.72
Key entry operators II	35	7.64	7.52	6.52– 8.42
File clerks	69	5.73	5.88	5.10– 6.27
File clerks I	66	5.63	5.56	5.10– 5.94
Switchboard operators	103	5.12	4.90	4.25– 5.92
Switchboard operator-receptionists	238	6.05	5.50	5.00– 6.36
Order clerks	307	7.18	7.50	6.54– 7.58
Order clerks II	208	7.39	7.50	7.50– 7.58
Accounting clerks	1,227	6.75	6.48	5.41– 7.45
Accounting clerks I	29	6.06	6.07	5.10– 6.89
Accounting clerks II	894	6.45	6.05	5.26– 7.27
Accounting clerks III	263	7.26	7.25	6.47– 8.19
Accounting clerks IV	34	10.44	10.25	8.71–11.34
Payroll clerks	174	7.72	7.21	6.07– 9.16
Computer systems analysts	227	16.94	16.87	14.65–19.62
Computer systems analysts I	34	14.52	14.57	12.23–16.88
Computer systems analysts II	63	18.04	18.87	16.30–19.99
Computer systems analysts III	39	19.37	19.69	16.98–21.19
Computer programmers	634	13.03	12.40	10.96–14.76
Computer programmers I	57	10.38	10.63	9.74–11.08
Computer programmers II	172	12.06	11.64	11.07–13.00
Computer programmers III	158	14.15	14.47	12.46–15.71
Computer programmers IV	87	16.59	16.50	15.15–19.09
Computer operators	324	8.79	8.00	7.10– 9.12
Computer operators I	66	7.25	7.86	6.24– 8.19
Computer operators II	121	7.42	7.30	6.49– 8.37
Computer data librarians	22	8.28	7.94	7.65– 8.76
Drafters	129	10.32	9.79	8.12–12.90
Drafters II	20	8.98	7.16	5.50– 7.70
Drafters IV	36	11.79	12.08	8.57–14.50
Electronics technicians	357	13.53	16.01	8.89–16.01
Electronics technicians III	21	16.42	15.54	15.47–18.04
Registered industrial nurses	15	12.31	12.45	11.83–12.74

Source: Reprinted from *U.S. Bureau of Labor Statistics Area Wage & Salary Survey*, p. 2, June 1989.

results would pay a nominal fee, perhaps $100, and would complete a survey questionnaire. The consultant would collect, analyze, and interpret the data and then report back to the participating practices, with each practice being identified by a code number. In this way, doctors could examine the data to see how their practice compares with other practices, yet complete anonymity would be maintained for all of the participating practices. An example of this type of survey report for a business manager position is found in Exhibit 4-1.

Exhibit 4-1 Coded Wage and Salary Survey for Business Manager (Direct Wages Only)

Job Description: The Business Manager handles the major day-to-day financial and supervisory duties in the practice. These include responsibility for at least three of the following: accounts receivable, accounts payable, insurance collection, checkbook, negotiation of patient payment arrangements, payment of taxes, supervision of clerical staff.

Rank	Code	Annual Salary ($K)	Rank	Code	Annual Salary ($K)
1	XO37	28.9	25	ER77	18.5
2	EK94	25.2	26	LL49	18.5
3	JK23	24.9	27	KK34	18.5
4	OI38	24.9	28	IO38	18.3
5	FI34	23.0	29	UT44	18.1
6	KL99	22.5	30	RR67	18.0
7	OF39	22.5	31	TW78	18.0
8	HL81	22.1	32	IQ37	18.0
9	JG88	22.0	33	OO99	17.7
10	BB12	22.0	34	PU38	17.3
11	CM31	21.7	35	HH78	17.0
12	XM44	21.5	36	RQ56	16.8
13	VM55	21.5	37	UT48	16.4
14	MM21	21.0	38	OW60	16.0
15	NN39	20.5	39	UW29	16.0
16	ZX94	20.5	40	NV39	15.9
17	AQ51	20.3	41	AQ29	15.8
18	PL81	20.0	42	QP51	15.5
19	PP79	20.0	43	XZ37	15.5
20	PU42	19.7	44	YT38	15.2
21	YT30	19.3	45	UW11	15.0
22	TT28	19.0	46	QQ55	15.0
23	YT23	18.8	47	LK38	14.8
24	UZ39	18.5			

MEAN = 19.30
STD DEV = 2.86
INTERQUARTILE RANGE = 21.5–16.8

A third alternative is to use published wage and salary surveys. This is probably the best alternative for most medical practices. There are several sources for published surveys. The U.S. Bureau of Labor Statistics publishes surveys for approximately 80 geographical areas, so it is likely that you will be able to obtain a survey containing data specific to your market. The surveys are available at most college libraries and larger public libraries. The BLS Area Wage Survey also contains data on benefits, including vacation time, sick leave, and insurance coverage. However, one problem with using government surveys, such as the BLS Area Wage Survey, is that they usually don't cover medical specialty jobs, such as nursing or medical technical specialties. Another problem with using government surveys is that the data may be old. If substantial inflation has occurred, this could cause the numbers to be misleading.

Other possible sources of published wage and salary data include your state employment commission or department of labor, your local chamber of commerce, and local trade and professional associations in both medical and nonmedical fields.[1] Finally, some consulting firms publish wage and salary survey data on a regular basis. Obtaining this information costs a fee, but this fee will be substantially less than the cost of commissioning a consultant to conduct a private survey for your practice.

Irrespective of the source of your survey, remember that the data it contains will to some degree be approximate due to the data collection method. When employers receive a request for data from the BLS or any other surveying organization, they also receive a set of job descriptions. Each employer selects the jobs in his or her company that most closely match the job descriptions provided by the surveyor, then reports the salary and benefits data for those jobs. Therefore, the salary data reported across a number of employers will be a blend of data for jobs that vary in their degree of closeness to the survey job descriptions. Thus, you should appreciate the need to adjust the salary survey figures based on your judgment of how similar the survey job descriptions are to your jobs.

The fourth method of obtaining external equity data is to contact a few major hospitals and colleagues in your area to obtain salary information on selected medical specialties. *This is not the same as conducting a survey.* Your data have none of the precision of data collected from a representative sample of employers. Since the data are not representative of the population of practices, you should not attempt to subject these data to any statistical operations, such as calculating a mean. Nevertheless, if you have a small practice, need data on only a few jobs, understand the concept of external equity, and can make some good intuitive inferences, this method can provide useful information. It certainly is a cost- and time-effective way of collecting information.

Many hospitals conduct wage and salary surveys. Some hospitals may provide you with these data if you are "one of the boys." Other hospitals will consider these data to be their property and will not share them. But you have nothing to lose by asking.

Finally, you can look at help wanted ads to get a sense of what some employers are paying for certain types of jobs. This method is very "coarse," because the wages that are being advertised may be above or below the wages actually being paid. In addition, many employers do not advertise their pay rates, and you will know very little about the job content other than the job title.

Almost certainly, the reality will be that by using published wage and salary surveys or contacting a local hospital and a colleague or two, you will be confident that you have good market rate data on some jobs but will also recognize that you have no good data on several other jobs. That is fine. Even very large organizations do not try to obtain market data for all jobs. Given the mechanics of conducting a survey, this would be an impossible task. Those jobs for which you can establish good market rates are called *benchmark jobs*. You will be able to use the benchmark jobs to anchor your compensation plan and to interpolate equitable compensation rates for the other jobs in your practice.

Internal Equity

Job evaluation is the process that is used to establish internal equity in a compensation plan and to assign a fair going rate for those jobs where it would be too difficult, too expensive, or impossible to obtain market data through a wage and salary survey or other means. Job evaluation methods measure the content of jobs in terms of compensable factors. Compensable factors are factors for which employers are generally willing to pay. Examples include education, experience, and supervisory responsibility. Generally, jobs that require more education or experience or require the incumbent to supervise subordinates are better paid. By using a job evaluation method, you can compare jobs with each other in terms of compensable factors. It is then possible to scale jobs based on their "compensability."

There are a number of different job evaluation methods. Small practices can use the simplest job evaluation method, which is called *ranking*. The object is to rank jobs on the basis of their overall value to the practice. The procedure is as follows:

1. Assemble all of the job descriptions to be covered in the compensation plan.
2. Read all of the job descriptions so that you are fully familiar with their contents.
3. Considering all issues covered by the descriptions, identify the job that is most important to the practice.

4. Next identify the job that is least important to the practice.
5. Of the jobs remaining, identify the one that is most important, then the one that is least important. Repeat this process until all jobs have been ranked.

Using the ranking process obviously requires an ability to evaluate subjectively the composite of compensable factors possessed by each job. For example, the business manager position may require more experience and supervisory skills than a nursing position, yet the nursing position may require more formal education and have greater responsibility. All of these are compensable factors, and it is the particular mix of the factors associated with a given position that will determine its internal equity ranking relative to other positions.

Next, examine the wage and salary survey data for the rank-ordered jobs and note the salary rates for the benchmark jobs. In Table 4-2, the secretary and business manager and computer operator positions are benchmark jobs. You can now use the ranking and the benchmark job salaries to determine equity for the nonbenchmark jobs. Obviously, this approach leaves considerable room for discretion. The salary for the nurse position could be anywhere between $15,179 and $21,388 and still be consistent with the ranking. The method restricts the salary range for the lab technician position much more severely.

The ranking procedure, combined with wage and salary information, should allow you to achieve internal and external equity for most of the positions in a small practice. Nevertheless, occasionally you will encounter an "outlier." Outliers are jobs that demand unusually high or low compensation due to temporary fluctuations or historic inconsistencies in the labor market. For example, the market rate in many parts of the country for nurses is below what job evaluations would project as equitable. Similarly, for many years geologists were paid at inequitably high rates by oil companies as a result of the oil crisis in the mid-1970s. Eventually, most of these market inequities work themselves out as the supply of candidates increases or decreases in response to prevailing salaries.

It is important, therefore, to know enough about the local market to know if a job or profession is an outlier. If it is, don't use it as a benchmark job, since it will

Table 4-2 Rank Ordering of Benchmark and Nonbenchmark Jobs

Rank	Title	Benchmark Rate
1	Business Manager	$21,389
2	Nurse	
3	Computer Operator	$15,178
4	Laboratory Technician	
5	Secretary I	$14,789

bias your estimates for other jobs. Wage and salary surveys, coupled with job evaluation, can give you good information on 85 to 90 percent of your jobs. The remaining 10 to 15 percent must be dealt with idiosyncratically and paid either what you can get away with, in the case of a low outlier, or what is necessary, in the case of a high outlier.

The ranking system has difficulty handling jobs that have some degree of complexity. We have seen that jobs are composed of factors, and obviously jobs can vary in value based on the mix and amount of certain factors. The ranking method evaluates jobs as wholes, so it is very difficult for the evaluator to take into account differences on individual factors. For example, if one job is high in responsibility and moderate in complexity and another is high in complexity and low in responsibility, how should the two be paid relative to each other? A point system will give you the capability of answering this question with more confidence.

In a point system, jobs receive points based on how much they possess of each compensable factor. An example of a point system is found in Appendix A. It is designed to assess jobs based on those compensable factors that often occur in medical practice jobs. Each factor is broken down into a number of different levels, which are called *degrees,* and point values are assigned to each degree. Jobs are then evaluated by comparing the job content to the degree definitions.

In order to do this effectively, you must be thoroughly familiar with the job content. Although the job description will be helpful, it is important to have a thorough knowledge of what job incumbents *really* do on a day-to-day basis. Second, remember that you are evaluating what is required by the job, not the characteristics of the particular incumbent. Many incumbents possess skills, education, or experience not required by the job. Since these are characteristics of the person and not job requirements, you should not pay for them and they should not enter into the evaluation of the job. For example, look at the degree choices (1–9) for education in Table A-1 (Appendix A). Now, suppose that you have a clerical position in which the demands of the job require a high school education. The incumbent happens to have a master's degree. Since the job only requires a high school education and some specialized courses, it would be evaluated at Degree 2 and would receive 135 to 255 points, depending on the number of years of experience required to adequately perform the job. The important thing to remember is that you are evaluating the worth of jobs, not people. Paying for irrelevant skills or experience that contribute nothing to your practice is simply a waste of money.

Let's examine how to use a point chart. Using the job description or your knowledge of the job, evaluate the job on each factor and calculate a point total. For example, Table 4-3 contains an evaluation for the job of computer operator/secretary (see Exhibit 2-1 for the job description). The job requires a high school education with experience of under one year, so it receives 110 points for the knowledge factor. The amount and nature of the job's nonsupervisory responsibility is best described by Degree 3C, so the job receives 185 points for this factor.

Table 4-3 Point Evaluation of Computer Operator/Secretary and Business Manager Positions

Factor	Computer Operator/Secretary		Business Manager	
	Degree	*Points*	*Degree*	*Points*
Knowledge	1A	110	1B	120
Nonsupervisory responsibility	2C	185	4E	320
Ingenuity	1B	115	3A	225
Personnel Management	1B	130	2B	140
Outside Relationships	3B	240	4B	430
Total Points		**780**		**1,235**

Given the evaluations for the other three factors, the job receives a total of 780 points. A similar evaluation of a business manager position produces a total of 1,235 points. *The point totals represent the relative worth of the jobs in terms of the compensable factors.*

The next step is to convert points into dollars. This is accomplished once again by identifying benchmark jobs. Table 4-4 contains data on the benchmark jobs of computer operator/secretary, business manager, and nurse practitioner. You can now derive the point-pay relationship in two ways:

1. Use regression analysis to derive the straight line formula for the relationship between points and pay.[2] In Table 4-4, this results in a y-intercept of $3,106.83, with each point worth $12.34.
2. Plot the relationship and "eyeball" a line that fits the data (see Figure 4-1). If you decide to eyeball a line, remember that measurement errors may cause your benchmark jobs not to line up perfectly. Once again, use your judgment. If you can eyeball a line that appears to do a reasonable job of describing the data, that will be sufficient.

Table 4-4 Determining Base Pay Using a Point System

	Salary	*Points*
Computer Operator/Secretary	$13,000	780
Business Manager	$18,000	1,235
Nurse Practitioner	$40,000	2,985
Nurse	$13,410.73 (projected)	835

Salary = $a + $b (points)
Salary = $3,106.83 + $12.34 (points)

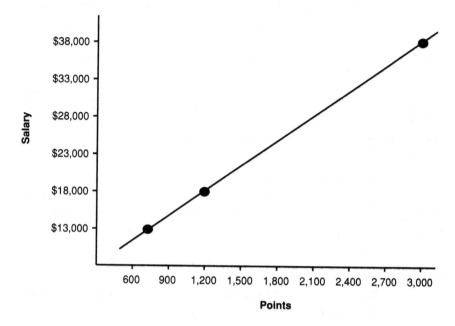

Figure 4-1 Eyeballed Line That Best Fits Benchmark Jobs

Since the line (either expressed as a formula or on paper) is based by definition on the equitable relationship of points and pay, any point on the line should represent equity. The line can be used, therefore, to calculate an equitable salary for other jobs. Table 4-4 illustrates this by showing a projected salary for a nurse position. The job description was evaluated using the point plan in Appendix A. The point total is 835. Using either the regression formula or a graph results in a projected base pay of $13,410.73.

Once you have determined equity for a position, you can then develop a range around equity, which is called a *spread*. Spreads can be useful for handling a number of compensation issues. For example, if $15,000 represents equity for a job, you may want the flexibility to pay somewhat above or below this amount to take into account differences between employees, such as their performance level and how long they have worked for you. There are no uncontestable ways of determining the correct size of a spread. Generally, rules of thumb are applied. At the low end of a pay scale, spreads may vary from 10 to 20 percent of equity. At higher pay levels, spreads may vary from 20 to 40 percent. Judiciously applying these rules of thumb to the positions listed in Table 4-4 might result in the salary structure found in Table 4-5.

Table 4-5 Job Salary Structure

		Range	
Job Title	*Midpoint*	*Percentage*	*Dollars*
Computer Operator/Secretary	$13,000	±10%	$11,700–$14,300
Nurse	$13,500	±10%	$12,150–$14,850
Business Manager	$18,000	±15%	$15,300–$20,700
Nurse Practitioner	$40,000	±25%	$30,000–$50,000

Realistically, pay levels substantially below equity will not be used very often because of the difficulty of recruiting at these levels. Labor markets, however, are not perfect, and the combination of job evaluation and wage and salary survey data provide you with only an estimate of equity. Employees and applicants will form their own equity judgments. As a result, you probably can hire applicants at below-midpoint salary levels. If you find resistance to these lower levels, then you will have to raise your salary offer. However, you may find that well-qualified applicants will accept below-midpoint offers.

The range above equity can be very useful as a control for excessive payroll expenses. When employees start to approach the top of the range for their job, it is time to do one of the following:

1. Increase the employee's duties and responsibilities in order to justify a higher salary. This option may be limited by the ability or willingness of the job incumbent to take on different duties or by the degree to which these changes would make sense given the various jobs in your practice.

2. Prepare the employee for a shift into another position in the practice. This option may be limited, once again, by employee ability and interest and by the availability of an appropriate higher paying position in the practice.

3. Tell the employee that, with the exception of cost-of-living adjustments to the whole salary structure, the employee will not be able to make more money in this job. If you do this, the employee may leave. Depending on other considerations, such as staff morale and the employee's job performance, it may be reasonable to risk the employee's resignation, for it could provide an opportunity to hire an acceptable replacement at a significantly lower pay level.

4. Continue to give the employee pay raises, fully recognizing that you are overpaying for the job. You may be able to justify this on the basis of staff morale or simply because it makes your life easier. However, any overpayment should be the result of a conscious, informed decision, and you should

be aware of the effect on your payroll and its potential for creating internal equity problems. At some point the overpaid employee will become costly enough in terms of dollar expenditures and equity problems that the inconveniences of turnover become more desirable than continuing to grant pay increases.

Finally, irrespective of how you derive your job rates, you should consider the effects of inflation. A year from now, your equitable rates may no longer be perceived as equitable due to inflation. You can adjust your salary line by the percentage increase in inflation to keep your compensation plan current. It is not advisable, however, to raise the salary line by the full increase in the cost of living, because you will have difficulty lowering salaries if the cost of living actually goes down. Cost-of-living adjustments, therefore, should lag cost-of-living increases by several points. If the cost of living increases 6 percent, you might adjust your salary line upward by 1 or 2 percent. Any increase that an employee receives above this level should be based on job performance or seniority.

Using a point system requires some degree of skill. At best it will provide you with guidance regarding how to integrate information across several compensable factors. It will also help you determine salaries for those jobs for which you don't have a sense of fair compensation rates. It can also be used to validate your assumptions about compensation levels for jobs, thereby increasing your confidence that you are not creating internal equity problems.

Individual Equity

Now that you have a pay range associated with a job, the next task is to decide where an employee fits in that range. The decision should be based on job performance, seniority, or some combination of the two. It is essentially a subjective decision, and in making it you will have to rely on your judgment of the employee and the employee's value to the practice. The discussion of performance appraisal in Chapter 3 gives you a number of ideas about how to obtain the performance data you need in order to make salary decisions on the basis of merit.

If you decide that you want to give merit pay increases, it is important to have wide enough pay ranges to make meaningful distinctions between employees. A merit system will be counterproductive if employees perceive that meaningful differences in performance are rewarded by trivial differences in compensation. This can be a particular problem at the low end, where the spread between low and high for a job might only be 20 percent. Under these circumstances, it is particularly important to make allowance in your pay ranges for increases in the cost of living. The problem is compounded by the fact that most people expect an annual salary increase.

You probably will find that it is best to base pay raises on a combination of seniority and merit. The seniority component might account for 1–3 percent, and it should be associated with, but not necessarily match, the rate of inflation. The merit component might account for an additional 1–10 percent.

PRACTICAL CONSIDERATIONS

The compensation process discussed in this chapter may sound like overkill for a small private medical practice. For most small practices, it *would* be overkill to implement complete external and internal equity procedures for all salaried positions. Medical practices are usually too small to make this financially justifiable, they don't have enough positions to make it technically feasible, and they usually don't have enough personnel with available time to undertake all of the necessary tasks. Understanding the theory and mechanics of compensation, however, will allow you to use a less formal approach and still achieve an equitable compensation plan.

For example, a cost- and time-effective strategy for a small practice might include obtaining the regional BLS Area Wage and Salary Survey to acquire data on some generic jobs, such as secretary and computer operator positions. Phone calls to a few hospitals and colleagues could provide ideas about the going rate for jobs with a medical content and in medical settings. The job evaluation system in Appendix A could then be used to calculate point totals for these positions as well as those for which you were not able to obtain market data. A "devil's advocate" pay line could be eyeballed. Salary spreads could be calculated and then adjusted based on your judgment of what makes sense for your practice. The time required for determining compensation for five positions might be as follows:

1.	Examining the BLS survey	15 min.
2.	Calling hospitals and colleagues	90 min.
3.	Using the job evaluation point system	30 min.
4.	Developing a pay line	20 min.
5.	Developing job spreads	20 min.
6.	Making adjustments based on practicalities	45 min.
	Total	**3 hrs. 40 min.**

This is a reasonable time investment. At a minimum, it will cause you to ask yourself penetrating questions whenever you make compensation-related decisions. It also has the potential of (1) saving you large amounts of money by controlling payroll costs and (2) avoiding employee problems due to complications resulting from perceptions of inequity.

As your practice grows in size, you will find that formal compensation methods give you confidence in your decisions. Eventually it may reach a size at which you can no longer deal effectively with each job on an individual basis. There simply are too many data and too many people and positions for you to be able to sub-jectively construct a compensation plan that works. At this point, more formal methods become necessary.

Whether you run a large or small practice, the compensation methods dis-cussed in this chapter are best used as a means of providing hypotheses. Formal methods can never replace good, sound management judgment. Formal meth-ods, however, can be used to force you to think and consider alternatives. If a wage and salary survey gives you answers that you don't like, then ask yourself why you don't like them. It is because you really don't want to hear that a fair salary for a position is $3,000 higher than you're willing to pay? Or is it because the survey was inaccurate or not really relevant? By forcing yourself to ask questions and investigate, formal compensation methods can help you to make better management decisions.

Who Should Construct Your Compensation Plan?

If you determine that you want to develop a compensation plan within your practice, you will have to do most of the work yourself. With the exception of some data-collecting tasks, such as obtaining published wage and salary surveys, the tasks should not be delegated to subordinates. The need for judgment, as well as the potential for influencing their own salaries, makes these decisions inap-propriate for your subordinates.

Hiring a consultant to construct a practice compensation plan can be an effec-tive strategy for three reasons. First, hiring an experienced consultant will give you the benefit of knowledge and perspective in a task where these commodities are obviously of great importance. Second, the objectivity that a consultant can provide will give your plan greater credibility with your employees and your partners. Finally, contracting this work to a consultant gets you out of the com-pensation business and back into practicing medicine. Most doctors would prefer to use their time to practice medicine, but the choice of what you should do is a matter of what suits you personally. If you do decide to use a consultant, be certain that you receive adequate training in the use and maintenance of the plan. The object is to have the consultant develop a plan that is usable by you and your staff and will not require the consultant's constant attention.

INCENTIVE PLANS

In an incentive plan, an employee receives compensation as a direct result of a change in a performance indicator. For example, a business manager who receives a percentage of the gross receipts as part of his or her compensation is receiving an incentive. Incentive plans appeal to most of us. After all, who can argue with the logic that employees will perform at their best if they directly benefit from their own performance? In addition, since the incentive payment is based on an objective index, both the employer and the employee have unambiguous commitments. There are no uncertainties such as those that characterize performance appraisals and merit compensation processes.

Incentive plans can provide motivation, but they can also be very dangerous. Employees will direct their performance toward maximizing their incentive payments. Often this is detrimental to other job performance areas. For example, the business manager who receives a percentage of the gross receipts may neglect or delay performing those duties that do not immediately affect the bottom line. Responding inadequately to patient inquiries, neglecting accounts payable duties, working on easy accounts while avoiding more difficult accounts, and so on, could all be dysfunctional results of an incentive plan. It is important, therefore, to anticipate dysfunctional reward contingencies. Some practices attempt to counteract dysfunctions by creating several incentives so that the employee cannot neglect a major aspect of the job. This quickly can become a cumbersome arrangement in which a crafty employee will meet the letter of the incentive agreement but still manage to avoid doing all that the job requires.

It is also important to remember that most performance indexes can vary for many reasons. It may be very difficult to say with certainty that one person is solely responsible for the increase or decrease of a performance index, such as gross receipts or insurance collections. Capital investment, effective employee selection, good marketing, an increase in the quality of services, and the hiring of additional physicians and employees can all contribute to raising objective indexes, even when an employee's performance remains the same on a comparative basis or is marginal when assessed using an absolute standard. Under these circumstances, an incentive arrangement will become very unfair to the practice, since employees will receive pay increases as a result of factors not under their control.

It is critical, therefore, to thoroughly think through the possible consequence of an incentive plan. If you still feel that an incentive is valuable, then try to build language into the employment contract that will protect you from the possible dysfunctional consequences. The object of this language is to reclaim your power to make appraisal and compensation decisions. For example, the contract may state that if management determines duties are not being performed adequately, the incentive payment is no longer payable. Another alternative is to put a cap on incentive payments or set a yearly maximum beyond which they cannot increase.

In summary, incentive payments can motivate behavior, but the behavior that is motivated may not be in the best interest of the practice. Incentive payments are not recommended for front office personnel. If, however, you determine that you want to use incentives, do so with caution and examine the arrangement from the employee's perspective to determine possible unintended consequences.

BENEFITS

Benefits are an important part of any compensation package. As with direct wages, the benefits you provide will affect the attractiveness of your practice to job applicants and influence employee satisfaction and job performance. Some benefits (e.g., vacation time) are simple and generally available, whereas others (e.g., retirement plans) are complex and require the consultation of a specialist. Data on many benefits can be found in wage and salary surveys. These benefits include vacation time, sick leave, holidays, and insurance (health, life, disability, and dental).

When considering the selection of benefits, look closely at the operation of your practice. For example, is the day before Christmas normally a slow day? If it is, consider making this a holiday; you would thereby provide a benefit to employees at little cost to yourself. Do you really want to work the day after Thanksgiving? If you do not intend to work, close the office. Once again, it will be a relatively inexpensive benefit. Do you want to keep employees for a longer time or do you prefer some turnover so as to keep salaries down? If the former, then you may want to offer retirement and education benefits. If the latter, then offering these benefits would be counterproductive.

Health insurance and sick leave are benefits that can have an important effect on your employees' productivity. Employees who delay medical treatment, don't take the time to get well, or are worried about their medical expenses will be less than fully productive. Good health insurance can also contribute to lower employee turnover, since it will tend to tie employees to your practice.

When considering which benefits to provide, it is important to determine the needs of your employees. You are simply wasting money if you spend it on unwanted benefits. Some companies have adopted what is called a *cafeteria plan*. A cafeteria plan allows employees some flexibility in choosing a set of benefits to meet their needs. Each employee is given a budget based on salary. Certain benefits are required, such as health insurance and a minimum number of vacation days. The employee may then use the remainder of the budget as he or she chooses. A cafeteria plan has the added advantage of familiarizing employees with the full cost of the benefits provided by the practice.

Retirement plans have a number of advantages for employers and employees. They not only provide a means of accumulating retirement income, but they can also be used to defer taxation and allow accumulation of funds at tax-deferred rates. For most doctors, their practice's retirement plan is one of the cornerstones of their personal financial plan. Because of tax and pension reform legislation, the provisions that govern your contributions and therefore your benefits are inextricably tied to the benefits offered to your employees. This can make a retirement plan a very expensive benefit.

Retirement plans can take on a number of different forms. A pension plan becomes a fixed obligation. Contractually, your practice is committed to make certain contributions to the plan. If you have agreed to a defined contribution plan, then you are obligated to make contributions for all qualified employees. If you have a defined benefits plan, then you are obligated to make contributions that will support the provision of benefits to employees upon retirement. The disadvantage of the pension plan approach to retirement planning is that your financial obligation does not vary with the success of your practice. This can be particularly burdensome for a young practice, where income may vary from year to year and substantial funds may have to be reserved for capital investment to support growth.

Profit sharing plans provide some of the same retirement and tax advantages. Contributions, however, are made out of profits. If there is no profit, the practice has no obligation to fund the plan. This is advantageous for young practices, because it provides discretion in the use of corporate funds. The theoretical disadvantage of this approach is that the amount of funds that can be sheltered in a profit sharing plan is less than in a pension plan. A careful analysis of your practice's financial needs, plus some personal introspection regarding your need for predictability and flexibility, are necessary before you can determine whether your retirement needs are best met by the pension or profit sharing strategy.

One option is to institute a 401K plan. A 401K plan can be used to amend a profit sharing plan so as to allow employees to contribute part of their salary to the plan. These contributions are deducted from the employee's taxable income and at the same time constitute a tax deduction for the practice. This can be advantageous, because employees, including you, can make contributions even if there is little or no profit available to fund the profit sharing plan. This flexibility is limited, however, by rules that govern the size of contributions and the ratio of contributions that can be made by high-salaried and low-salaried employees.

Retirement planning has developed into a profession. The taxation issues and the IRS rules that have been developed to determine whether a plan qualifies for preferential tax treatment are very complex and change on an annual basis. It is essential, therefore, that you consult an advisor who specializes in retirement plans. In addition, you should remember that creating a retirement plan is like creating a new child. It is going to be with you for the remainder of your professional life. It will be continually consuming time and resources. There are annual IRS statements and financial reports that must be constructed. The plan will have to be updated from time to time to comply with current law. Finally, someone will have to administer the plan and make investment decisions. Employees will come and go, and some will leave their vested money in the plan whereas others will withdraw it. In each case, documentation and management will take time and effort. Unless you are particularly interested and skilled in this area, you will have to pay someone to administer the plan and invest the funds.

In summary, a retirement plan can have great financial advantages for both you and your employees. A retirement plan should only be adopted after careful consideration of the overall financial effects on the practice in both good and bad times. It should also be undertaken with the advice of a professional whom you have educated regarding both your personal financial objectives and your practice's objectives.

CASE APPLICATIONS

Dr. Early

Dr. Early was an internist with a growing group practice. After Dr. Garland joined the practice, the amount of clerical work in the front office began to dramatically increase. Dr. Early employed a business manager, Ralph, whose primary responsibilities were to handle the accounts receivable and accounts payable. Dr. Early also employed Louise as a full-time secretary. Her duties included typing, filing, transcribing, greeting patients, scheduling appointments, and answering the telephone. Finally, Brenda worked four hours each afternoon as a part-time receptionist. When she arrived, she replaced Louise at the front window and took over the role of greeting patients, scheduling appointments, and answering the telephone. Louise was then able to work uninterrupted on typing, filing, correspondence, and so on.

Within a few weeks of Dr. Garland's arrival, it became obvious that the clerical staff could not handle the additional work. Dr. Early decided that the best way to manage the increased front office workload was to change the part-time receptionist position into a full-time position and restructure the secretarial position. The secretary would no longer perform receptionist duties, such as greeting patients, answering telephones, and scheduling appointments. The secretary would instead concentrate on typing, correspondence, filing, recordkeeping, and other clerical duties.

Dr. Early offered the full-time receptionist position to Brenda at the same pay ($5.75 an hour) that she had been receiving for the past four months. She refused to take the job, stating that she was only interested in part-time work. Dr. Early now had to find someone to fill the position. He was worried about two issues. First, he was somewhat concerned that Brenda might have turned down the job because the pay was too low. He had assumed that if Brenda was already working for $5.75 an hour, this would be a fair pay for the same work done full-time. Second, he was concerned about Louise's reaction if he reduced the pay differential between her job and the receptionist position. Because of both these issues, he undertook a compensation study.

First he consulted a BLS Area Wage and Salary Survey. None of the job descriptions in the survey exactly matched either the secretary or receptionist position. He felt, however, that two positions in the survey were close enough to allow him to work with the figures: The Secretary III position in the survey could be used as a basis for his secretary position, and the Secretary I position could be used for his receptionist position. The $5.75 an hour that he was currently paying his receptionist was well under the median of $8.01 an hour and even well under the low end of the midrange for Secretary I. Louise's salary of $17,100 was very close to the Secretary III median of $17,430 ($8.38 × 2,080 annual hours). In addition, Louise had been in the position for a little over two years. Her initial salary was $14,800. She received a $1,000 increase at the end of her first year and a $1,300 increase at the end of her second year. Dr. Early also thought that Louise's position had fewer responsibilities than the survey's Secretary III position.

Dr. Early could find no job in the BLS survey that was similar in content to his business manager position. He decided to ask three of his colleagues what they were paying their business managers. He wasn't certain how confidential his peers would regard this information, so he decided to ask them in terms of the following pay ranges:

Less than $18,000
$18,000–$20,000
$20,001–$22,000
$22,001–$24,000
More than $24,000

He also decided to ask for the number of years the incumbent had been in the position. Two colleagues stated that their business managers were in the $20,001–$22,000 range. Both managers had more than two years of experience. The other colleague indicated her business manager was in the $18,000–$20,000 range and had three years of experience. Ralph had been Dr. Early's business manager for almost three years, and his current salary was $21,750.

Dr. Early formed some initial hypotheses. He felt that he was probably going to have to increase the salary for the receptionist. Although he had not previously considered the concept of a pay range for a position, it appeared that both the secretary and business manager salaries were within reason. He concluded that if he did formally construct pay ranges for these two positions, the current salary of each incumbent certainly would be within the relevant pay range.

He now attempted to validate his conclusions. Using a point system, he evaluated the secretary, business manager, and newly defined receptionist positions. His results are reported in Table 4-6. The projected salary for the receptionist was $14,752.13. Eyeballing this result, he felt that this was a little high. A call to one of his colleagues, plus his increasing familiarity with the medical practice market, indicated that a fair rate would be closer to $14,000. In addition, he recalled that his secretary position seemed to carry fewer responsibilities than the BLS Secretary III position, so that in general his compensation rates appeared to be on the low side. Taking $14,000 as a midpoint, he decided to construct a devil's advocate pay range of plus or minus 10 percent. This resulted in a pay range for the recep-

Table 4-6 Point and Pay Evaluations of Dr. Early's Employees

	Salary	Points
Business Manager	$21,750	1,550
Secretary	$17,100	1,005
Receptionist	$14,752 (projected)	730

tionist position of $12,600–$15,400. In addition, since he was only remixing duties that Louise already performed, he saw no need to change her pay as a result of the reorganization.

Dr. Early decided that the receptionist job required no special medical background, so he placed his advertisement in the general classified section of the local newspaper. Careful questioning of several of the best applicants revealed that the realistic market minimum was about $13,500. He hired the best of the applicants for a starting salary of $13,600. He did so with confidence that neither Louise nor Ralph would feel the new receptionist's pay was unfairly high. This was very important to Dr. Early, since both Louise and Ralph were good employees. They would be instrumental in the new receptionist's training, and turnover in either of their positions at that time would have been a serious problem.

Dr. Early drew several conclusions from this episode. He knew that he could have called a few colleagues, looked at some relevant help wanted ads, and talked to his own employees to get an indication of what the receptionist salary level should be. In fact, he had done all of these things. He concluded, however, that using survey and job evaluation data made him much more confident about his decision. The fact that several pieces of independent information all pointed in the same direction was very reassuring. He also liked being reasonably sure that by solving one problem he was not creating a whole new set of problems. Finally, he felt a sense of satisfaction from knowing that he had done everything using the best tools and information available to him. This feeling was somewhat similar to how he felt when he combined several pieces of test and examination information to arrive at a clinical diagnosis.

Ramona's Equity

Dr. Phillip Hendricks was an owner and the managing physician of a group family practice. He received a resumé from Ramona for his vacant business manager position. Ramona had previously worked for Dr. Johnson's group radiology practice at a salary of $45,000. When Dr. Johnson retired, the remaining partners eliminated Ramona's position and her entire staff, with the justification that it would be more economical to use a billing service. Ramona's experience was excellent, and at the interview she gave the impression of being a calm, mature 50-year-old woman who knew that she could do the job.

Dr. Hendricks had some reservations about hiring Ramona. The salary for the business manager position was $20,000, which he knew was a fair salary, perhaps even somewhat above the median salary for this type of position. Dr. Hendricks sensed that Ramona's real job at Dr. Johnson's practice had been to supervise an overstaffed office and that she hadn't been in the trenches actually billing insurance companies, posting payments, and so on, for many years. He knew that in his practice, the business manager was in the front line and had to personally bill companies, follow up on problem claims, and negotiate payment plans with delinquent patients, among other things. Dr. Hendricks was concerned that the combination of more demanding work and substantially lower pay would result in perceptions of inequity, irrespective of the fact that he had given Ramona a realistic job preview and that she was voluntarily taking a job at a lower salary. Ramona, however, insisted that she knew that she would have to take a pay cut and that it was important to her to work for people with whom she felt some affiliation. As a result of two interviews with Dr. Hendricks and his staff, she felt that she would enjoy working at his practice. Ramona was the most qualified applicant in Dr. Hendricks' selection pool, he needed to fill the position as soon as possible, so he hired her in spite of his reservations.

Ramona's tenure turned out to be unsettling to all involved. She quickly grew frustrated with the demands of the job. Her frustration manifested itself in temper tantrums and insubordinate comments and actions towards Dr. Hendricks and the other associates. She resigned after four months of employment. Dr. Hendricks had these comments:

> It started to go wrong right from the start. She was used to a country club atmosphere in which she was also overpaid. She quickly grew to resent realistic job demands at a realistic salary. She treated me like it was *my* fault that she was in this situation—that she was no longer employed by a sugar daddy practice! Toward the end, she even tried to manipulate me into firing her, so that she wouldn't have to take the responsibility for her circumstances!

> She never did get her equity equation readjusted to reality. Her comparison "other" was this image of herself at the previous practice, which had no grounding in the real world. How can I fight that? The answer is that I can't, and I should have realized this, despite her assurances to the contrary. Dr. Johnson's largess made her largely unemployable. It would be a rare individual who has the self-awareness to be able to take a career step backwards of this magnitude. Ramona couldn't do it, and I

suppose that I shouldn't hold that too much against her. At the same time, however, I've learned that you can't fight unrealistic equity perceptions. In her mind her previous employment situation was equitable, and only she can change that perception. If she doesn't find another sugar daddy practice, she will eventually have to adjust her expectations. I have sympathy for any practice which she encounters between now and then. I'll never hire a person under these circumstances again. I've learned my lesson.

CONCLUSION

Making good compensation decisions is more of an art than a science. The most significant message of this chapter is the importance of achieving equity. The tools that were described are essentially aids for achieving equity. Some smaller practices may find that understanding the objectives of individual, internal, and external equity at the conceptual level will allow them to make good compensation decisions. Other practices may find it preferable to use compensation tools, such as wage and salary surveys, ranking or point job evaluation plans, and pay ranges, to achieve these objectives. You should be wary of incentive plans and always consult a knowledgeable professional regarding complex benefits, such as a retirement plan. Finally, consultants can be particularly useful in designing compensation plans because of the importance of experience in making good compensation decisions.

NOTES

1. Surveys conducted by nonmedical trade and professional associations would be very useful for jobs that cut across types of organizations, such as clerical positions.
2. In order to use regression analysis, it is important to have enough data points to be certain that the data are essentially linear. Regression will fit a straight line to any data, including curvelinear data. If the underlying data are not generally linear, the use of regression analysis can be misleading.

Chapter 5

Motivation and Leadership

CHAPTER OBJECTIVES

This chapter will help you understand what motivates your employees and how best to lead. As a result, you will be able to

1. motivate your employees to achieve practice objectives
2. understand how to select and modify rewards so that employees will work toward practice goals
3. evaluate the leadership situation so that you can choose the most appropriate leadership style

INTRODUCTION

Providing motivation and leadership is critical for the success of your practice. Motivating and leading employees are related but separate skills. Motivation is concerned with persuading employees to work toward practice goals by giving them the rewards that they desire. If the rewards are truly valued and properly presented, then employees will work toward achieving practice goals because they will simultaneously be achieving their own personal goals. Leadership is concerned with obtaining the voluntary cooperation of employees to achieve practice goals. Providing leadership involves more than appealing to the self-interest of employees. It is concerned with influencing your employees' behavior through your personal words, actions, and interactions with them.

To some extent your motivational skills and your leadership skills can compensate for each other. For example, employees who are only moderately motivated by your ability to satisfy their needs may nevertheless work very hard if you are an effective leader. Similarly, a well-designed reward system may compensate for a substantial lack of interpersonal skills on your part. Obviously, neither of these situations is optimal. In order to obtain the most productivity from your employees, it will be necessary to learn both how to motivate employees and how to lead them.

MOTIVATION

Why does an employee work? You may have thought that this question was addressed in the chapter on compensation. It was, but only partly. Your compensation plan, important as it is, only determines what you should pay your employees. It does not address such questions as these:

- What is the relationship between the rewards that an employee receives from the practice and the employee's non-job-related goals?
- Does the employee think that he or she will be able to perform successfully?
- How does the employee perceive the relationship between performance and rewards?
- What things, in addition to money, does each employee desire?

You might respond to this list of questions by saying, "Well, I really don't care!" You *should* care, because knowing the answers to these questions can help you to obtain better job performances from your employees.

Obtaining the knowledge necessary to answer these questions requires taking the time to learn something about each employee. Time, of course, is one of your most valuable commodities. It is largely what you sell to generate your practice's revenue. You won't want to make the same investment for all employees. Employees in less critical positions may merit little or no time investment. Employees in very critical positions may merit a substantial investment. Once you learn how to motivate employees, you can then make an intelligent, informed decision regarding whether you want to try to influence an employee's motivation.

The questions listed above were not randomly selected. Instead, they related to the elements of expectancy theory, a well-developed theory of motivation designed by Victor Vroom[1] at Yale University. Expectancy theory has become one of the dominant theories for understanding and directing work behavior. Vroom observed that the rewards that we obtain from a job are often only intermediary benefits that will be used to satisfy other more fundamental needs. For example, a nurse works for a salary, which is then used to buy a car, go on vacation, continue her education, and so on. Her motivation, or *force* to perform, is a function of

1. her *expectancy* (subjective probability) that by acting in certain ways she will obtain certain work-related outcomes, such as a salary increase, expressions of satisfaction with her performance, and so on

2. the *valence* (anticipated satisfaction) that would be derived from the work-related outcomes

This can be expressed symbolically as

$$F_i = \Sigma(E_{ij}V_j) \tag{5-1}$$

where

F_i is the force on the individual to perform act i, which is job-related behavior
E_{ij} is the strength of the expectancy that act i will be followed by outcome j, which is the reward that you provide
V_j is the valence, or anticipated satisfaction arising out of job-related outcome j

It is possible, therefore, to restate the nurse's motivation in the following manner. Her effort or work level (F_i) is a function of both her anticipated satisfaction from a pay raise and any other job-related rewards you might provide (V_js) and the subjective probabilities (E_{ij}s) that if she performs at a certain level you will in fact provide these rewards. Her effort or work level is equal to the sum of all of the $E_{ij}V_j$ combinations for all of the work outcomes that she perceives. What determines her valence (V_j) for the pay raise? That is a function of

1. the *instrumentality* of the pay raise for satisfying *other needs in her life, and*
2. the *valence* (anticipated satisfaction) that she will derive from satisfying these other life needs, such as a car, a vacation, a master's degree, a personal sense of control over her life, and so on.

This can be expressed symbolically as

$$V_j = \Sigma(V_kI_{jk}) \tag{5-2}$$

where

V_j is the valence, or the anticipated satisfaction that would be derived from the first-level work-related outcome j
V_k is the valence, or the anticipated satisfaction that would be derived from the second-level personal outcome k
I_{jk} is the instrumentality or subjective correlation between the first-level work-related outcome j and achieving the second-level personal outcome k

It is possible, therefore, to restate the nurse's valence (V_j) for a pay raise or any other first-level outcome offered by your practice as a function of both her valences for second-level personal life goals that she seeks (V_ks) interacting with how instrumental (I_{jk}s) she perceives the first-level rewards provided by your practice for achieving her second-level personal life goals. Restated more simply, if your rewards help the employee achieve what she really wants to achieve in her personal life, then these rewards will motivate the employee.

Examination of formulae 5-1 and 5-2 will show that the ultimate value of any reward is related to second-level goals. If you offer rewards that contribute little toward achieving these second-level goals, they will have a correspondingly small motivational value. Your first objective, therefore, is to understand what an employee ultimately desires.

The expectancies and instrumentalities define the paths that your practice provides an employee for reaching his or her personal goals. Once you understand the employee's personal goals and his or her perception of these paths, you can then increase the employee's motivation to perform.

Expectancy theory suggests several points at which you can influence an employee's motivation. First, however, you must understand the employee's goals and perceptions, in particular, the employee's second-level goals and instrumentality and expectancy perceptions. Of these, the second-level outcomes are the most critical for you to understand. Since the second-level outcomes are personal and out of your control, you must direct your efforts toward enhancing the perceived *relationship* between the rewards you do provide and the achievement of these outcomes. This can be accomplished in three ways:

1. You can provide first-level outcomes (js) that have high valences for the employee.
2. You can influence the employee's expectancy perceptions.
3. You can influence the employee's instrumentality perceptions.

Before investigating how these three strategies can be used to affect motivation levels, let us consider a few general observations that are useful for understanding the motivational implications of expectancy theory:

1. If either expectancy or instrumentality is low, then the employee's motivation will be low.
2. An employee is motivated by the *anticipated* satisfaction (valence) of a reward, not by the ultimate satisfaction received.

Even if you provide excellent rewards, there will be little or no motivation to act in the ways you want if the relationship between the desirable job behaviors and receiving the rewards is not perceived. For example, suppose you pay an employee well, but he continues to be discourteous to your patients. The fact that he is currently well paid and instances of the inappropriate behavior have already occurred will prevent him from seeing his compensation as linked to patient courtesy. You may tell him that they are linked, but your actions have amply demonstrated that this is not true. As a result, the desired behavior doesn't occur.

Finally, all of us work for rewards based on what we imagine they will be like. Our actual satisfaction may be far different from what we anticipate. The reality of receiving a reward only affects the perceptions of future valence judgments.

First-Level Outcomes

Providing first-level outcomes that are directly related to an employee's ultimate goal is an effective strategy for increasing employee motivation. For example, a retirement plan will have a high valence to an employee who has long-term financial security as an ultimate goal. On the other hand, a retirement plan that reduces immediate discretionary income would have a negative instrumentality for an employee whose life goals were strongly oriented toward satisfying present material needs. Providing schedule flexibility or educational benefits could have a high valence for some employees and a valence approaching zero for others. A four-day workweek is a benefit that many employees can use to meet their own idiosyncratic second-level goals. In the case of any benefit, you must determine whether the expense or inconvenience of providing the benefit is too burdensome.

The variability of employees' second-level goals is responsible for a corresponding variability in the valences of first-level outcomes. Since salary can be used to satisfy so many different needs, it is a safe motivational tool. However, because salary is not the only requisite for achieving life goals, your ability to use it to motivate employees is limited. Many people who have written about motivation have discussed the nonmonetary reasons why people work. For example, Abraham Maslow discussed self-actualization, or the desire to grow and express creativity, David McClelland described a need for achievement, and Fred Herzberg et al. concluded that employees were motivated by a number of factors, including recognition and responsibility.[2]

These nonmonetary motivators are very real, and they can be particularly attractive because their nonmonetary nature means that they don't cost you anything. Stated very simply, it doesn't cost you a dime when you reward an employee by fulfilling his need for self-respect, accomplishment, recognition, or becoming the best of which he is capable.

Self-actualization, achievement, recognition, and responsibility certainly qualify as "life goals" and can therefore be second-level outcomes (as defined in expectancy theory). The nice thing about them is that you can directly help employees achieve these goals by providing appropriate first-level outcomes. Stated another way, the instrumentality of many nonmonetary rewards will be exceedingly high because they are so closely related to corresponding second-level outcomes. If an employee has the goal of feeling respected, then showing respect will have high motivating value.

Not all employees are motivated by nonmonetary rewards. It is important, therefore, for you to obtain a sense of each employee's need for these types of rewards. In addition, it is important to remember that even those employees who are motivated by nonmonetary rewards will still be strongly motivated by financial rewards. You cannot compensate for inadequate financial rewards by providing a sense of achievement and recognition. Appropriate use of nonmonetary re-wards, when coupled with *adequate* financial rewards, can result in a highly mo-tivating work environment.

Expectancy

Expectancy is the employee's subjective estimate of the probability that his or her actions will lead to certain outcomes. Changing employee perceptions of ex-pectancy is one of the more effective motivational strategies. Perhaps the most important systematic way of influencing expectancies is by conducting thorough performance appraisals and distributing rewards on the basis of merit. Providing immediate feedback is another way of raising expectancies. If employees are rou-tinely told when their performance is adequate or inadequate, this tells them that their performance is noticed and that it matters. When this is coupled with a merit compensation plan, all of the parts are in place for very strong expectancy linkages between desired behaviors and rewards. Correspondingly, you will also establish weak expectancy linkages or none at all between undesirable behaviors and re-wards. That is, employees will perceive that inadequate performance will have a low probability of being rewarded.

The valences of nonmonetary rewards are particularly susceptible to manipula-tion through expectancies. For example, you know that an employee is especially desirous of personal recognition. You say to her, "I will consider it to be an out-standing, personal achievement if you manage to solve our computer billing problem. In addition, the ideas that you have proposed to fix it seem like they should work. All that it will now take is your hard work and concentration to fix this problem." You have in effect told the employee that there is a high probability that her actions will lead to the desired work-related outcome. Your pep talk has encouraged the employee to give it a try. Upon successful completion of the task, you should then personally congratulate the employee, document the incident in the employee's critical incident file, and verbally recognize her achievement at the next staff meeting.

Discussions in which you encourage employees or try to strengthen their confi-dence that they can achieve an objective essentially attempt to increase motivation through altering expectancies.

Instrumentality

Instrumentality is the correlation that an employee sees between the rewards that you provide and the life goals that the employee desires. If you understand what the employee ultimately seeks, you can point out how your rewards will facilitate the achievement of these goals. If the employee is logical and intelligent, he or she will have already discerned this relationship, and your ability, therefore, to influence motivation by exploring instrumentality may be inversely related to an employee's introspectiveness. Nevertheless, it does not hurt to point out the instrumentality relationships to an employee.

Another approach to using instrumentality to motivate employees is to select rewards based on the likelihood that they will have high instrumentalities for an employee. For example, suppose that your computer operator has second-level achievement and recognition needs. By expanding the opportunities to obtain these on the job, you will increase the instrumentality of work outcomes and second-level outcomes. You could do this by providing the employee with additional training or opportunities to troubleshoot computer problems or design computer solutions for problems before you call on a consultant or intervene yourself. As a result, there will be a high degree of instrumentality between achieving the work objectives and the personal second-level outcomes of achievement and recognition.

Physician Motivation

Understanding the concepts discussed above is particularly important for motivating associates. Professionals often work on extended reward contingencies. They are willing to make sacrifices in the present to achieve long-term goals. If you understand their ultimate objectives, then you can structure your rewards so that they contribute more effectively to the attainment of these objectives.

This can be especially important if you have associates who are not owners. For example, consider how an associate's need for recognition, responsibility, and respect is satisfied by your practice. Once again, your response may be, "I really don't care. It's enough that he earns a good income with me and that I provide a nice place to work."

Ultimately, you don't have to give another doctor recognition, for example, or opportunities for achievement, and you certainly don't have to do it to your own detriment. Understanding what the other doctor needs and then using the information to better achieve your own objectives is the goal. Whether to ignore or to take into account another doctor's needs should be a conscious choice, not a decision that has been blundered into because you don't understand the reasons for your own or your associate's actions.

Motivational Strategies

You motivate employees by understanding their ultimate goals in life and the contingent relationships between job performance, the rewards you can supply, and the employees' attainment of their goals. Obtaining the level of knowledge necessary to affect the motivation of employees may take some time. Talking with employees about their life objectives and how their work at the practice might lead to the realization of those goals is an important motivational strategy. This strategy should be supplemented with a healthy dose of unobtrusive observation. Sometimes, idly made comments can also reveal a second-level goal, instrumentality, or expectancy. A secretary who whimsically states that he always wanted to go to college may be making a profoundly important statement. You may be able to use this information to structure practice rewards so that you motivate the employee to achieve his objectives while simultaneously meeting practice needs.

Correspondingly, you can also understand when you won't be able to motivate an employee. For example, you notice that an employee's performance is inadequate or marginal, and this does not result from inadequate training. You know from previous discussions with the employee that his or her second-level objectives are inconsistent with the first-level outcomes that you can provide. Formula 5-2 predicts that when the instrumentality is low (or perhaps even negative), the anticipated satisfaction with the first level outcomes that you provide (V_j) is low (or aversive). If the anticipated satisfaction is low (V_j), then the Force (F_i) as defined in formula 5-1 will be low. Under these circumstances, you will not be able to motivate the employee to meet the needs of the practice. Pep talks or threats of progressive discipline will simply be a waste of time and delay the inevitable. It would be best to cut your losses, and replace the employee.

Getting to know your employees on a more personal level has some inherent dangers. It is important never to allow your interest in the goals and desires of an employee to develop into friendship. Employees can never be friends, because the employer-employee relationship has adversarial aspects to it. If you begin to look upon an employee as a friend, you expose yourself to the risk of manipulation and disappointment when the employee acts in his or her own interest. Similarly, if the employee perceives you as a friend, he or she will inevitably be disappointed and resentful when you must act as a supervisor. Getting to know your employees' personal goals should take place, therefore, at an arm's length.

LEADERSHIP

Leadership is the process of getting subordinates and peers to voluntarily work toward your vision of the practice. Sometimes it is easier to identify a successful leader than it is to understand what he or she does to be a successful leader. Bennis[3] has noted that successful leaders seem to have some characteristics in common.

- They use exceptional communication skills to make ideas and visions tangible to others.

- They generate trust through clear, consistent behavior.
- They have a realistic sense of their limitations.
- They reject the notion of failure.

How do you become a successful leader, and how do you know what to do so that subordinates and peers will perceive you as a leader? Originally, management scientists thought that leadership was a personality characteristic: Leaders were essentially born with an innate skill to lead others. When research studies found too many exceptions to this theory, it was then proposed that leadership was a set of behaviors. For example, researchers at Ohio State University concluded that leaders exhibited varying amounts of concern for employees' welfare, which was called *consideration,* and concern for getting the task accomplished, which was called *initiating structure.* Once again, too many exceptions were found to conclude that behaviors per se were the essence of leadership.

A more recent approach to understanding leadership focuses on examining leader attributes and behaviors in the context of specific situations. Successful leaders seem to be able to choose certain behaviors or decision-making styles that are appropriate *given the situation at the time.* This is called a *situational* approach to leadership. Sometimes a leader has to make decisions like a dictator, sometimes delegate decisions to subordinates. There are also many situations in which a leader will be most effective if he or she uses methods somewhere between these two extremes. The successful leader knows *when,* for example, to delegate, and *when* to make decisions himself.

There is considerable research and practical evidence supporting the validity of the situational approach to leadership. Imagine, for example, the model Marine Corps drill instructor. He or she certainly would typify the directive leader. Imagine, however, if this very successful leader of Marines was to direct the efforts of a volunteer church organization using the same behaviors used with recruits! It is obvious that the result would be a disaster. Conversely, leadership behaviors that would bring success to the volunteer church organization would be equally inappropriate for leading Marine recruits. The key is to match the leadership style to the situation. There are very few organizations in which a leader can be successful using only one leadership style. The truly successful Marine Corps sergeant will on occasion have to delegate decisions or involve subordinates or peers in the decision-making process. Once again, the skill is to know *when* to choose a particular decision-making style.

The following discussion presents a way of *thinking* about leadership. You won't want to use this method every time you make a management decision. On the other hand, it provides a way of playing devil's advocate and challenging your natural decision-making inclinations. In addition, over a period of time you will learn about the environmental circumstances that should influence your leadership strategy.

Exhibit 5-1 contains a range of leadership or decision-making behaviors that you can use. These five styles differ in type and quality of subordinate involvement. *A* stands for autocratic, *C* stands for consultative, and *G* stands for group (style GI is not used in this application, so it is not presented in this discussion). In some types of situations, several of the styles will result in reasonable decisions, while in other situations only one style will be truly effective.

Most managers, doctors included, have the ability to use a range of behaviors. Each manager has a predisposition toward favorites but is usually capable of exhibiting a variety of leadership styles. Research conducted by Victor Vroom and Phillip Yetton shows that effective leaders choose a decision-making style that

1. protects the quality of the decision
2. protects the acceptance of the decision
3. makes a decision in a minimum of time
4. makes a decision that will develop the skills and abilities of their subordinates

Although effective leaders may not consciously understand why they make decisions in a certain way, they nevertheless somehow have learned to act so as to

Exhibit 5-1 Different Leadership Styles

AI (Autocratic 1): You solve the problem or make the decision yourself using information available to you at that time.

AII (Autocratic 2): You obtain the necessary information from your subordinates, then decide on the solution to the problem yourself. In getting the information from them, you may or may not tell your subordinates what the problem is. The role played by your subordinates is clearly to provide the necessary information to you rather than to generate or evaluate solutions.

CI (Consultative 1): You share the problem with relevant subordinates individually, getting their ideas and suggestions without bringing them together as a group. Then you make the decision, which may or may not reflect your subordinates' advice.

CII (Consultative 2): You share the problem with your subordinates as a group, collectively obtaining their ideas and suggestions. Then you make the decision, which may or may not reflect your subordinates' advice.

GII (Group): You share the problem with your subordinates as a group. Together you generate and evaluate alternatives and attempt to reach general agreement on a solution. Your role is much like that of a chairperson. You do not try to influence the group to adopt "your" solution, and you are willing to accept and implement any solution that has the support of the entire group.

Source: Adapted from *Leadership and Decision Making* by V. Vroom and P. Yetton, p. 13, with permission of the University of Pittsburgh Press, © 1983.

achieve the objectives noted above. Vroom and Yetton[4] have developed a decision-making model that can provide guidance for selecting a decision-making style that will secure quality, acceptance, timeliness, and employee development. Their decision-making model is presented in Figure 5-1.

A situation can be defined by asking seven questions. The flow chart in Figure 5-1 will guide you through the questions, which are discussed in greater depth below. Based on your answers to these questions, you will define a set of feasible decision-making strategies. Some situations can be successfully addressed with any of the decision-making styles, whereas other situations are best addressed

---

A. Is there a quality requirement?
B. Do I have sufficient information to solve the problem?
C. Is the problem structured?
D. Is acceptance of the decision by subordinates critical?
E. If I make the decision myself is it reasonably certain that it would be accepted by those involved?
F. Do participants share the organizational goals?
G. Is conflict among participants likely?

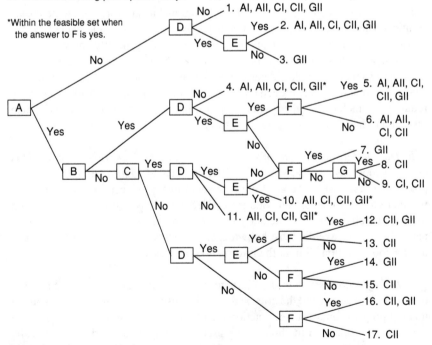

Figure 5-1 Decision-Making Flow Chart. *Source:* Reprinted, by permission of the publisher, from *Organizational Dynamics*, Spring 1973, © 1973. American Management Association, New York. All rights reserved.

with only one or two. In those situations where more than one approach is feasible, the alternatives are listed in order of timeliness. If making a decision quickly is important, then use the first style in the set. For example, in Situation 1 in Figure 5-1 (top branch of the flow chart), any decision-making style is feasible; however, the AI style will result in the quickest decision. On the other hand, if employee development is important, then work from the other side of the set, such as style GII in Situation 1.

By learning how this model works, you can sharpen your decision-making and leadership abilities. By answering the seven questions, you will be able to define the decision-making situation and identify a subset of appropriate decision-making styles. The questions you use to define the decision-making situation are summarized in Figure 5-1 and discussed below in more detail.

A. Does the problem possess a quality requirement? This question concerns the importance of identifying a high-quality solution *irrespective* of the need for subordinates to accept the solution. If a problem does not possess a quality requirement, you would be indifferent to any proposed solution. Generally, if a problem does not possess a quality requirement, this means that there are two or three obvious solutions and there are no technical or rational means for picking the "best" solution. The primary consideration is that *some* solution be implemented.

Most problems do possess a quality requirement, and generally you will answer yes to this question. Problems (or processes) with quality requirements include developing a marketing plan, determining which brand of x-ray equipment to purchase, and making clinical decisions. Problems that might not possess a quality requirement include whether to paint the waiting room beige or white and which weekend to have the office Christmas party.

B. Do you have sufficient information to make a high-quality decision? This question concerns whether you have sufficient technical information to solve the problem yourself without consulting your subordinates or peers. The main issue is whether you have enough knowledge to understand all aspects of the problem and to solve it technically, not whether you have more knowledge than your subordinates. You may have the most knowledge, yet lack sufficient knowledge to produce a good solution without the information possessed by others.

C. Is the problem structured? A structured problem is one in which the alternative courses of action and the criteria that will be used to evaluate whether you are making progress on a course of action are obvious. For example, once you have identified the selection methods to be used in filling a secretarial position, the problem is structured. At that point, someone can mechanically apply the methods to a group of applicants and make a selection decision. Developing a comprehensive community care system for AIDS patients, including family, medical, and financial issues, would be an unstructured problem, since there is no existing "game plan" indicating all of the issues to be considered, their relative importance, and potential sources of funding.

D. Is acceptance of the decision by subordinates important or critical for effective implementation? Even a technically correct solution can fail if those who must implement it are resistant or opposed to it. The issue is whether, *irrespective of how the decision is made,* subordinate acceptance is critical to implementing the decision. When judging whether a solution has an acceptance requirement, consider (1) whether your subordinates' initiative, judgment, or thinking will affect their execution of your orders; and (2) whether your subordinates are likely to disapprove strongly enough to actively oppose the solution. The question here is whether they will do what you want, not whether they like it. If a problem does not require your subordinates to be involved in the execution of the decision, there is no acceptance issue. Similarly, if subordinates are likely to be indifferent, there is also no acceptance issue.

E. If you were to make the decision yourself, are you reasonably certain that it would be accepted by your subordinates? If subordinate acceptance as defined by Question D is important to the successful implementation of the solution, then you certainly want to use a decision-making process that will increase the chance of acceptance. If you allow subordinates to participate in the decision, this can further their acceptance. On the other hand, if you are viewed as the person who legitimately *should* make the decision, or as someone who has the *expertise* to make the decision, then autocratic methods also may be acceptable.

F. Do subordinates share the organizational goals to be obtained by solving this problem? Employee self-interest can be incompatible with the goals of your practice. Our discussion of motivation makes it clear that people may work for many reasons that have nothing to do with the goals of your practice. Employees are not altruistic. If their personal goals are incompatible with your practice's goals, they will work to achieve their personal goals.

G. Is conflict among subordinates likely in preferred solutions? This question concerns whether employees are likely to disagree on the best way to solve a problem. This is different from Question F, since it is possible for employees to share organizational goals but to disagree on how best to realize them.

The flow chart in Figure 5-1 can be used in several ways. First, the questions themselves should sensitize you to issues that merit consideration in your day-to-day relations with your peers and subordinates. Obviously, you would not and should not consult this chart for daily decision making. Being sensitive to the issues raised, however, is helpful in any interpersonal situation.

Second, when you are confronted with a major decision requiring considerable thought, you may want to use Figure 5-1 to play devil's advocate vis-à-vis the position you are inclined to take. If, for example, the chart says to delegate but your gut intuition is to be autocratic, then you have the basis for a dialogue with yourself regarding the two approaches. No matter what you finally choose to do, your decision will be based on considerable thought.

A CASE APPLICATION

Larry Johnson owns a radiology practice. He has one associate, Phil Downs, who shares expenses but does not yet own part of the practice. Both Larry and Phil are doing very well, their appointment slots are usually filled, and it is Larry's intention to have Phil become a partner in the future. Recently, Larry decided that he would bring in a new associate. He was uncertain how much he should involve Phil in the selection process. Larry analyzed the decision-making situation by using the Vroom and Yetton model presented in Figure 5-1. He came to the following conclusions.

Question A: Yes. The problem certainly does have a quality requirement. He could hire someone who was deficient in the appropriate clinical skills or was unable to get along with himself or Phil.

Question B: Yes. Larry believed that he knew more about hiring people, as well as the personal characteristics that he desired, than did Phil, and he also believed that he knew enough to make a decision by himself. After all, he went through this process when he hired Phil.

Question D: Yes. If Larry hired someone who Phil thought was incompetent or greatly disliked, there was always the chance that Phil would eventually leave. Larry didn't think that this was probable, but it was important to Larry that Phil like the new associate.

Question E: Yes. Larry felt that as sole owner it was his prerogative to make hiring decisions. In addition, he sensed that Phil would recognize his legitimate right as owner to make these decisions.

Question F: No. Phil, as an associate, did not have the same interest in the success of the practice as Larry. In addition to being interested in short-term issues, Larry was very concerned about the long-range future of the practice. Phil was certainly concerned about his own long-range prospects as a radiologist, but whether he would continue as an associate of Larry's was an open question. For example, Phil might perceive the new associate as a competitor and therefore seek a nonthreatening associate.

According to Larry's analysis, the selection process should either be autocratic or involve consultation with Phil. Larry should not, however, share the ultimate decision making with Phil.

Larry informed Phil before the hiring process began that he would be consulted but that he would have no part in the final decision making. Larry eventually decided that he would do all of the initial screening himself and eliminate those applicants whom he did not like for one reason or another. Larry allowed Phil to interview four candidates and sought his opinions. He then combined Phil's opinions with his own and by himself reached the decision to hire Jay Jones.

Larry decided to create a new technician position two months after Jay joined the practice. He analyzed the decision-making situation in the following manner.

Question A: Yes. Once again, Larry could hire someone who was incompetent or hard to get along with.

Question B: Yes. Once again, Larry felt that he would be able to find a replacement by himself.

Question D: Yes. The new technician would be working with both Phil and Jay. If they did not like the new technician, it could result in dissension.

Question E: No. Since the technician would be working with all three of them, Larry felt that both Phil and Jay would be resentful if they were not included in the hiring process. Would they actually take it out on him if he did make an arbitrary decision? Larry didn't really know, but he felt that it would be safer to assume that they would.

Question F: Yes. Unlike in the hiring of an associate, Larry thought that he, Phil, and Jay would have the same goals. The difference in their roles should not affect their decision making.

The analysis pointed to GII as the only appropriate form of decision making. Larry met with Phil and Jay, and they decided that the business manager should do the initial screening and interviewing of applicants. Each of the three shared in the interviewing and work sample testing of the final four candidates. Due to their schedules, Larry evaluated two applicants and Phil and Jay evaluated one each. They had a group meeting and decided that two of the applicants really stood out. Both were scheduled for a final group interview with Larry, Phil, and Jay after business hours. After the final interview, they reached a consensus on whom to hire. Larry had this to say after the whole process was completed: "The Vroom-Yetton way of thinking about how to lead was helpful, because it made me think about important considerations related to *how* I make a decision. I might well have come up with the same decision-making processes on my own. At least I like to think that I would. At a minimum, this process gave me confidence that my gut intuition regarding how to proceed was valid."

CONCLUSION

Much of the work performed in your practice will be accomplished through your employees. If your employees are not motivated in ways that are consistent with your objectives or if they don't share your vision of the future, then your practice will be less productive than it could be.

Knowing how to search for the life goals of your employees, as well as their expectancies and their perceptions of instrumentalities, can help you motivate them to perform at higher levels. This chapter outlines a strategy for motivating employees by structuring your practice so that employees achieve their own personal goals in the process of working toward the achievement of practice goals.

Leadership involves conveying a vision of what you want and inspiring employees to work toward that vision. The way in which you make leadership decisions will have a profound effect on the willingness of employees to follow. This chapter provides a method of examining decision-making situations and determining how best to lead. It also shows how to arrive at high-quality decisions that are accepted by subordinates and peers and are consistent with time constraints and employee development needs.

NOTES

1. Victor Vroom, *Work and Motivation* (New York: Wiley, 1964).

2. Abraham Maslow, "A Theory of Human Motivation," *Psychological Review* (1943): 370–96; D. McClelland, *The Achieving Society* (New York: The Free Press, 1961); F. Herzberg, B. Mausner, and B. Snyderman, *The Motivation to Work* (New York: Wiley, 1959).

3. W. Bennis, "The Four Competencies of Leadership," *Training and Development Journal,* 1984, 15–19.

4. V.H. Vroom and A.G. Jago, *The New Leadership* (Englewood Cliffs, N.J.: Prentice-Hall, 1988).

Chapter 6

Organizational Issues

CHAPTER OBJECTIVES

This chapter covers four organizational issues that will affect the productivity of your practice. You will learn how to design training programs for new employees and determine appropriate training methods. You will also learn how to design jobs so that they form logical units and are consistent with financial controls. You will learn how the structure of your practice will directly affect your administrative tasks and when various organizational structures are most appropriate. Finally, you will learn why employees and partners sometimes resist organizational change and what strategies can be used to overcome their resistance.

INTRODUCTION

This chapter discusses several issues that you will need to address if your practice is to succeed. Training is the process of familiarizing new employees with your office procedures and facilitating the learning of necessary new skills. Job design is the process of determining exactly what tasks should compose a job. Occasionally tasks will be included in a job when they really could be more effectively performed by someone else in your practice. This can result either from tasks being placed in the wrong job to begin with, or as a result of changes that occur over time. It is important, for reasons of efficiency and financial control, to look closely at how tasks are divided among employees. The practice structure is the way in which the jobs in your practice fit together. An effective practice structure will give you more time to work with your patients while still keeping you informed and involved in the management of your practice. Large practices must be more concerned about their structure and the division of tasks among employees. If your practice only consists of you and your secretary, whatever you don't do is obviously done by the secretary, and vice versa. Nevertheless, even with such a small practice, the division of labor is not a foregone conclusion. For example, there are several financial tasks that your secretary could perform but that, for financial control and security reasons, you should either perform yourself or contract out to a consultant.

Finally, all practices undergo change. Changes in employees, policies, laws, insurance regulations, and your personal preferences, to name a very few, can have effects throughout your practice. Often, change will be resisted by some employees and partners. Understanding and overcoming resistance to change is important to organizational survival and growth.

TRAINING

The object of training is to make a new employee an effective member of your practice as soon as possible. Although you hire an applicant because he or she will bring many skills to the job, there will be other skills that the new employee must learn. Some may be technical, such as knowing how to use your practice's computer hardware and software, whereas others may be procedural. Procedural skills might include knowing how to answer the telephone properly, how to take a referral, where to place lab reports, what to do in an emergency, how to handle a patient who asks a clinical question, and so on. Eventually new employees learn the finer points of practice operations. The question is how dysfunctional they will be during the learning process. An effective training procedure will minimize problems and allow a new employee to be fully functional as quickly as possible.

Effective training begins with defining what the new employee must learn. The first step is to make a list of all of the areas that must be covered in the training program. Each of these areas can then be broken down into finer detail. The resulting list of learning objectives is called a *training plan*. A sample training plan for a secretarial position is found in Exhibit 6-1. The same training plan can be used indefinitely for the position as long as job content does not change.

The training plan can be used in two ways. One approach is to use it as a checklist for developing a training program. A training program is a detailed document that describes the specific content that must be learned by the new employee. It is analogous to a lesson plan that a teacher prepares to be certain that the appropriate information will be logically and effectively communicated to students.

A second use of a training plan is as a checklist for training. Often current employees of a medical practice are familiar with the information that a new employee must learn. There is no need to write a detailed training program. Instead the training strategy is to have appropriate employee-trainers talk with the new employee. The training plan can be used to determine the appropriate employee-trainers and the best training sequence. Employee-trainers can then use the items

Exhibit 6-1 Training Plan for a Secretarial Position

JoAnn Harrison's Training Program

The name(s) after a training subject indicate who will be providing the training. These people can also be used as a resource if you have a question. The person(s) responsible for training in a subject area will initial the subject area after the training has been provided. After you feel that you have developed proficiency in or a sense of comfort with an area, initial it. If at any time you have any questions or feel that you need additional instruction, go first to those who have the responsibility for training in the appropriate area.

J.H.

I. Interaction with patients (Dr. White)
    A. Greeting patients
    B. Attitude toward patients
II. Scheduling appointments
    A. Dr. White's appointment book (Julie, Dr. White)
    B. Idiosyncrasies of various physicians' schedules (Julie, Nancy)
    C. Late cancellation fees (Julie, Dr. White)
    D. Dr. Raymond's appointment book (Nancy, Dr. Raymond)
    E. Completion of appointment cards (Julie)
    F. Notifying physicians of changes (cancellations, changed appointments, or anything that could affect their professional lives) (Julie, B.J.)
    G. Informing patient of cancellation charge if less than 24 hours notice (Julie, B.J.)
    H. Who uses which office and when (Julie, Nancy)
    I. Condensing schedules to take advantage of cancellations, changes, etc. (Julie, B.J.)
III. Telephones (Julie)
    A. How to use the telephone equipment
    B. How to answer the telephone
    C. Taking messages, informing physicians, etc.
    D. How and when to forward calls to answering service
    E. How to take phones off of answering service
    F. Emergency on-call schedule
    G. How to deal with an emergency (Dr. White)
    H. What not to tell patients (when physician is leaving, personal information, information about other patients, etc.)
    I. Nasty or inappropriate calls
IV. New referrals
    A. Collecting information and use of new referral form (Julie)
    B. Familiarization with fee structure (Julie, Larry)
    C. How to handle the discussion of fees (Julie, Dr. White)
    D. Insurance and copayments (Julie, Larry)
    E. Assignment of referrals to physicians (Dr. White)
    F. What to do when a new patient arrives for first appointment (Julie, B.J.)
        1. Method of payment form (Julie)
        2. Intake questionnaire (Julie)
V. Patient chart organization (Julie)
    A. What charts are used for
    B. What goes where in a chart
    C. Chart notes paper

continues

Exhibit 6-1 continued

      D. Pulling and distributing charts
      E. Collecting charts
      F. Chart security
      G. Release of chart information and release form
  VI. Fees
      A. Collecting fees (Julie, Dr. White)
      B. Using the day sheet (Julie, Larry)
      C. Refusals to pay and difficulties getting payment (Julie, Larry, Dr. White)
          1. Distributing collection envelope
          2. Informing patient of office policy that copayment must be paid before next visit
      D. Receipt of
          1. Cash (Julie, Larry)
          2. Checks (Julie, Larry)
          3. Credit cards (Julie, Larry)
 VII. Confidentiality (Dr. White)
      A. On telephones
      B. Release of records
      C. How a patient can put you in the position of breaching confidentiality
      D. Contacting patients
      E. Use of -2275 telephone number
VIII. Use of Macintosh and office equipment
      A. General orientation (Bob)
      B. Typing documents (Bob, Julie)
      C. Using the printer, copier, dictaphone, etc. (Julie, Nancy)
      D. MediMac orientation (Bob, Julie)
      E. Keeping track of new referrals (Bob, Julie)
      F. Backing up your documents (Bob, Julie)
  IX. General office procedures and responsibilities (Larry)
      A. General orientation on insurance, copayments, etc.
      B. Office policy on work priorities
      C. Who you report to (Dr. White)
      D. Opening up in morning
          1. What to do if Nancy is sick
      E. Closing up at night
      F. Alarm system
          1. What to do when the alarm goes off!
          2. Arming and disarming the alarm
      G. Where things are kept
      H. What supplies we stock and where they are (Julie)
      I. Opening mail and stamping checks
      J. Familiarization with
          1. Nancy's job (Nancy)
          2. Larry's job (Larry)
          3. Melinda's job (Melinda)
      K. Familiarization with file cabinets and their contents (Julie)
          1. Clinical charts
          2. Business charts
          3. Business records
          4. Templates

continues

Exhibit 6-1 continued

> L. The importance of keeping coworkers informed (Dr. White, Larry)
> M. Orderly transfer to Melinda at 5:30 (Melinda)
> N. Keys and orientation to security (Larry)
>   1. Locking of doors
>   2. Awareness of strangers
> O. Sick leave, vacation time (Dr. White, Larry)

listed in the training plan to guide their discussions and to ensure that all training subjects are covered. The training plan in Exhibit 6-1 was developed to be used in this manner. In this example, the employee-trainers are instructed to place a mark next to each subject after it has been taught. The trainee is also instructed to indicate when he or she feels comfortable with each subject. The training plan thus becomes a useful record of training progress.

Use your judgment when determining who should conduct the training. Generally, the best trainer is the previous job holder. If, however, the previous job holder has been forced to leave, or is leaving under bad circumstances, he or she *should not conduct the training.* There is too much opportunity for the departing employee to poison the relationship between the new employee and the practice. Use another employee as the trainer, do the training yourself, retain a consultant, or let the new employee muddle through, but *never* use a disgruntled employee to conduct training.

The trainer must determine how to conduct the training. Most training in medical practices occurs on the job. This can be a very effective way of training a new employee. The trainer provides some preliminary instruction regarding what will be happening and then gives a demonstration. After the new employee observes the trainer performing the tasks, he or she then does the task while the trainer observes and coaches.

Another effective training method is formal instruction. This can be useful in cases of detailed content, such as policies and procedures, word processing programs, clinical procedures, and computer hardware and software. This type of training should be conducted away from any distractions. It is always tempting to conduct formal instruction where the trainer can answer the telephones, cover the window, and do those things that he or she would normally do. This can make the formal training take longer, and the inevitable interruptions will interfere with the new employee's ability to learn. Structure the training time and location to avoid or minimize interruptions. Smaller practices and practices that are very thinly staffed, however, may have to compromise training effectiveness in order to ensure operational coverage. This is a situation in which the realities of running a business must be balanced against the objective of effective training.

Often the most neglected training method is reading. Training manuals for your office equipment and computer software can be very effective training tools. The trainer must understand what preliminary training must occur before the new employee can fully benefit from a manual. In addition, the trainer can greatly facilitate the process by reviewing the manual and only assigning those parts that (1) are useful given how the equipment or software is used in your practice, or (2) are necessary in order to understand a subsequent part of the manual that does contain job-relevant material.

It also is important to isolate new employees from distractions so that they can read and understand the material in the training manual. Trainees also should have access to the equipment or software while they are studying the manual so that they can practice what they are learning. There is often a temptation, which should be avoided, to make new employees "useful" while they are learning, such as placing them next to a telephone while they are supposed to be studying a training manual. Access to the trainer for questions and answers while studying the manuals can also be very helpful. Finally, the trainer should follow training with opportunities to practice what has just been studied.

The following training schedule shows how the ideas noted above can be combined to provide effective word processing training:

1. Trainer provides initial orientation to and overview of word processing program.
2. New employee is isolated and given a computer and word processing manuals to work with.
3. Trainer performs his or her normal job but is available for questions.
4. Following training, trainer gives new employee a real document to prepare.
5. Trainer remains available while performing normal job and answers new employee's questions on an "as needed" basis.
6. Trainer examines completed document, provides feedback to new employee, and uses completed document to develop content of next training session.

One final training strategy to consider is use of an outside trainer. This can be especially helpful in the case of technical training, such as word processing, computer software, and laboratory equipment training. If practice personnel do not have the time or the ability to provide effective training, you will do better to send the new employee to a few hours of training by the appropriate software or equipment specialist. After the training is completed, be certain to provide plenty of opportunity to practice the new skill as well as sufficient access to the software or equipment and the manuals.

Irrespective of the particular training methods used, the trainer must examine the training process through the eyes of the trainee. The trainer must "unlearn" what comes naturally so that he or she can see the components that must be presented to the trainee separately. For example, answering the telephones may involve all of the following: (1) using an appropriate greeting; (2) knowing the types of services provided by the practice; (3) knowing how to schedule appointments; (4) understanding insurance benefits; (5) understanding patient confidentiality policies; (6) understanding practice payment policies; and (7) technical use of telephone equipment. A trainer who cannot break down complex tasks into simple constituent elements will provide frustrating, ineffective training. Recollecting what it was like to learn the tasks, as well as adopting a reasonable time schedule, will greatly facilitate training.

The doctor's role in training varies with the type of job and the size of the practice. With front office jobs in larger practices, the doctor's role is to be certain that the business manager or trainer has in fact created a training plan and is proceeding in a reasonable manner. This can be handled as part of the normal supervision of top-level office staff. In smaller practices, the doctor may have to pay closer attention to the actions of the trainer, provide more written and verbal guidance, and perhaps even take the time to conduct some of the training personally.

JOB DESIGN

The content of jobs can evolve for reasons that have little or nothing to do with logic or work efficiency. It is important, therefore, to look at the content of jobs every now and then to reestablish their legitimacy. Controlling job content is also an important element in preserving the financial security of your practice. By effectively dividing the financial responsibilities between two or more positions, you can create safeguards against the diversion of funds. As your practice grows and changes, the workloads of different employees may change. Your bookkeeper might have time to spare, whereas a word processing position might have gradually become overloaded. Finally, adjusting the design of jobs can result in increased employee satisfaction. Employees who strive for recognition and a sense of achievement will be more satisfied if their jobs provide these. To some extent you may be able to alter the content of jobs to increase the likelihood employees will be more satisfied. Since satisfaction is related to reduced turnover, this can help you to control your recruiting, training, and hiring costs.

Assuming that you have two or more front office positions, you can reduce the chances of theft by a careful division of the financial responsibilities. There are three points at which the diversion of money can occur: (1) when it comes into the practice, either in the form of cash or checks received from patients at the time of service or in the form of checks sent in the mail by patients or insurance companies; (2) at the time of posting to your computer or bookkeeping system; and (3) at the time of posting to the checkbook. These critical points can also act as a control if they are kept in the hands of separate personnel. For example, if funds are diverted by an employee as they come into the practice, then eventually the person who does posting and manages your accounts receivable will notice that the accounts are not being paid. He or she will then contact the "delinquent" patient or insurance company, who will state that the fee was in fact paid, thereby disclosing the diversion. If the money is diverted by the person posting payments, then either (1) reports generated by your accounting system will not balance with deposits to the checkbook, or (2) reports generated by your medical office management software will show an increase in receivables (money owed by patients). In either case there will be a warning signal indicating that something unusual is happening. Finally, if the person managing your checkbook is diverting funds, then the checking account will not balance against the reports of gross receipts from your medical office management software.

In order to have good, although not foolproof, financial security, the handling of practice funds needs to be distributed among three separate positions. The incumbents of these positions can perform other duties. The main functions are (1) intake of funds, (2) posting of funds, and (3) checkbook and depositing of funds.

In a small practice, the intake of funds could be handled by the receptionist. The receptionist would open the mail and stamp "For Deposit Only" on the back of each check and also collect cash and checks at the window. These funds would then be passed to a second employee, perhaps called the bookkeeper, who would post the payments to the appropriate accounts and prepare deposit slips. In this system, the doctor would manage the checkbook. The doctor would receive the checks from the bookkeeper, log them into the checkbook, and make the deposit. The doctor would keep control of the checkbook, write the checks, and reconcile the checkbook against reports from the bookkeeper's patient accounts ledgers. If the secretary embezzles, then the bookkeeper will notice, and if the bookkeeper embezzles, then the doctor will notice.

Most doctors will not want to maintain the checkbook, since this task consumes time that could be used to generate revenue. As a result, this task should be contracted out to a consulting bookkeeper or accountant. If that is the case, the doctor's role is to review financial reports (see Chapter 7) generated by the contracting bookkeeper or accountant. Managing the checkbook should never, however, be given to the employee responsible for posting payments, since the employee's ability to cover the diversion of funds would simply be too great to justify this arrangement. Unfortunately, the division of tasks will not protect you against collusion between several employees.

Finally, you want to design your jobs so that the incumbents are fully occupied without being overloaded. You need to look for signs that you are overworking your employees. Too many duties assigned to a job will result in frustration, uncompleted work, and employee turnover. There is no magic formula for determining when a job is overloaded. If an employee is not completing the work, you must determine whether the job would be too demanding for *anyone* or whether the employee is not skilled enough to plan or perform the work properly. If the fault lies with the employee, then terminate the employee and find a suitable replacement. If the job is simply too demanding, then reassign some of the tasks to other employees or create a new position.

If you notice that your employees aren't constantly busy, this may mean that you are overstaffed. Eliminating unneeded employees will obviously have an impact on the profitability of your practice. A good time to consider the necessity for a position is when an employee resigns or is terminated. Use this as an opportunity to look at all of the jobs in the practice to see if the open position's responsibilities could be divided among other positions. Give particular consideration to reassigning duties in conjunction with purchasing new equipment. Even very expensive computers and office equipment are generally far less expensive than employees. They don't take vacations, you don't have to pay FICA for them, and they work as long as you ask. There are no rules of thumb to determine the feasibility of replacing a position through reassignment of duties and automation. You have to use common sense and logic to be certain that you will not overload the remaining positions.

STRUCTURE

The structure of your practice defines the reporting relationships among your employees. The structure you choose will also affect your own management role. If you employ only one other person, the structure is very simple, since that person must report directly to you. If you have several employees, you have some choice regarding the reporting relationships. All too often, practice structures come into existence for no logical, considered reason. A poor structure can result in an excessive payroll as well as less effective office operations.

One choice would be to have all employees report directly to you. This is called a *simple practice structure* (Figure 6-1). One feature of the simple practice structure is that you will be the focus of all of the upward and downward communication in your practice. If Secretary A has a problem, you are the one he will tell. You will then have to do something about it, even if it is nothing more than telling Secretary B to help A do some of the word processing. Assuming that you listen to your employees and that they feel you are responsive to reasonable requests, this type of structure will provide you with a lot of information about the daily operations of your practice. It will give you the opportunity to become involved in the smallest details of your practice's operations. It will also give you the responsibility of *integrating* the work performed by your employees. This means that *you* will be personally responsible for making certain that each employee's contributions fit together, so that the totality of your employees' efforts result in a smooth-run-

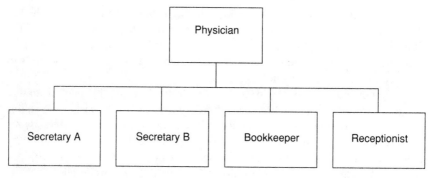

Figure 6-1 Simple Practice Structure

ning, coordinated, and productive team effort. In addition, your management responsibilities will also include making practice policies and plans, including strategic plans, marketing plans, and personnel plans.

If your response to this scenario is, "My time is too valuable to be listening to secretaries argue about who should do what," then you need another type of practice structure. Figure 6-2 presents the office manager structure. In this structure the "bookkeeper" takes over some of the management responsibilities that were previously assumed by you. This office manager–bookkeeper will of course have to

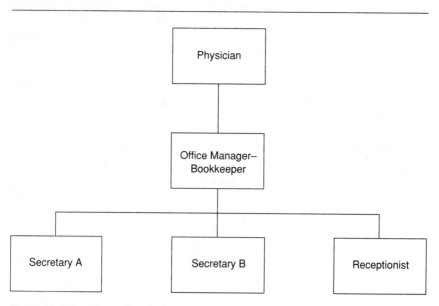

Figure 6-2 Office Manager Practice Structure

be paid more than a simple bookkeeper. The $2,000 to $4,000 salary increase, however, can be easily justified if, by being freed of some management responsibilities, you are able to perform additional clinical work. For example, if the additional clinical time amounted to two hours per week and that time could be sold at $100 per hour, this would result in an additional $9,600 of revenue per year (assuming 48 workweeks).

In the office manager structure, your office manager performs the front line management functions. This includes directing the daily activities of office staff, setting priorities, implementing standard office policies, and integrating the efforts of the front office to produce coordinated, effective group performance. Your role is to supervise the office manager and focus on long-term planning and policy decision making.

In this structure, effective communication between you and the office manager is essential. In addition, the office manager must have very good communication skills so that you will be informed about the state of your organization. It is a good idea to have a weekly meeting with the office manager. The agenda should include a discussion of developing office issues and allow time for you to provide guidance. When your decisions evolve into policies or procedures requiring implementation, you will make them operational through your office manager. For example, if the accounting reports indicate that expenditures for supplies seem to be rising, you would tell the office manager to determine the reasons why and propose solutions. The office manager would also be responsible for implementing changes and keeping you informed of any progress made in controlling these expenditures.

A possible disadvantage of this structure is that you are removed from the day-to-day operations of your practice and are dependent upon the skill and ability of your office manager. If the office manager thinks as you do, then the structure can be successful and time-effective. If, on the other hand, your office manager is not capable of making decisions that are generally consistent with your management philosophy, then you will have the worst of both structures. You will find yourself constantly reviewing your office manager's daily decisions, and overriding those that you find to be inadequate. You will effectively be operating as though there were no office manager, yet you will be paying a salary for one! In addition, the office manager will come to resent your "interference," and the office manager's subordinates will realize that he or she is a figure head. All of this will tend to create dissension and dissatisfaction.

If you find yourself in the position of reviewing all of a business manager's decisions, you must ask yourself some hard questions. Are you perhaps too perfectionistic? Are you able to recognize that there may be more than one effective solution to a problem? Is it possible that the office manager's solutions to problems could be as effective as your solutions? If your answers to these questions are yes, no, no, then you must consider whether you *really* want to use an office manager structure. If you can honestly answer these questions with a no, yes, yes, then you need a new office manager. Similarly, if you find that many of the daily details are not being attended to, then you need a new office manager. Unfortunately, with this type of practice structure, you will not notice that the daily details are going unattended until a major problem develops. The delegation of power and authority through an office manager structure can provide you with great power, because it effectively multiplies your presence. Unfortunately, delegation is a double-edged sword that can wound you seriously if your office manager is inadequate.

The office manager structure will suffice for most private practices. Larger practices, however, may find it necessary to evolve additional structural elements to deal with the complexity and quantity of policy decisions that must be made in such functional areas as production, marketing, and personnel. A functional structure (Figure 6-3) can be used effectively in very large practices and in practices with more than one owner. This kind of structure divides management responsi-

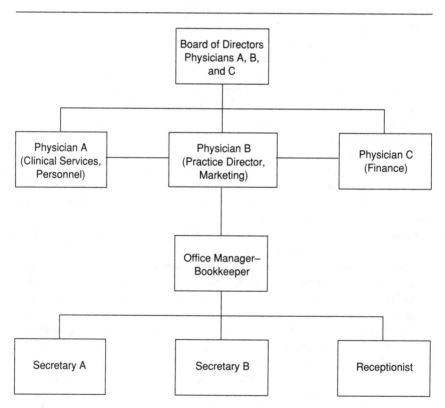

Figure 6-3 Functional Practice Structure

bilities along functional lines. In the structure outlined in Figure 6-3, the owners have divided the senior-level management responsibilities so that they do not become excessive for any one physician. Physician B has primary responsibility for the marketing of all of the practice's services and is the director for matters related to the type and quality of clinical services and for personnel matters. Physician C has the primary responsibility for the financial affairs of the practice. By dividing the management responsibilities in this manner, the partners achieve two objectives:

1. They reduce the amount of time that each partner devotes to practice management so that no one is unduly burdened.
2. Each partner develops a relative degree of expertise in one or two functional areas. As a result, the practice as a whole acquires more total management expertise. For example, Physician C, by specializing in the financial affairs of the practice, becomes very knowledgeable about and comfortable with that functional area.

The division of responsibilities could be based on personal interest, seniority, or any other reasonable basis. With this type of structure, it is important for the partners to integrate their actions. Each functional area must be coordinated with all the others. On occasion, the partners must meet together as a "board of directors." In these meetings they discuss and set policy and objectives for the practice as a whole and for the specific functional areas. In addition, each partner familiarizes the others with what is happening in his or her functional area of responsibility.

In a functional structure, the business manager will report to one of the partners (practice director) on a daily basis. Depending on what the partners prefer, this direct supervisory responsibility can be rotated on an annual basis or can be considered a permanent part of one partner's management responsibilities.

Irrespective of the type of practice structure you choose, it is important to make a conscious choice and to stick with it—unless, of course, the structure, as opposed to specific employees, is obviously causing a problem.

CHANGE

Change is as inevitable for organizations as it is for humans. Organizations, including medical practices, have to adapt to changes in their external and internal environments if they are to survive and prosper. The external causes of change include medical technology, peer competition, legal and insurance regulations, the local and national economies, standards of practice, advertising, and real estate and property rental prices. Internal sources of change include the growth and success you experience, the amount of revenues collected, the abilities of your employees and peers, and your preferences regarding type and amount of clinical work. Any of these forces can create circumstances that require a change in practice operations, policy, personnel, plans, and so on. Problems can arise when you, your employees, or your peers become resistant to necessary changes.

Why would anyone resist a change that is necessary for practice survival or growth? One reason why employees and partners resist change is that they anticipate losing something as a result of the change. This will occur whenever organizational and personal goals are divergent. For example, you decide that the office has grown to such an extent that it is necessary to move from a simple practice structure to an office manager structure. As a result of this, a secretary who previously reported directly to you and who was allowed considerable autonomy sees that she will (1) lose the status of reporting directly to you, and (2) be more closely supervised and have less discretion regarding the utilization of her time.

A second major reason that people resist change is fear. The current situation is a known commodity, whereas the state of affairs after a change will always be uncertain to some degree. For example, a psychiatrist decides to hire a clinical social worker to conduct group therapy and thereby offer her patients an alternative treatment modality. Clinically, this will provide a nice complement to the medical treatment and individual psychotherapy she provides. In addition, she can schedule the group meetings in the evening, thereby utilizing office space at a time when it has been unutilized. The psychiatrist's clinical psychologist, however, may be very fearful of the change. Does this mean that he won't get as many referrals? Does this mean that he will also be expected to work in the evenings? If the clinical social worker's groups do very well, does this mean that the clinical psychologist will be out of a job?

Finally, people also resist change to save face. They may view the change as a personal criticism of their job performance or a rejection of their opinions. For example, your partner recommended a year ago that the practice should construct a 3,000-square-foot addition. He was anticipating that both of you would be working to capacity and would want to bring in an associate. You opposed the idea because you didn't really think that the practice would do this well. But it has. Once again your partner proposes the construction of an addition. Once again you resist the change, arguing that you are not sure that you should enlarge at this time. However, are you arguing for this because you are convinced that it is the best strategy or because you are trying to avoid admitting you made the wrong decision last year?

Given that employees will resist change, why should you be concerned? After all, this is still *your* practice. If the fools stand in your way, you can always fire them! Unfortunately, the things employees do to thwart change can be subtle and devious. Although on occasion resistance will be expressed as open rebellion, usually it will be expressed in subtle, passive-aggressive ways. For example, the secretary in the first example might think this: "So he's going to give me a supervisor. Well, I wonder how much a supervisor will help when I leave my computer on during electrical storms. That will fix him!"

The clinical psychologist in the second example may have the following thoughts: "Going to replace me with a clinical social worker, huh? Going to force me to work at nights, huh? Well, I think that the next five hospitalizations that I make will have to go to St. Michael's Hospital for clinical reasons instead of the boss's floor at Lakeview. And I will probably never see a patient who is appropriate for our social worker's group, except for an occasional one with no insurance and no money!"

The physician with the expanding practice may think to himself, "Going to embarrass me by throwing that addition idea in my face again, are you? Well, I've got just the contractor for you. George Michael will talk your ear off. He'll chew up so much of your time that you'll wish that you never dreamed of that idea. To Bill, 'Hey Bill, if you want to pursue the addition idea, go ahead, but you have to take the lead. Call George Michael. He's an old patient of mine and a hell of a good contractor.' "

In all of these cases, the resistance to change would be costly, but it would be expressed in a subtle manner and so might not even be recognized as resistance. This being the case, what can you do to reduce or eliminate resistance to change? Over the years, a number of tactics have been devised to introduce change in ways that will overcome resistance. These strategies vary in terms of (1) how quickly they implement change, (2) the amount of planning required, (3) the amount that others are involved in the change process. Following are a number of change strategies proposed by Kotter, Schlesinger, and Sathe.[1]

Coercion

When you use coercion, you try to force employees to accept the change by informing them that if they don't like it they can quit, be fired, lose additional benefits or power, or be passed over for promotions or pay raises. The advantage of using coercion is that it is *fast*. If you must put a plan in place tomorrow, then coercion will allow you to overcome immediate resistance quickly. This is a risky way to introduce change, however, because people resent being coerced. The long-term consequences are less predictable than with some other change strategies.

Manipulation

Manipulation is a matter of attempting to influence behavior covertly. It often involves selectively revealing information. You tell others only enough to get what you want or get them to do what you want. Once again, the downside of this strategy is that it can eventually result in reprisals. You may find yourself justifying its use by the thought, "I have to get this change implemented now. I'll worry about the consequences later." If you don't have the power to coerce and you need to get something done quickly, manipulation can be a very effective strategy.

Co-optation

When you co-opt someone, you make the person part of the change process by giving him or her a desirable or visible role in the change process. The danger here is that the co-opted person may use his or her role to influence the change in a direction that you did not anticipate. On the other hand, co-optation can be a quick, effective way to overcome resistance. In the first example above, the secretary who contemplated flying a kite from her computer during a lightning storm might feel very differently if she was selected to be the new office manager. Assuming that the person is qualified for the position, co-optation can be a very effective way to overcome resistance to change.

Negotiation

Negotiation amounts to buying out the opposition. In effect, you give the resisters something they want in exchange for something you want. This of course implies that you have some bargaining chips. Negotiation can be very effective when it is obvious that the change is going to result in an employee clearly losing something of value. For example, the psychiatrist above now tells one of her secretaries that she will have to provide coverage until 7:30 PM Monday through Thursday. In exchange, however, she offers her a four-day workweek with a paid lunch hour. Keep in mind that negotiation sets a precedent that you will "pay" for change, and this may or may not be desirable.

Facilitation and Support

This approach to diffusing resistance to change involves providing training and support for employees so that they will be able to adjust to the new circumstances. For example, if you are intending to introduce new technology into your office or laboratory, you can reduce resistance to it by making it clear that you will be providing extensive and effective training as opposed to throwing your employees in a room with the training manuals and saying, "Okay, go to it!" This approach is obviously most appropriate when employees anticipate problems adjusting to the change. The disadvantage of this tactic is that it can take time and can be expensive.

Participation

In this approach, potential resistors are allowed to participate in the design and implementation of the change. The risks here can be large. Participation can lead to changes that you didn't anticipate or that don't meet your demands. Participation can lead to poor solutions and the participation process can absorb large amounts of time. Participation also has some potential advantages. If you don't have all of the information that you need to design the change, participation allows you to obtain additional information from others. It can also be valuable when implementing the change will depend on employees' good will.

Education and Communication

This tactic relies on familiarizing potential resistors with the reasons behind the change. This tactic is particularly effective when resistance is based on erroneous or insufficient information. Relying on education and communication to reduce resistance can take time. It also means that potential resistors must trust you. If they do not, they will simply dismiss the information as propaganda. The psychiatrist in the example above might well have reduced her clinical psychologist's resistance by explaining the reasons behind hiring a social worker and by discussing any possible changes in their working relationship. If the psychologist trusted the psychiatrist, then he probably would accept the explanation at face value and any resistance would be attenuated or eliminated.

The best reason to choose a particular change tactic is that it will most likely achieve *your* objectives. Don't decide, for example, to use the tactic of employee participation simply because it may be the nice thing to do. Similarly, don't decide to use coercion because "that is how doctors are supposed to run their practices." The object is to implement change successfully, not fit a socially appropriate stereotype. Here are some pointers offered by Jay Lorsch regarding choice of change strategies:[2]

1. The greater the anticipated resistance, the more consideration should be given to using slow change methods. Greater levels of resistance are more difficult to overwhelm. Lower levels of resistance can be blitzkrieged.
2. The greater your power, the better your relationship with your employees and peers and the more they accept the legitimacy of your acting unilater-

ally, the easier and more productive it is to use fast change methods. If your position is weak relative to the potential resistors, such as relative to your peers in an equal partnership, then you should use slower methods.

3. The more you will need others to help you to design or implement the change, the more you should rely on slow change methods. For example, if you know that you need new word processing equipment but don't really know what its characteristics should be, the secretaries will have to be consulted. There is great potential for resistance if you purchase the "wrong" equipment. Delegating the change process to your business manager and allowing the possibility of an arbitrary decision would probably be an undesirable strategy. You would do best to employ one or several slow change methods that directly include the users of the equipment.

4. The greater the immediate threat to organizational survival, the more you will have to rely on fast change methods. If the immediate stakes are not high or if the negative effects of postponing change will not occur for some time, then you may be able to afford to use slower methods.

John Kotter has summarized the advantages and disadvantages of the various change tactics. His summary is found in Table 6-1. The change tactics are arranged in descending order from the most time consuming to the least time consuming.

CONCLUSION

Training employees, structuring your practice, and planning for the implementation of change will help your practice to run more effectively. This chapter should have made you aware of the need to plan for how employees will be trained. You should also now be aware of the need to consciously determine the reporting relationships between employees so that their tasks make sense and their work is coordinated and integrated. Finally, you should now understand why employees and partners sometimes resist change and how to introduce change so that it is most likely to succeed.

Table 6-1 Six Strategies for Overcoming Resistance to Change

Tactic	Purpose	Advantages	Disadvantages
Education/ Communication	Resistance based on lack of information or inaccurate information and analysis.	Once persuaded, people will often help with the implementation of the change.	Can be very time consuming if large numbers of people are involved.
Participation	Situations in which initiators do not have all the information needed to design the change and where others have considerable power to resist.	People who participate will be committed to implementing change, and any relevant information they have will be integrated into the change plan.	Can be very time consuming. Participants could design an inappropriate change.
Facilitation and Support	Dealing with people who are resisting because of adjustment problems.	No other tactic works as well with adjustment problems.	Can be time consuming, expensive, and still fail.
Negotiation	Situations where someone or some group will clearly lose out in a change and where the losers will have considerable power to resist.	Sometimes is a relatively easy way to avoid major resistance.	Can be too expensive in many cases. Can alert others to negotiate for compliance.
Co-optation	Very specific situations where the other tactics are too expensive or are infeasible.	Can help generate support for implementing a change (but less than participation).	Can create problems if people recognize the co-optation.
Manipulation	Situations where other tactics will not work or are too expensive.	Can be a relatively quick and inexpensive solution to resistance problems.	Costs initiators some of their credibility. Can lead to future problems.
Coercion	When speed is essential and the change initiators possess considerable power.	Speed. Can overcome any kind of resistance.	Risky. Can leave people angry with the initiators.

Source: Reprinted from *Organization: Text, Cases, and Readings on the Management of Organizational Design and Change,* 2nd ed., by J.P. Kotter, L.A. Schlesinger, and V. Sathe, p. 359, with permission of Richard D. Irwin, Inc., © 1986.

NOTES

1. J.P. Kotter, L.A. Schlesinger, and V. Sathe, *Organization: Texts, Cases, and Readings on the Management of Organizational Design and Change*, 2nd ed. (Homewood, Ill.: Irwin, 1986), 349–62.

2. Jay Lorsch, "Managing Change," in *Organizational Behavior and Administration*, ed. Paul Lawrence, Louis Barney, and Jay Lorsch (Homewood, Ill.: Irwin, 1976), 676–78.

Chapter 7

Management Accounting

CHAPTER OBJECTIVES

This chapter provides information that you need in order to be an informed *consumer* and *user* of accounting information. This means that you will be able to use accounting information to make management decisions. When you have completed this chapter you will be able to

1. create financial controls to ensure the accuracy of your patient financial records
2. evaluate the effectiveness of your collection procedures and the performance of your collection personnel
3. devise cash controls that will deter, prevent, or identify the diversion of funds
4. implement cash accounting methods that will tell you the cash status of your practice, where you are spending money, and your ability to meet your cash obligations
5. assess the financial health of your practice and determine how well it is doing in comparison with past years
6. evaluate capital decisions, such as the decision to purchase additional equipment, enlarge your facility, and so on
7. determine whether you should lease or purchase equipment
8. use a budget to help you guide the financial future of your practice
9. evaluate the financial consequences for the practice when an associate physician wants a better contract
10. identify your most appropriate role in the management of your practice's finances as well as the most appropriate roles for your business manager, accountant, and so on

INTRODUCTION

In order to run a successful practice, you must develop ways of understanding and controlling its finances. By examining your practice's financial and accounting data, you will be able to make informed management decisions and respond quickly and appropriately to economic issues. The object of this chapter is to educate you in the use of financial and accounting concepts so that you can make informed decisions. The object is not to train you to perform rote accounting calculation tasks, which can be better and less expensively performed by your accountant or bookkeeper, or by accounting software.

The relationship that you should have with your accountant is analogous to that between an architect and an informed client with opinions regarding the qualities and characteristics of his home. By having a very clear, measurable and objective understanding of your specific needs, you will be able to most effectively work with the accountant, so that the accountant can best utilize his or her professional skills. By understanding financial and accounting concepts, you will be able to maximize the use of your accountant's professional skills.

Accounting data are to your practice what current and historical medical test results are to you when you are treating a patient. They indicate the current and past states of the practice and allow you to make reasonable and rational management decisions. The object of using management accounting information is to manage your practice proactively and make appropriate changes. It is not to amass numbers that describe a problem after it has occurred. By identifying symptoms and trends in the present—before they develop into a crisis—you can actively manage your future or at least prepare for it. You can also evaluate the effects of past actions. A well-conceived set of management and accounting reports will allow you to direct your practice so that you can

1. make decisions based on their future financial implications
2. obtain information about the effects of previous management decisions
3. manage your practice based on an understanding of its current financial status
4. establish financial controls, thereby deterring theft

In order to effectively utilize your limited management time, it is important to understand what your role should be. Let's start with the assumption that if you wanted to be an accountant, you would have studied accounting instead of medicine. Given that assumption, when should you use the services of an accountant and what tasks should you use an accountant for? Generally, it will be a misuse of your staff's time to perform specialized tasks that accountants develop proficiency in over a period of years. For example, use an accountant for tasks that require skilled or timely financial or accounting knowledge, such as the preparation of tax returns or the development of a pension or profit sharing plan. Also, use an accountant to get an expert's perspective. For example, if you are evaluating the financial health of your practice, you may want to have an accountant examine your financial data and provide you with an interpretation that takes into account other practices and organizations. Similarly, you may want to retain an accountant to create your financial procedures so that you produce accounting data in a form that is most useful for preparing your tax returns and generating financial reports.

There are many pieces of accounting information that you or your staff can collect and interpret in an efficient and cost-effective manner. It is important to remember that this is *your* practice and that you are the *only* person who will consistently look out for your own welfare. The data you should examine on a routine basis have the potential for revealing many positive and negative things about your practice. They can divulge that disaster is imminent or that you should plan now for the consequences of success. They can indicate that bringing on an associate is a reasonable gamble or that an employee may be stealing funds. As a consequence, relying on another party to examine the accounting data might be inefficient, ineffective, or even disastrous, since the other party's point of view or self-interest might not be consistent with your own. For example, a business manager with an incentive compensation contract might benefit if you bring in additional colleagues, and hence might interpret the financial data in a biased manner. Similarly, a business manager who is on a flat salary might have an interest in keeping the practice small in order to minimize work. Your bookkeeper might be diverting funds and would be only too pleased to tell you that the accounting reports indicate all is well. An accountant may simply be *uninterested* in why expenditures for supplies have been steadily growing over the last two years. He or she might assume that it is a result of practice growth, whereas you would be likely to wonder whether your staff has been wasteful. In summary, it is important to remember that others may waste your wealth if it in some measure will increase their own wealth. Although easily obtainable accounting information can allow you to identify the consequences if others are wasteful, you probably will have to examine and interpret this information personally in order to secure your own interests.

Your staff can routinely use accounting information to help them perform their jobs. This information relates to the daily operation of your practice, and it can be used to ensure that mistakes such as posting errors, wrong charges, missed procedures, and assignment to incorrect producers will be identified and corrected. In addition, accounting data can provide checks on employees' performance, so that they will be less likely to hide problems from you. Finally, accounting data can provide you with important employee performance indicators, which can be especially useful when you are conducting employee performance appraisals.

In order to produce accurately and easily the accounting data that will be discussed, it is essential that patient accounts be based in a computer. Computers and medical practice management software provide doctors with so many benefits that their utilization is justified in even the smallest private practice. The selection of specific medical office management software and appropriate computer hardware will affect your ability to manage your practice's financial affairs. This chapter describes the types of financial reports that your software and hardware should be able to produce. In addition, you may want to use accounting software to generate additional data and reports. These are also described in this chapter. The process of selecting medical office management and accounting software is discussed in Chapter 11.

MAINTAINING SHORT-TERM FINANCIAL CONTROL

Short-term financial control involves generating financial and production reports that tell you how well your practice is functioning. Although the reports you should examine can be produced without a computer, using a computer makes it feasible to produce them on a routine basis. One consideration in selecting medical practice management software is that it be capable of producing reports similar in nature to those discussed below.

The following sections describe a number of reports that will help you to maintain financial control. Many of the reports will be used on a daily basis by your staff. Nevertheless, you must be familiar with the significance and use of these reports so that you can be certain subordinates are using them properly and so that you can use them yourself to assist with management decisions.

Daily Receipts/Adjustments

This report (Table 7-1) provides you with the information necessary to determine whether the posting of payments to patient accounts is accurate. It should be run either at the very end of each day or at the beginning of each day on the transactions for the previous day. It provides you with the ability to audit, or verify, the accuracy of the following critical pieces of information:

1. the amount of each payment
2. the type of each payment (e.g., insurance payment, check, cash, credit card, etc.)
3. the totals for each type of payment

The contents of this report should be checked against the actual receipts for that day. Receipts must *exactly* match the totals reported in the daily receipts/adjustments report. If there is a discrepancy, it must be immediately resolved.

Table 7-1 Daily Receipts/Adjustments (7/13/88)

Number	Name	Transaction	Amount
21-G	Mills Joe	» Check Payment	500.00
21-G	Mills Joe	» Cash Payment	310.00
21-2	Mills Candace	06/10/87 Full-Thick Skin Graft to Lip/Mouth	
21-G	Mills Joe	» Card Payment	600.00
21-3	Mills Jeff	06/10/87 Closure of Nasal Sinus Fistula	
23-G	Hernandes Tim	» Positive Adjustment	150.00
23-G	Hernandes Tim	06/10/87 » Positive Adjustment	
23-G	Hernandes Tim	Uncollectible Write-off	191.80
23-2	Hernandes Christine	06/10/87 Corneal Transplant—Not Other Spec	
23-2	Hernandes Christine	06/10/87 Tatooing of Cornea	
10-G	Snyder David	» Card Payment	85.00
10-1	Snyder David	06/10/87 Cisternal Puncture	
10-1	Snyder David	Δ Aetna Life & Casualty	210.00
10-1	Snyder David	06/10/87 Other Diagnostic Procedures on Skull	
10-G	Snyder David	» Money Express	45.00
10-2	Snyder Shari	06/10/87 Other Cranial Puncture	
10-G	Snyder David	» Cash Payment	35.00
10-G	Snyder David	» Welfare Check	50.00
20-G	James Jim	» Check Payment	90.00
20-1	James Jim	06/10/87 Suture of Corneal Laceration	
20-G	James Jim	» Negative Adjustment	96.80
20-G	James Jim	» Welfare Check	126.55
20-1	James Jim	06/10/87 Thermokeratoplasty	
2-G	Prokesh David	» Cash Payment	55.00
2-3	Prokesh David Jr.	06/10/87 Myringotomy w/Insert of Tube	
2-G	Prokesh David	» Welfare Check	150.50
2-3	Prokesh David Jr.	06/10/87 Myringotomy w/Insert of Tube	
2-G	Prokesh David	» Negative Adjustment	90.00

Total Checks	590.00
Total Cash	400.00
Total Credit Cards	685.00
Total Insurance	210.00
Total Uncollectible Write-offs	191.80
Total Adjustments (+)	150.00
Total Adjustments (−)	186.80
Coupon	45.00
Welfare Checks	327.05
Two-Party Check	0.00
	0.00

Source: Reprinted from *MediMac Users Manual* courtesy of Healthcare Communications, Lincoln, NE.

This report is important for several reasons. First, if you ensure the accuracy of your accounts on a daily basis, any problems identified are more easily resolvable, since the problems must have occurred on the date of the report. If you wait a longer period of time, such as a week, between audits, you will have to examine five reports to find the problem, which is a more complex auditing task.

Second, using this report on a daily basis acts as a deterrent to some types of theft. If funds are being diverted by the employee who receives them, this will be detected when the funds posted do not balance against the funds on hand. In order for this control to be effective, both the posting of funds and the verification of the posting must be separated from the task of receiving funds. Running this report each day ensures that any employee whose theft could be detected by this report will only have access to funds for one day.

This report should be run daily.

Daily Activity by Producer

This report (Table 7-2) provides you with a summary of clinical work performed each day. If you have a solo practice, this report will ensure that all of your work has been entered into the patients' accounts. If your practice has more than one producer, this report also will ensure that the proper doctors have been credited for their work. This report should be run either at the end of each day or at the beginning of each day on the procedures for the previous day.

The report should indicate the name of the patient, the procedure that was performed, the producer who performed the procedure, and the fee that was charged. The contents of this report should be checked against the appointment book or some other independent record, such as the day sheet, to ensure that all services have been properly entered. If the day sheet, however, was used as the source to enter procedures into the computer, it would not be appropriate to use, since errors on the day sheet would be then be entered into the computer and produced on the report. Alternatively, the producers can be given copies of this report so that they can determine for themselves if their procedures have been correctly entered into the computer.

This report can also be used to deter theft. An employee might try to cover up the diversion of funds by simply not entering the funds or the procedures that generated them into the computer. Comparison of this report with the appointment book or some other independent record of procedures could defeat this strategy. In order for this control to be effective, the person reviewing the report would have to be someone other than the person who enters data into the computer. Once again, having producers review this report will serve as a deterrent.

This report should be run daily.

Table 7-2 Daily Activity by Producer (7/13/88)

Number	Patient Name	Diagnosis	Procedure	Prd	Fee	Bal
21-4	Mills Heather	995.5	21.22	D6A6	250.60	250.60
21-4	Mills Heather	682.2a	21.71	D4A4	382.98	633.58
21-3	Mills Jeff		22.71	D1A1	600.00	600.00
21-3	Mills Jeff		22.11	D1A1	274.60	874.60
21-2	Mills Candace	781.2	27.55	D3A3	306.32	306.32
23-2	Hernandes Christine	303.93	11.60	D2A2	91.80	91.80
23-2	Hernandes Christine		11.91	D2A2	100.00	191.80
10-1	Snyder David	793.2	01.01	D3A3	83.75	83.75
10-1	Snyder David		01.19	D3A3	210.00	293.75
10-1	Snyder David		01.24	D3A3	150.00	443.75
10-2	Snyder Shari	781.2	01.12	D2A2	284.75	284.75
10-2	Snyder Shari		01.09	D2A2	45.00	329.75
20-1	James Jim	303.9	11.51	D5A5	89.25	89.25
20-1	James Jim		11.74	D5A5	126.55	215.80
20-2	James Bonnie	704.00	02.02	D5A5	471.00	471.00
2-3	Prokesh David Jr.	272.2	20.01	D2A2	205.50	205.50
2-3	Prokesh David Jr.		20.22	D2A2	390.00	595.50

Total for Producer(s)	4062.10
D1A1 Joe Carter	874.60
D2A2 Mary Kramer	1117.05
D3A3 Stephen Webb	750.07
D4A4 Anne McConnell	382.98
D5A5 Joseph Harris	686.80
D6A6 Bob Lovette	250.60

Source: Reprinted from *MediMac Users Manual* courtesy of Healthcare Communications, Lincoln, NE.

Gross Receipts

This report (Table 7-3) gives you a summary of gross receipts for any given time period. Gross receipts are defined as revenue actually received by your practice. Understanding how much money your practice is actually collecting over any given time period is obviously important to evaluating its financial health. For example, Table 7-4 contains a practice's monthly gross receipts for the past 21 months. The data reveal that gross receipts are clearly seasonal: The summer has been a slow time for the past two years. The data also reveal that gross receipts are consistently down when compared with the same time period in the previous year. This finding should immediately generate an investigation. For example, is the decline due to fewer patients? Perhaps the ability to collect the revenue that was generated has declined. This would show up as an increase in receivables. Ex-

Table 7-3 Gross Receipts by Time Period (7/1/89 to 7/31/89)

Description	Amount Received
Checks	$21,239.37
Cash	$2,405.75
Credit Card	$978.80
Insurance	$32,547.13
Total Receipts	**$57,171.05**
Write-offs	$18,966.90
Positive Adjustments	$69.30
Negative Adjustments	$0.00

amination of a receivables report (to be discussed later) would support this hypothesis. Examination of the data in Table 7-4 should have precipitated an investigation into the declining gross receipts no later than the beginning of April, when the March figures would have become available. Sometimes it is easier to see an emerging trend when it is presented as a picture. Figure 7-1 presents the data from Table 7-4 in graph form.

The gross receipts report also can serve as a deterrent to theft. The gross receipts for a month should balance against bank deposits over the same time period. If the gross receipts report does not reconcile against the deposits to your bank account, as indicated on your monthly bank statement, then it is possible that the person responsible for managing your checking account or making deposits is diverting funds. In order to make this reconciliation easier, the posting of payments to pa-

Table 7-4 Comparison of Gross Receipts across 21 Months

Month	Gross 1988	Gross 1989
January	$15,172.38	$15,387.52
February	$14,271.56	$13,117.53
March	$16,865.42	$14,576.23
April	$15,982.75	$14,578.21
May	$13,554.61	$12,812.45
June	$10,568.43	$8,991.57
July	$9,852.53	$9,005.73
August	$11,552.35	$10,788.54
September	$11,985.54	$10,185.78
October	$14,889.35	
November	$16,557.97	
December	$16,855.18	
Total	**$168,108.07**	**$109,443.56**
Total thru Sep	**$119,805.57**	**$109,443.56**

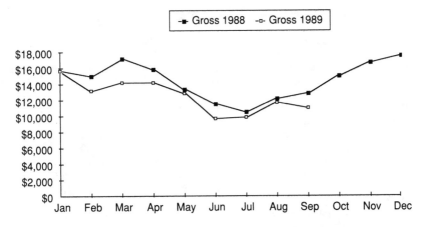

Figure 7-1 Graph of Gross Receipts Data

tient accounts should be coordinated with deposits into the bank account, so that all payments posted for a calendar month will appear on the bank statement for the same month.

This report should be run at the end of each month. If your practice has fairly consistent cash flow from one week to the next, you may want to run this report weekly or biweekly. In this way you will detect collection trends more quickly than with a monthly report. If your collections tend to vary significantly from week to week, then the monthly report would probably cover the shortest time period that would allow meaningful comparisons.

Detailed Production Report

This report (Table 7-5) gives you details and a summary of all of the procedures performed for a specific time period. The data contained in this report should include the type of procedure, the number of times each procedure was performed, and the fees generated by each procedure. The fees generated (revenues) are a very important indicator of the financial status of your practice, especially if you do a lot of work that is billed to insurance. The term *revenue* will be discussed in more detail in the section entitled "Accrual-based Accounting." At this point it is sufficient to understand that revenue is earned when you provide a service irrespective of whether the patient actually pays for the service at that time. The revenue figures tell you what you are putting into the "pipeline." Unless you put revenues into the pipeline, you cannot get payments out. This truism is important, because it will allow you to spot changes well before their cash impact. For example, if you are tracking revenues and you notice that they suddenly decline, you can be certain that cash will decline several weeks later. This lag can be predicted with some

Table 7-5 Detailed Production Report (7/1/88 to 7/13/88)

Procedure	Description	Cnt	% Cnt	Fees	% Fees	Lab	% Lab
01.01	Cisternal Puncture	4	15.38	336.79	8.64	5.00	1.97
01.02	Ventriculopuncture/ Implanted Catheter	1	3.85	83.21	2.13	30.00	11.85
01.09	Other Cranial Puncture	1	3.85	45.00	1.15	0.00	0.00
01.11	Diagn Procedures/Skull, Brain, Cerebrum	1	3.85	268.96	6.90	12.00	4.74
01.12	Other Biopsy of Cerebral Meninges	1	3.85	269.00	6.90	15.75	6.22
01.14	Other Biopsy of Brain	1	3.85	99.75	2.56	31.50	12.44
01.15	Biopsy of Skull	1	3.85	236.25	6.06	10.50	4.15
01.18	Other Diag Proc/Brain & Cerebral Meninges	2	7.69	350.00	8.97	26.00	10.27
01.19	Other Diagnostic Procedures on Skull	2	7.69	424.44	10.88	31.00	12.24
01.22	Removal/Intracranial Neurostimulator	2	7.69	585.00	15.00	40.00	15.79
01.23	Reopening of Craniotomy Site	2	7.69	199.75	5.12	10.50	4.15
01.24	Other Craniotomy	1	3.85	150.00	3.85	0.00	0.00
02.02	Elevation of Skull Fracture Fragment	1	3.85	450.00	11.54	21.00	8.29
02.92	Cisternal Repair	1	3.85	92.58	2.37	0.00	0.00
03.31	Spinal Tap	1	3.85	100.00	2.56	0.00	0.00
03.92	Injection of Other Agent into Spine	1	3.85	39.29	1.01	20.00	7.90
03.98	Removal of Spinal Thecal Shunt	1	3.85	78.00	2.00	0.00	0.00
04.03	Divis/Crush of Other Cranial Nerve	1	3.85	48.29	1.24	0.00	0.00
04.43	Release of Carpal Tunnel	1	3.85	43.93	1.13	0.00	0.00
Totals		**26**		**3900.24**		**253.25**	

D1A1 Joe Carter
D2A2 Mary Kramer
D3A3 Stephen Webb
D4A4 Anne McConnell
D5A5 Joseph Harris
D6A6 Bob Lovette

Source: Reprinted from *MediMac Users Manual* courtesy of Healthcare Communications, Lincoln, NE.

accuracy by knowing the normal delay in payment by your insurance companies. If you know now that revenues are down, then you can plan for the decline in cash by curtailing and delaying spending, arranging for credit, and so on.

A decline can arise from many different causes, and it should always generate an investigation. For example, revenues will decline if there has been a shift from higher paying procedures to lower paying ones. Similarly, a decline in the absolute level of work will also generate reduced revenues. One practice identified a software problem in its billing procedures by noting a decline in revenues. The billing program was not recognizing some procedures as billable, and as a result it did not send bills that would have generated an increase in revenues.

Lower revenues can also be a symptom of theft. If the person collecting fees is pocketing the money and not entering the sessions in your computer in order to cover the theft, then revenues will decline. Similarly, if an employee enters a session to generate an insurance check and then removes the session so that he or she can keep the check when it is received by your office, this will also result in a decline in revenues. If you have split the fee collection and posting duties, a decline in revenues may indicate collusion between the two employees.

Revenue data can be assembled into a separate database so that you can more easily detect changes in revenue trends. An example of a report produced from such a database is found in Table 7-6. It can be seen that this practice is undergoing very rapid growth, in terms of both revenues and procedures. The 90801 procedure is an initial evaluation. Since this code is only used for the patient's first visit, it is a precursor of growth in other procedures. In this case the practice's revenue growth is driven by an increase in demand for the 90844 procedure. The revenue growth could be predicted, however, by the 90801 growth.

This report should be run at the end of each month. In addition, any associated databases should be revised and examined each month. If your production is fairly consistent from week to week, you may want to run the report on a weekly or biweekly basis. If your activity tends to vary significantly from week to week, then the monthly report would probably cover the shortest period of time that

Table 7-6 Database Report Constructed from Detailed Production Report

Month	Revenue	Procedures				
		90801	90844	90815	90853	All Others
Jan	$60,584	18	608	8	47	12
Feb	$64,378	27	640	17	49	3
Mar	$70,720	35	701	11	55	7
Apr	$75,618	40	745	15	54	9
May	$79,450	35	779	25	55	12
Jun	$84,456	42	815	27	63	18
Jul	$86,076	45	830	25	63	20
Aug	$92,508	52	876	35	69	25

would allow meaningful comparisons. Since this report is a predictor of future collections, it is important to run it.

Aging Analysis

Effective utilization of an aging analysis report (Table 7-7) is critical to the financial success of your practice. This report tells you which patients owe you money and how long they have owed it to you. In addition, it indicates how your practice is doing as a whole in collecting on its accounts. There are many reasons why this type of report is crucial to managing your financial affairs. As accounts become older, the probability of collecting the money decreases. People move and change jobs and as a result become more difficult to trace. In addition, as the service that you provided to the patient recedes into the hazy past, they become more reluctant to pay. They forget the pain you relieved or the comfort you provided; they can only see their bank account declining. Finally, the dollar you collect today is worth more than the dollar you collect in the future, since you can invest the dollar you collect today and earn interest on it.

A good aging analysis report should have several characteristics. First, it should give you an aging breakdown by patient account so that you can see exactly which accounts are delinquent. Normally, this is done in time periods of 30 days. When accounts are in the first 29 days, they are considered to be current. When a charge goes unpaid for 30 days it will appear in the 30-day column, which means that it is between 30 and 60 days past current. The report should also tell you when the patient's last payment was made and the size of the payment. This will help you to identify those accounts that need immediate action. For example, in Table 7-7 the Lichte account has $500.00 over 150 days old and no payment has been made for almost seven months. This patient should be contacted immediately and arrangements should be made to settle the account. On the other hand, Beeris has recently made a large payment on his account. You certainly want to follow the Beeris account, but it has a lower priority than the Lichte account.

A good aging analysis report will allow you to select a minimum balance. For example, if you find that your report becomes cumbersome because it contains many insignificant balances, then you want to be able to run a report that only contains accounts larger than some arbitrary figure, such as $25. In addition, an aging analysis report that contains telephone numbers can save your collection person a lot of time.

The degree to which you take assignment of insurance will have an impact on your aging figures. For example, if you do a significant amount of Blue Cross work and it takes Blue Cross an average of six weeks to process a claim, then you should expect to see a significant part of your revenue sitting in both current and 30 days. In this situation, you want to be monitoring the proportion of revenue in each category. For example, if historically the 60-day receivables category has

Table 7-7 Aging Analysis

Acct	Name	Current	30 Days	60 Days	90 Days	120 Days	150+ Days	Total
1592-G	Ferguson, Ralph	$2,270.75	$308.00	$77.00	$0.00	$0.00	$0.00	$2,655.75
			Last Pmt.	$100.00	Date	12/4/90		
1624-G	Delock, Ike	$281.17	$890.00	$0.00	$0.00	$0.00	$0.00	$1,171.17
			Last Pmt.	$438.83	Date	9/24/90		
1287-G	Beeris, Ray	$199.00	$527.00	$0.00	$0.00	$0.00	$331.90	$1,057.90
			Last Pmt.	$350.50	Date	12/28/90		
1191-G	Marston, Del	$568.00	$235.00	$110.00	$16.25	$0.00	$0.00	$929.25
			Last Pmt.	$234.00	Date	11/12/90		
1896-G	Jones, Ed	$560.23	$221.20	$0.00	$0.00	$0.00	$0.00	$781.43
			Last Pmt.	$110.00	Date	11/18/90		
1480-G	Stanton, Anita	$0.00	$500.00	$0.00	$40.00	$77.00	$77.00	$694.00
			Last Pmt.	$57.60	Date	9/24/90		
1111-G	Smith, Elwood	$160.00	$240.00	$100.00	$0.00	$8.00	$54.50	$562.50
			Last Pmt.	$10.00	Date	9/18/90		
1474-G	Corry, Allison	$0.00	$0.00	$72.00	$144.00	$216.00	$72.00	$504.00
			Last Pmt.	$18.00	Date	7/9/90		
1323-G	Lichte, Lauren	$0.00	$0.00	$0.00	$0.00	$0.00	$500.00	$500.00
			Last Pmt.	$15.00	Date	5/1/90		
1570-G	Mercer, Robert	$144.00	$236.00	$72.00	$0.00	$0.00	$0.00	$452.00
			Last Pmt.	$236.00	Date	10/1/90		
1575-G	Schwill, Bruce	$72.00	$144.00	$216.00	$0.00	$0.00	$0.00	$432.00
			Last Pmt.	$18.00	Date	9/20/90		
1424-G	Brown, Bobby	$45.00	$0.00	$0.00	$45.00	$135.00	$35.00	$260.00
			Last Pmt.	$45.00	Date	10/3/90		
1435-G	Richards, Robert	$77.00	$0.00	$0.00	$0.00	$45.00	$136.40	$258.40
			Last Pmt.	$13.00	Date	9/17/90		
1406-G	McDougal, Gil	$32.50	$65.00	$65.00	$90.00	$0.00	$0.00	$252.50
			Last Pmt.	$45.00	Date	10/1/90		

continues

Table 7-7 continued

Acct	Name	Current	30 Days	60 Days	90 Days	120 Days	150+ Days	Total
1238-G	Sheldon, Rollie	$0.00	$0.00	$0.00	$0.00	$0.00	$192.75	$192.75
			Last Pmt.	$44.38	Date	4/30/90		
1278-G	Turner, Mark	$0.00	$0.00	$0.00	$0.00	$0.00	($74.30)	($74.30)
			Last Pmt.	$26.42	Date	4/30/90		
1188-G	Arrington, Arlo	$0.00	$0.00	$0.00	$0.00	$0.00	($86.60)	($86.60)
			Last Pmt.	$52.00	Date	7/18/90		
1010-G	McCord, Floyd	$0.00	$0.00	$0.00	$0.00	$0.00	($124.60)	($124.60)
			Last Pmt.	$19.20	Date	8/31/90		

Net Current	$4,409.65
Net 30 Days	$3,366.20
Net 60 Days	$712.00
Net 90 Days	$335.25
Net 120 Days	$481.00
Net 150 Days	$1,399.55
Net Accounts Receivable	$10,703.65
Total Credit Balance	($285.50)
Report Date	Jan. 13, 1991

Source: Reprinted from *MediMac Users Manual* courtesy of Healthcare Communications, Lincoln, NE.

contained 25 percent of your revenue and for each of the past two months that percentage has risen to 35 percent, you should start asking questions. This may be a sign that something is not working properly. It may be that your claim forms are not being generated or properly completed. Perhaps your front office staff has become lax in collecting copayments at the time of service. It may also mean that a major insurance carrier is having internal problems processing and paying its claims. In any event, a change in the normal pattern of receivables should generate immediate action.

A standard for the size of your receivables is that your total accounts receivable should not exceed two times the sum of the current and 30-day receivables balances. For example, if current contains $20,000 and 30 days contains $10,000, then the total accounts receivable across all aging categories should not exceed $60,000.

Rule-of-thumb standards, however, should be examined in the context of your particular practice. For example, if you are running an oncology practice with long billing-payment cycles, then this standard might be unrealistic. If the typical billing-payment cycle is 75 days, then you should be more concerned with watching the amount in the 90 days category and making certain that it does not begin to grow. A practice in which patients largely pay at the time of service, with insurance reimbursement going directly to the patient, might find "two times current plus thirty" to be a lax standard. In this practice, anything that isn't paid while it is in current is probably indicative of a collection problem, and a rise in 30-day receivables would be a sign that something is wrong.

Interpretation of exactly what an aging pattern means must be based on additional sources of information. There is nothing in the aging data alone to indicate whether any particular hypothesis is correct. If the practice is in fact growing, this should be reflected in other areas of the practice and subsequently in other reports. An examination of revenues and number of procedures and a close examination of high-paying procedures might clarify the situation. If one or more of these variables are growing, this could indicate that receivables are growing for a reason that need not be a source of worry.

Ultimately, the best way to assess your practice's performance in collecting receivables is to qualitatively examine your old accounts. If an examination of old accounts makes it apparent that there are many actions that could have been taken well before now, then you have reason to be critical of your collections effort. For example, if insurance was not billed or should have been rebilled, if secondary insurance was not filed, or if collection letters were not sent, then you have reason to be critical. If you examine an old account and you find that you provided many services after the patient or the insurance company was seriously delinquent, then you also have reason to be critical of your collection effort. If you find instead that the actions taken to collect were reasonable but took place too slowly, then you should examine two other possibilities:

1. You have a procedural problem. The person responsible for revenue collection needs to review accounts more frequently, generate collection letters sooner, cut off services quicker, take legal action more promptly, and so on.

2. You have a workload problem. Ask yourself whether it is reasonable for your collections person to manage this volume of accounts given your computer system, other job responsibilities, and so on. For example, does the employee take too many rest or smoke breaks? Do his or her working habits, time management skills, and ability to set priorities leave something to be desired? If you answer yes to both questions, then you should improve your supervision or consider making a personnel change. If you answer no, then you must increase your collections efforts. This may mean hiring more full-time or part-time personnel or acquiring additional or more efficient computer hardware or software.

A separate database should be constructed from the aging report totals, and periodic reports should be run from it. These reports will allow you to spot trends in the aging of various categories. An example of this type of report is found in Table 7-8. This particular practice did a considerable amount of insurance work. As a result, management felt that 90 days was a reasonable amount of time to collect on a procedure. Management created a "beyond tolerance" column ("120–180+ Days"). The data in Table 7-8 indicated that the practice was growing, as evidenced by the increase in the "Current" column. The growth in the "beyond tolerance" category precipitated an examination to determine whether this was due simply to practice growth. A qualitative examination of the business manager's actions indicated that her management of revenue collection had been haphazard. The database report provided the "red flag" to the practice's owners, indicating that something might be going wrong.

In summary, the aging analysis report is useful to you and to your collections personnel. Your collections personnel can use the report to direct their efforts toward the most rewarding accounts. You can use it to obtain a picture of your collections effort and to generate other reports to reveal trends that may be indicative of changes in collection effectiveness.

An aging analysis report should be run each week. Since this report is an obvious control for the collection function, it is important to run it often, even if you only personally examine it on a biweekly or monthly basis. If your practice is having a collection problem, then you should closely examine this report each week. In addition, any related databases, such as in Table 7-8, should also be updated at least monthly.

Uncollectible Write-offs

An uncollectible write-offs report (Table 7-9) will indicate the amount of bad debt written off in a given time period. Once again, the most important use of this

Table 7-8 Aging History Report

Date	Current	90 Days	120 Days	150 Days	180+ Days	120–180+ Days
8/19/88	$50,337.71	$10,848.94	$7,808.98	$7,367.05	$13,133.66	$28,309.69
9/1/88	$50,662.18	$12,553.90	$9,316.42	$5,821.28	$16,796.44	$27,691.60
9/8/88	$45,168.16	$11,917.86	$10,072.02	$6,188.59	$17,316.72	$33,577.33
9/16/88	$44,391.19	$11,100.43	$10,558.39	$6,448.95	$17,404.32	$34,411.66
9/23/88	$46,590.00	$11,261.68	$11,392.22	$7,220.92	$17,900.17	$36,513.31
10/1/88	$44,213.02	$12,888.17	$10,106.40	$8,144.31	$17,650.38	$35,901.09
10/8/88	$50,995.77	$13,960.67	$10,278.99	$8,887.63	$16,988.79	$36,155.41
10/20/88	$52,224.71	$15,564.54	$8,929.06	$8,673.35	$17,979.17	$35,581.58
10/31/88	$52,893.07	$13,872.83	$10,933.86	$7,764.96	$18,678.98	$37,377.80
11/11/88	$51,042.84	$11,861.86	$12,372.18	$8,545.72	$19,477.86	$40,395.76
11/16/88	$56,353.12	$11,233.73	$13,329.26	$7,880.51	$18,820.92	$40,030.69
11/23/88	$56,918.49	$10,269.26	$12,861.16	$5,818.36	$19,801.99	$38,481.51
11/30/88	$54,111.96	$10,368.25	$11,315.71	$7,339.91	$20,091.09	$38,746.71
12/7/88	$56,878.04	$9,530.61	$12,226.70	$7,419.02	$21,086.99	$40,732.71
12/21/88	$58,209.00	$9,699.90	$9,558.29	$9,991.87	$19,730.74	$39,280.90
12/28/88	$56,851.92	$10,561.54	$9,861.57	$9,251.78	$23,662.41	$42,775.76
1/11/89	$44,365.88	$15,368.72	$8,017.26	$8,312.27	$24,480.69	$40,810.22
1/25/89	$51,291.50	$17,920.38	$9,215.53	$7,672.12	$25,599.25	$42,486.90
2/2/89	$52,428.12	$19,180.18	$10,213.47	$7,690.16	$27,296.92	$45,200.55
2/22/89	$56,697.74	$15,610.55	$15,598.89	$7,075.35	$25,485.00	$48,159.24
3/8/89	$53,696.79	$16,538.98	$16,055.50	$9,189.50	$27,179.17	$52,424.17
5/11/89	$57,707.94	$11,786.93	$8,260.40	$10,561.27	$34,407.16	$53,228.83
5/24/89	$52,550.12	$12,584.63	$8,089.75	$9,761.48	$36,362.00	$54,213.23
6/20/89	$62,099.38	$13,994.78	$9,657.96	$6,154.00	$40,096.60	$55,908.56
7/6/89	$63,470.52	$14,751.89	$9,494.78	$7,456.28	$41,387.89	$58,338.95
7/10/89	$60,828.01	$16,570.60	$9,129.24	$8,190.20	$42,778.60	$60,098.04
7/19/89	$58,256.31	$14,958.84	$10,003.03	$7,688.08	$42,295.48	$59,986.59
8/11/89	$48,444.09	$11,753.63	$10,831.80	$5,795.95	$34,785.62	$51,413.37
8/29/89	$62,533.46	$14,226.72	$9,193.01	$6,449.50	$34,508.65	$50,151.16

report is examining patterns over time. If your write-offs are increasing, it could be a sign that you have truly incurred more bad debt. This could be due to a number of causes, including inadequate collection efforts on the part of your staff, a change in your clientele, or deteriorating economic conditions. On the other hand, an increase in write-offs could simply mean that you are doing more work. For example, you will certainly notice an increase in your write-offs if (1) you are a participating physician with an insurance company and you agree to accept their usual and customary rate (UCR) as payment in full for your service; (2) the insurance carrier's UCRs are less than your standard fees, and (3) you are treating more patients who insure with this carrier.

Once again, the numbers simply provide you with information that you must interpret. If the increase in write-offs is in fact due to a growth in rate-capped patients, then you need to evaluate the desirability of this situation. You must

Table 7-9 Uncollectible Write-offs (7/4/88 to 7/10/88)

Guarantor Name	Home Phone	Work Phone	Amount	Balance
Hansen Doug	(402) 464-8982	(402) 471-7725	20.50	100.50
Lichte Lauren	(976) 972-6475		29.00	533.73
Swanson Kris	(892) 849-5823	(325) 834-5834	2.34	69.02
Total for Producer(s)	**51.84**			
D1A1 Joe Carter				
D2A2 Mary Kramer				
D3A3 Stephen Webb				
D4A4 Anne McConnell				
D5A5 Joseph Harris				
D6A6 Bob Lovette				

Source: Reprinted from *MediMac Users Manual* courtesy of Healthcare Communications, Lincoln, NE.

decide whether changing to a nonparticipating status would allow you to generate more in revenue than you would lose due to patients who would not come to you as a result of a higher copayment.

This report should be run monthly.

Cash Receipts and Disbursements

Cash receipts are the monies your practice actually collects, and cash disbursements are the payments you make to others. Cash receipts and disbursements journals are records of original entries. The receipts and disbursements can be tabulated into a number of separate accounts. Exhibit 7-1 contains a chart of accounts for one private practice. Table 7-10 contains an example of a practice's monthly cash receipts journal. The document column is used to record the deposit slip number. The accounts column lists the accounts that have been debited and credited in the transaction. All accounts have two sides, which always must be in balance. The left side is referred to as the debit side and the right side as the credit side. Assets are increased by a debit and decreased by a credit, while liability accounts are increased by a credit and decreased by a debit. Therefore, when you add funds to checking (an asset account), these funds are listed as debits, and they show as a credit in the liability account that they are also posted to. For example, for deposit 2312, the checking account (1010 Cash in Checking) has been debited $2,339.57 because the receipts were added to it, and the income account (4100 MediMac Income) has been credited for the deposits made for collections on January 2 and 3 for $2,339.57. Table 7-11 contains a practice's cash disbursements journal. The documents column contains the check number, and the account col-

Exhibit 7-1 Chart of Accounts

Current Assets	6250 Bank Service Charges
1010 Cash in Checking	6275 Interest Expenses
1020 Cash in Savings	6300 Conference Expenses
1100 Accounts Receivable	6350 Conference Travel
1200 Prepaid Expenses	6360 Travel—Not Conference
	6370 Dues
Fixed Assets	6380 Licenses—Professional
1620 Furniture and Equipment	6390 Licenses—Business
1820 Accumulated Depreciation	6400 Entertainment
	6500 Food
Current Liabilities	6550 Food—Entertainment
2100 FICA Tax Payable—Employer	6600 Legal Expenses
2210 FICA Tax Payable—Employee	6650 Accounting Expenses
2220 Federal Withholding Taxes Payable	6670 Other Professional Expenses
2230 Virginia Withholding Taxes Payable	6680 Other Office Expenses
2240 Federal Unemployment Taxes	6700 Rent—Office Space
2250 Virginia Unemployment Taxes	6750 Rent—Equipment
2300 Employee Deductions	6800 Office Supplies
2400 Stockholder Loans Payable	6810 Medical Supplies
	6820 Lab Supplies
Owners' Equity	6850 Payroll Taxes—Employer Total
3000 Common Stock	6900 Postage
3020 Retained Earnings	7100 Health Insurance
	7150 Professional Liability Insurance
Income	7175 Insurance—Other
4000 Cash Payments	7200 Repairs
4100 MediMac Income	7300 Salaries—Professional Staff
4200 Interest Income	7400 Salaries—Front Office Staff
4300 Other Income	7500 Commissions—Contractors
	7600 Fees—Billing Staff
Operating Expenses	7650 Wages
6100 Advertising—Marketing	7700 Telephone—Regular Service (C&P)
6150 Advertising—Personnel	7750 Telephone—Long Distance Service (MCI)
6180 Advertising—Yellow Pages	7760 Telephone—Answering Service
6200 Credit Card Discounts	

umn indicates the accounts that were credited and debited as a result of each transaction. For example, check 1674 was written on or credited to account 1010 (Cash in Checking), and used to pay or debit the rent account 6700 (Rent–Office Space).

By classifying transactions in this manner it is possible to track where your receipts and disbursements come from and go to. The accounts which you choose to use are entirely up to you. In the extreme you only need two accounts—receipts and disbursements. The object, however, is to create a more precise set of receipt

Table 7-10 Cash Receipts Journal (1/1/91 to 1/31/91)

Document (Deposit Slip)		Acct				Debits	Credits
2312	1/4/91	1010	1/3			$2,339.57	
		4100	1/3				$2,324.25
		4100	1/2				$15.32
2313	1/6/91	1010	1/6			$2,354.67	
		4100	1/6				$2,354.67
2314	1/10/91	1010	1/10			$727.31	
		4100	1/7				$12.34
		4100	1/8				$458.65
		4100	1/10				$256.32
2315	1/15/91	1010	1/15			$2,161.73	
		4100	1/12				$654.57
		4100	1/13				$657.84
		4100	1/15				$849.32
2316	1/20/91	1010	1/20			$3,578.66	
		4100	1/18				$1,009.34
		4100	1/20				$2,569.32
2317	1/25/91	1010	1/25			$3,307.32	
		4100	1/20				$3,307.32
2318	1/30/91	1010	1/30			$482.40	
		4100	1/26				$298.35
		4100	1/27				$58.69
		4100	1/30				$125.36
				1010	Cash in Checking	$14,951.66	
				4100	MediMac Income		$14,951.66
					Total	**$14,951.66**	**$14,951.66**

and disbursement classifications for greater understanding and control of your practice's finances. Typical disbursement accounts for a medical practice include office expenses (rent, electricity, water, and so on), advertising, office supplies, medical supplies, interest payments, lab fees, legal and accounting fees, payroll, payroll taxes, corporate taxes, insurance, and so on. Receipt accounts might include patient receipts from the practice and/or a hospital, and medical test receipts. Work with your accountant to develop a system of accounts which will provide you with the most useful reports. In addition, the Medical Group Management Association[1] has developed a chart of accounts for medical practices, and most accounting software will come with suggested charts of accounts. Monthly cash receipt and disbursement journals can help you control the flow of cash through

Table 7-11 Cash Disbursements Journal (1/1/91 to 1/31/91)

Document (Check Number)	Date	Acct	Item Description	Debits	Credits
1674	1/3/91	1010	Blair Associates		$5,765.99
		6700	Rent	$5,765.99	
1675	1/3/91	1010	UPS		$8.99
		6800	Mailing	$8.99	
1676	1/10/91	1010	Frank Johnson		$1,619.33
		7500	Frank Johnson	$1,619.33	
1677	1/10/91	1010	Gray Medical Supplies		$879.56
		6810	Gray Medical Supplies	$879.56	
1678	1/12/91	1010	Postmaster		$75.00
		6800	Stamps	$75.00	
1679	1/12/91	1010	Microage		$43.96
		6800	Computer Supplies	$43.96	
1680	1/15/91	1010	VISA		$408.03
		6800	VISA	$25.96	
		6550	VISA	$125.75	
		6300	VISA	$200.00	
		6400	VISA	$56.32	
1681	1/17/91	1010	Price Club		$52.65
		6800	Price Club	$52.65	
1682	1/18/91	1010	C&P Telephone		$754.25
		7700	C&P Telephone	$387.36	
		6180	C&P Telephone	$366.89	
1683	1/18/91	1010	MCI		$29.65
		7750	Long Distance	$29.65	
1684	1/19/91	1010	Dictograph		$66.00
		6680	Security Monitoring	$66.00	
1685	1/19/91	1010	Rockies Water		$23.65
		6680	Water	$23.65	
1686	1/19/91	1010	Wooden Boat Magazine		$24.00
		6800	Subscription	$24.00	
1687	1/19/91	1010	The Copy Store		$232.95
		7200	Copier Repair	$232.95	
1688	1/20/91	1010	Media Paging		$59.64
		7760	Media Paging	$59.64	
1689	1/20/91	1010	Town Club		$276.32
		6680	Monthly Fee	$60.00	
		6500	Town Club	$216.32	

continues

Table 7-11 continued

Document (Check Number)	Date	Acct	Item Description	Debits	Credits
1690	1/20/91	1010	Virginia Pilot		$425.68
		6100	Display Ad	$425.68	
1691	1/20/91	1010	BCBS		$897.86
		7100	BCBS	$897.86	
1692	1/20/91	1010	Griffin Insurance		$237.89
		7175	Workers Compensation	$237.89	
1693	1/20/91	1010	Larry Eldridge		$489.56
		7600	Collections	$489.56	
		1010	Cash in Checking		$12,370.96
		6100	Advertising—Marketing	$425.68	
		6180	Advertising—Yellow Pages	$366.89	
		6300	Conference Expenses	$200.00	
		6400	Entertainment	$56.32	
		6500	Food	$216.32	
		6550	Food—Entertainment	$125.75	
		6680	Other Office Expenses	$149.65	
		6700	Rent—Office Space	$5,765.99	
		6800	Office Supplies	$230.56	
		6810	Medical Supplies	$879.56	
		7100	Health Insurance	$897.86	
		7175	Insurance—Other	$237.89	
		7200	Repairs	$232.95	
		7500	Commissions—Contractors	$1,619.33	
		7600	Fees—Billing Staff	$489.56	
		7700	Telephone—C&P	$387.36	
		7750	Telephone—MCI	$29.65	
		7760	Telephone—Answering Service	$59.64	
			Total	**$12,370.96**	**$12,370.96**

your practice by allowing you to examine in detail the sources of your receipts and disbursements.

Cash receipt and disbursement journals and reports can be constructed using accounting software. It also is possible to construct these journals and reports using spreadsheets, such as Lotus 1, 2, 3 and Excel. Spreadsheets are not recommended, however, because they lack the internal checks and controls that are built into good accounting software.

Journal-level data can then be assembled into reports, which can be helpful for tracking changes to accounts over time. Table 7-12 contains a cash receipt and disbursement report that has been assembled from journal-level data. Reports of this type can be used to assess receipt and disbursement trends over time and to

Table 7-12 Cash Receipts and Disbursements Report

	January	February	March	Year to Date
Cash Receipts				
Fees Collected	$60,046.06	$33,082.35	$68,746.74	$161,875.15
Interest Income	$61.49	$59.73	$48.56	$169.78
Total Income	$60,107.55	$33,142.08	$68,795.30	$162,044.93
Cash Disbursements				
Salaries—Management	$0.00	$6,812.22	$7,322.70	$14,134.92
Salaries—Administrative	$1,735.79	$4,016.14	$6,429.97	$12,181.90
Salaries—Physician	$7,536.15	$30,723.40	$22,976.23	$61,235.78
Temporary Help	$401.85	$619.20	$0.00	$1,021.05
Employee Benefits	$236.98	$445.70	$440.00	$1,122.68
Building Rent	$5,789.95	$7,021.41	$5,492.48	$18,303.84
Equipment Rental	$0.00	$836.74	$418.37	$1,255.11
Utilities	$447.95	$381.69	$626.91	$1,456.55
Maintenance and Repairs	$0.00	$46.25	$40.50	$86.75
Advertising	$0.00	$570.25	$407.34	$977.59
Office Overhead	$1,409.03	$656.80	$1,804.09	$3,869.92
Professional Services	$500.00	$700.00	$250.00	$1,450.00
Billing Service	$0.00	$0.00	$321.00	$321.00
Insurance	$1,060.01	$455.06	$877.99	$2,393.06
Interest	$0.00	$0.00	$0.79	$0.79
Credit Card Discounts	$30.50	$84.29	$53.53	$168.32
Bank Service Charges	$0.58	$0.39	$0.61	$1.58
Dues and Subscriptions	$97.47	$58.00	$51.47	$206.94
Auto and Travel	$0.00	$0.00	$178.00	$178.00
Meals and Entertainment	$626.49	$146.35	$318.99	$1,091.83
Taxes and Licenses	$739.03	$1,375.27	$1,969.83	$4,084.13
Fines and Penalties	$0.00	$0.00	$10.00	$10.00
Depreciation	$294.00	$294.00	$294.00	$882.00
Amortization	$5.00	$5.00	$5.00	$15.00
Total Disbursements	$20,910.78	$55,248.16	$50,289.80	$126,448.74
Net Income	$39,196.77	($22,106.08)	$18,505.50	$35,596.19

evaluate the financial health of the practice. Cash receipts and disbursements journals and reports tell you how well you are meeting your cash needs, and this determines whether you will be around long enough to collect your receivables.

Cash receipts and disbursements journals and reports should be prepared each month.

Accrual-Based Accounting

The cash-based accounting that has been described above is essential for operating your practice. It gives you the control necessary to collect the cash and pay the bills. You can operate a practice on the basis of cash-based accounting. Once you have established your cash-based accounting procedures, you can obtain a deeper insight into your practice's finances by utilizing additional accounting concepts. For example, suppose that you pay an annual liability insurance premium of $12,000 in April. If you record this transaction on a cash basis, then the effects could be somewhat misleading. If total disbursements for April were $50,000 and total monthly receipts were $45,000, then on a cash basis you would be showing a $5,000 loss for the month. The insurance payment is an *annual* premium, however, and so you are distorting the April results by allocating all of the insurance expense to that month. In order to gain a better understanding of how the practice really performed in April, you should make an adjustment for the fact that you really only used one-twelfth of the premium ($1,000) during April.

These adjustments are characteristic of *accrual-based accounting*. Accrual-based accounting allows you to construct a number of useful financial statements, such as balance sheets and income statements, that more accurately reflect the financial condition of your practice than cash-based accounting. When using accrual-based accounting, expenses are incurred in the time period when the items that generate them are *used* or *consumed* and revenues are recognized when they are *earned* as opposed to when the cash is actually collected.

In the example above, the cash receipt and disbursement analysis for April indicated that you would have a $5,000 loss for the month. An accrual analysis would reveal the following:

Revenue		
All Sources		$45,000
Expenses		
Noninsurance	$38,000	
Allocated Insurance	1,000	$39,000
Net Income		$6,000

In a similar way, the net income picture for May would be somewhat misleading unless you make an adjustment for one-twelfth of the annual insurance expense, since with cash-based accounting you would allocate none of the annual insurance premium to May.

Accrual-based accounting will allow you to make adjustments for four circumstances that otherwise would distort the financial picture of your practice:

1. *Revenue collected in advance but not yet earned (deferred revenue).* Mr. Johnson sees you on January 23 for a sinus infection. You treat him and tell him to return in two weeks. Mr. Johnson pays $25 for today's appointment and an additional $25 to cover the future visit. In this case, the cash that was collected for the future visit preceded the recognition of revenue, since you have not yet provided the service. Mr. Johnson's payment for the future

appointment would appear as a balance sheet liability, since it is a debt or obligation that you owe to Mr. Johnson. For example, it might appear under the category "Prepaid Patient Fees" (see Exhibit 7-2).

2. *Revenue earned but not yet collected (accrued revenue).* When you provide services today but patients pay at a future time, the monies are recorded *now* on your books as revenue. Revenue is recorded when you provide the service irrespective of whether the service is paid for immediately in cash or whether you extend credit in the form of a promise to pay or a bill to an insurance company. Some revenue will translate into future cash, some will not, such as revenue that will be written off as bad debt or insurance company contractual write-offs. Revenue that will be paid at a future time can be listed as an asset in the form of an "Accounts Receivable" item (see Exhibit 7-2). Notice that the balance sheet shown in Exhibit 7-2 makes a provision for bad debts and contractual write-offs.

3. *Expenses paid in advance but not yet incurred (deferred expenses).* Expenses that are paid in advance must be deferred to the future time periods to which they apply. These prepaid items appear as assets on a balance sheet. The "Prepaid Expense" item in Exhibit 7-2 could include annual insurance premiums, computer service contracts, and so on. Usually, you will have no choice regarding the prepayment of these items. The insurance company, for example, may want the whole annual premium now. From a cash receipt and disbursement perspective, this can create real cash flow problems. Examining this situation from an accrual perspective will not make the insurance company's "bite" any less painful, but it will put it into perspective so that you can see the real balance between your assets and your liabilities.

4. *Expenses incurred but not yet paid (accrued expenses).* Expenses in this category must be recorded in the time period in which they were incurred irrespective of when you actually pay them. For example, using the previous insurance example, suppose your insurance company bills you a year in *arrears.* Your cash analysis will show no insurance payments for 11 months and one $12,000 payment in the 12th month. Accrual-based accounting, however, would allocate $1,000 to each month, since you were actually "consuming" the insurance and incurring some debt monthly. Once again, cash-based accounting would be deceptive, and if you had not made a provision for the big insurance bill at the end of the year, you could have a cash flow problem. (It is likely that you have an intuitive understanding of the concept of accrual-based accounting. For example, if during the course of the year you say to yourself, "I've got a big insurance bill due at the end of the year and I should reserve some cash each month so that I will be able to pay it," you are making a provision for an expense incurred but not yet paid.)

Exhibit 7-2 Balance Sheet for Arnold Bennett, M.D., P.C., December 31, 1989

Assets			
Current Assets			
Cash	$40,589.00		
Accounts Receivable ($145,664 less allowance for participating write-offs and 10% allowance for bad debt)	$101,965.00		
Marketable Securities	$3,572.00		
Prepaid Expenses	$7,325.00		
Inventory of Medical and Office Supplies	$3,589.00		
		$157,040.00	
Property and Equipment			
Building and Leasehold Improvement	$109,237.00		
Land	$40,896.00		
Medical and Office Equipment, Office Furniture	$87,567.00		
Less Accumulated Depreciation and Amortization	($23,879.00)		
		$213,821.00	
Total Assets			$370,861.00
Liabilities			
Current Liabilities			
Accounts Payable	$14,897.00		
Refunds Due Patients	$879.00		
Commissions Due Providers for 12/89	$29,875.00		
Prepaid Patient Fees	$527.00		
Payroll Taxes Due	$5,010.00		
Commissions Due on Accounts Receivable	$61,179.00		
Salaries Due Employees	$13,582.00		
		$125,949.00	
Long-Term Debt			
Loan from Sovran for Capital Equipment	$40,500.00		
		$40,500.00	
Total Liabilities			$166,449.00
Owner's Equity			
Contributed Capital at Start-up	$20,000.00		
Retained Earnings	$184,412.00		
Total Owner's Equity			$204,412.00
Total Liabilities and Owner's Equity			$370,861.00

Balance Sheet and Income Statement

A balance sheet (Exhibit 7-2) and an income statement (Exhibit 7-3) are standard financial reports used to describe the condition of a practice at a given point in

Exhibit 7-3 Income Statement for Arnold Bennett, M.D., P.C., for the Year Ended 12/31/89

Revenues		
Clinical Services	$700,689.00	
Laboratory Services	$40,897.00	
Total Revenues		$741,586.00
Expenses		
Clerical Salaries	$62,984.00	
Prof. Compensation	$462,454.74	
Payroll Taxes	$22,740.00	
Rent	$50,000.00	
Advertising	$5,123.26	
Office Supplies	$42,895.00	
Medical Supplies	$22,330.00	
Interest	$4,860.00	
Local Taxes	$8,758.00	
Insurance	$18,957.00	
Education	$2,350.00	
Telephone	$3,645.00	
Depreciation	$11,207.00	
Total Expenses		$718,304.00
Pretax Income		$23,282.00
Income Tax Expense		$8,148.70
Net Income		$15,133.30

time and the performance of a practice over a period of time respectively. Both provide a standard, accepted way of presenting and summarizing important financial data that are informative in their own right but that can also be used as the basis for additional analyses. For example, it is possible to construct ratios between several of the financial variables found in the balance sheet and income statement. These ratios can be used to assess the financial progress of a practice over time.

A balance sheet (Exhibit 7-2) shows the financial condition of your practice on a given day. It summarizes your practice's assets, its liabilities, and your equity as an owner. The balance sheet is based on the following accounting model:

$$\text{Assets} = \text{Liabilities} + \text{Owner's Equity}$$

Your practice's assets are the resources owned by the practice, including cash in the checking account, office equipment, receivables, and so on. Your practice's liabilities are the debts or obligations owned by the practice, including loans, supplies purchased on credit, taxes owed but not yet paid, and so on. Owner's equity is the difference between assets and liabilities. Your owner's equity arises from two sources. One is the capital that was contributed to start the practice. The other is retained earnings, or the accumulated wealth that has been kept in the practice.

An income statement (Exhibit 7-3) reports performance for a stated time period, normally one year. An income statement is based on the following accounting model:

$$Income = Revenues - Expenses$$

Revenues reflect the acquisition of wealth, and they can be generated by clinical services, laboratory fees, or any other product or service that you provide. Expenses are all of the costs incurred by your practice in order to generate the revenues. These include clerical and professional salaries, rent, depreciation, taxes, and so on.

Preparing balance sheets and income statements involves a number of accounting decisions regarding adjustments to revenues, expenses, assets, and liabilities. These tasks can be complex, and a failure to properly take adjustments into consideration can result in misleading balance sheets and income statements. Often, substantial accounting experience is required. Two strategies are worth considering to obtain these skills: (1) have your accountant prepare your balance sheets and income statements, or (2) obtain the necessary accounting knowledge in the form of accounting software. When using accounting software, cash-based reports are virtually a no-cost byproduct of paying bills and collecting receipts. If the person using the software is capable of making accrual adjustments, or if the software is sophisticated enough to be programmed for accrual decisions, then useful accrual-based reports can be produced within the practice at virtually any time.

Ratio Analyses

Data from the balance sheet and the income statement can be used to assess a practice's liquidity, solvency, and profitability. Ratios can also be used to help you examine your practice's financial performance over time and observe developing financial trends.

Liquidity is the ability to use assets to meet currently maturing debts. Tests of liquidity evaluate the degree to which a practice's current liabilities can be met using its current assets. Current liabilities are defined as obligations or services that a practice owes or will have to fulfill within the next year. Examples include wages payable, income tax payable, and credit card balances. Current assets are resources owned by the practice that are currently in cash form or could be converted into cash within the next year. Examples include cash savings, shares in publicly traded common stock, and a reasonable (defined as likely to be collected) proportion of accounts receivable.

Liquidity Ratios

A commonly used test of liquidity is called the *current ratio*, which is defined as follows:

$$\text{Current Ratio} = \frac{\text{Current Assets}}{\text{Current Liabilities}}$$

Referring to the data in Exhibit 7-1, the current ratio for Dr. Bennett's practice is

$$\text{Current Ratio} = \frac{\$157,040}{\$125,949} = 1.25$$

This indicates that Dr. Bennett has $1.25 of current assets for each dollar of current liabilities. Stated another way, this indicates that Dr. Bennett has about a 25 percent "cushion" to deal with his liabilities. This cushion is helpful given that revenue may flow unevenly into his practice. If Dr. Bennett's current ratio was 1.50 at this time last year, then he should begin to investigate the change.

A more demanding test of a practice's liquidity is called the *quick ratio* or the *acid test ratio*:

$$\text{Quick Ratio} = \frac{\text{Quick Assets}}{\text{Current Liabilities}}$$

Quick assets are cash or other current assets that can be easily converted into cash, such as stocks, bonds, certificates of deposit, accounts receivable, and prepaid expenses. Dr. Arnold Bennett's quick ratio is as follows:

$$\text{Quick Ratio} = \frac{\$153,451.00}{\$125,949.00} = 1.22$$

All of Dr. Bennett's current assets except his inventory are considered to be quick assets, since they could be readily converted into cash. Dr. Bennett's quick ratio indicates that his practice has $1.22 worth of readily available assets for each dollar of current debt.

An additional perspective on liquidity is gained by considering how quickly a practice's receivables are turned into cash. An index of this can be calculated by examining the average daily billings and the average collection period, which are defined as follows:

$$\text{Average Daily Billings} = \frac{\text{Net Billings}}{365 \text{ Days}}$$

$$\text{Average Collection Period} = \frac{\text{Accounts Receivable}}{\text{Average Daily Billings}}$$

By using the data in Exhibit 7-2 and Exhibit 7-3, we can calculate these ratios for Dr. Bennett's practice:

$$\text{Average Daily Billings} = \frac{\$741,586}{365} = \$2,032$$

$$\text{Average Collection Period} = \frac{\$101,965}{\$2,032} = 50.18$$

This indicates that on average Dr. Bennett collects his receivables in 50.18 days, or 20.18 days past current. This figure can be used for two purposes. First, it can help in determining whether the collections performance is acceptable. What is required is a qualitative evaluation in which Dr. Bennett examines the 50.18-day average in the context of his revenue sources. If, for example, he does a large amount of insurance work, then an average collection period of 50.18 days might indicate a high level of efficiency. On the other hand, if a large proportion of Dr. Bennett's patients are supposed to pay at the time of service, then 50.18 days might indicate a collection problem, since his patients would clearly not be paying at the time of service. Under these circumstances, Dr. Bennett could improve the liquidity of his practice and his ability to deal with expected and unexpected expenses by changing his collections procedures.

A second use of the average collection period ratio is as a gauge of liquidity over time. By tracking this ratio over the years, Dr. Bennett will be able to assess how his practice's liquidity is changing and to examine whether changes in his clientele, the services he provides, insurance company policies and procedures, and so on, may be affecting its liquidity.

Solvency Ratios

A practice's solvency is its ability to meet its debt obligations. A common statistic used to assess solvency is the debt-to-equity ratio (DER). The data used to compute the debt-to-equity ratio are contained in the balance sheet (Exhibit 7-2). The ratio is computed as follows:

$$\text{DER} = \frac{\text{Total Liabilities}}{\text{Owner's Equity}}$$

Both the current and long-term practice liabilities are included in this ratio. Dr. Bennett's DER is as follows:

$$\text{DER} = \frac{\$166,449}{\$204,412} = .81$$

This means that for every dollar of equity owned by Dr. Bennett, there are 81 cents worth of liabilities. The use of debt involves risk, since interest may have to be paid on some of it and eventually the principal must be repaid. Typically, young medical practices have high debt-to-equity ratios, since large capital expenditures are required for equipment and income levels are relatively low at the start-up.

Profitability Ratios

Return on owner's investment (ROI_o) is a measure of a practice's profitability. It indicates how well the owner's equity is being used to generate income. Stated another way, the equity that you have in your practice could be "cashed in" and invested in other ways, such as in treasury bills or the stock market. Given that this money is invested in your practice, what return are you receiving on this investment? In a sense, evaluating your practice's profitability requires you to take off your physician's hat and look at your practice as a stockholder. Are your investment funds being well used? ROI_o is calculated using the following formula:

$$ROI_o = \frac{\text{Pretax Income}}{\text{Owner's Equity}}$$

Dr. Bennett's ROI_o is as follows:

$$ROI_o = \frac{\$23,282}{\$204,412} = .11$$

It is important to remember when examining Dr. Bennett's ROI_o that his salary and his net income are inversely related. If Dr. Bennett increases his salary, then the net income of his practice will decline. In order to evaluate the profitability of your practice as a *business*, you must assign, therefore, a fair market rate to your own professional and administrative services. Looking at it another way, Dr. Bennett wears two hats: On the one hand, he is an employee-physician-administrator; on the other hand, he is a stockholder-investor. In order for him to evaluate his success as a stockholder-investor, he must compensate himself fairly as an employee, just as he would compensate any other person who would perform the same administrative and medical duties with the same level of competence. In summary, Dr. Bennett's ROI_o of 11 percent is meaningful only to the extent that his compensation as an employee-physician-administrator is equitable. (A tax reality is that many physicians will pay their practice's profit to themselves before the end of a tax year to avoid double taxation. To the extent that this occurs, the ROI_o can still be meaningful if the calculations are made taking this tax adjustment into account.)

Another way of assessing profitability is to examine the relationship between total assets and the income used to generate them. This ratio is called *return on total investment* (ROI_t). ROI_t is defined as follows:

$$\text{ROI}_t = \frac{\text{Pretax Income} + \text{Interest Expense}}{\text{Total Assets}}$$

Dr. Bennett's ROI$_t$ is as follows:

$$\text{ROI}_t = \frac{\$23,282 + \$4,860}{\$370,861} = .08$$

Stated another way, Dr. Bennett's practice earned 8 percent on the total resources that it used during the year. Conceptualized in this manner, investment is defined as the total resources provided by both the owners and the practice's creditors (e.g., the bank that lent Dr. Bennett money). The denominator, therefore, contains both the pretax net income and the interest expense incurred by Dr. Bennett.

A third gauge of profitability is the profit margin. The profit margin is defined as follows:

$$\text{Profit Margin} = \frac{\text{Income}}{\text{Total Revenues}}$$

Dr. Bennett's profit margin is as follows:

$$\text{Profit Margin} = \frac{\$23,282}{\$741,586} = .03$$

This says, in effect, that for each dollar of service provided by Dr. Bennett's practice, the practice makes an average of three cents profit. It is important to remember when evaluating the profit margin that this statistic does not take into account the amount of resources invested to generate this profit. Obviously, a practice that has a 3 percent profit margin but has required only a $10,000 investment is performing better than a practice that has the same profit margin but has required a $50,000 investment. The profit margin is a part of the profitability picture, but since it omits the very important investment component, it should be considered in conjunction with ROI statistics.

After examining the above ratios, you may well be wondering how to use them. Ratios are useful as screening devices to highlight possible practice problems and strengths. They are particularly useful for making comparisons over time. If you notice, for example, that your profit margin has declined from the previous year, this should stimulate you to investigate why this happened. Have expenses risen without your making an appropriate adjustment to fees? Are you conducting a greater proportion of lower profit procedures? If you find that your quick ratio is more favorable this year than it was last year, then you might give yourself a pat on the back. On the other hand, you might conclude that you could be investing your funds in other more profitable ways, which might make the funds less liquid and could reduce your quick ratio. Perhaps your quick ratio is in fact too high.

Ratios, therefore, are useful tools for stimulating thought about your practice. They do not provide answers by themselves. Instead they allow you to focus and direct your inquiries.

If you decide to proceed with accrual-based accounting, then a balance sheet and income statement, along with associated ratios, should be compiled at least annually.

Summary: Accrual-Based Accounting

Balance sheets, income statements, and associated ratios can be very useful indicators of how your practice is performing relative to last year and how it is performing against a projected budget for this year. These reports and statistics are not as critical to the day-to-day running of your practice as the cash-based receipt and disbursement report and the other reports discussed above in the section "Maintaining Short-Term Financial Control." In a sense, accrual reports and the information they provide constitute the "next step up" in obtaining financial control. They are appropriate to consider after you have developed good cash-control procedures and cash-accounting reports.

BREAK-EVEN ANALYSIS

A break-even analysis (BEA) will tell you whether your practice is financially viable. It is particularly informative for practices that are young or undergoing substantial growth or decline. A break-even analysis also will assist you in making various management decisions, including decisions regarding the following:

1. *Expansion.* The analysis will indicate whether the combined revenue and expense effects of an expansion will result in additional profits.
2. *Capital Equipment Purchases and Automation.* You can use the analysis to evaluate the effects on profitability of purchasing new equipment or substituting computers, equipment, or software for personnel.
3. *New Services.* The analysis will help you examine how expenses and revenues associated with new services combine to have an effect on profit.

In a BEA you determine whether your net revenue can cover your *fixed costs.* (Some revenue will not be collected, e.g., insurance company write-offs and patients who do not pay. Net revenue is the revenue that is eventually collected.) *Fixed costs do not vary with the number of patients that you treat.* Fixed costs include your rent, the clerical payroll, clerical payroll taxes, liability insurance, and so on. Within a broad range of business activity, your fixed costs will remain the same irrespective of the number of patients that you treat. This range of business activity is called the *relevant range*. Obviously, there are limits to the relevant range. If your practice becomes considerably smaller, you may be able to reduce some fixed costs, such as by eliminating a clerical position. Similarly, if your practice grows considerably, your fixed costs may increase due to the related need for additional personnel and office space. Nevertheless, the relevant range is usually quite wide, and fixed costs, therefore, tend to rise or fall in discrete steps. Fixed costs are also a measure of your risk in doing business, since they must be paid whether or not you generate revenue.

In addition to fixed costs, your practice incurs *variable costs*. Variable costs are *proportional* to the level of business activity. They fluctuate with the number of patients treated or the amount of revenue generated by your practice. Variable costs include lab fees, clinical supplies, payments to associates on commission contracts, profit-sharing benefits, taxes based on gross receipts, and so on.

Mixed costs are costs that have both fixed and variable attributes. If you pay a fixed fee for your telephone answering service and an additional fee for each call handled, the basic fee is a fixed cost and the per-call fee is a variable cost. Mixed costs must be broken down into their fixed and variable components in order to consider them in a BEA.

Finally, the *contribution margin* is the amount remaining after you subtract your variable costs from your revenue. The contribution margin can then *contribute* to covering your fixed costs, and after your fixed costs have been covered, it can contribute to profits. For example:

Revenue	$250,000
Variable Costs	100,000
Contribution Margin	$150,000
Fixed Costs	140,000
Net Income	$10,000

Stated another way, if 40 cents of each dollar of revenue ($100,000 ÷ $250,000) must be consumed in order to generate that revenue, then your practice must be able to cover its fixed costs on the remaining 60 cents of each dollar. If it cannot, then your contribution margin cannot support your fixed costs. If the contribution margin matches your fixed costs, then you are at the break-even point, and if the contribution margin exceeds your fixed costs, you will make a profit.

In the following discussion of break-even analysis, three reasonable assumptions are made:

1. You can determine if a given cost is fixed or variable.
2. You will not change your fees based on the volume of business.
3. There is a consistent linear relationship between costs and some measure of your practice's activity, such as the number of patients treated or the amount of revenue.

Exhibit 7-4 contains a BEA for a medical practice, and it illustrates why this type of analysis can be important. In this example, a large proportion of the practice's expenses are variable, since its producers are paid a percentage of the fees collected from their patients. On average, the practice's variable costs are 61.34 percent of revenue. Therefore, the percentage of collected fees retained by the practice (38.66 percent) must cover the fixed costs if the practice is to break even and must exceed the fixed costs if the practice is to show a profit. In this example, the practice had revenue of $270,229.47, and after variable costs had been paid, the contribution margin was $104,470.71. Unfortunately, the practice had fixed costs of $115,283.91, so it showed a loss of $10,813.20 for the year, or $901.10 per month.

In a situation like this, a BEA can be more than an after-the-fact autopsy. It can be used to assist management in discovering a solution. The strategy for controlling fixed costs is different from that for controlling variable costs. Since fixed costs are constant throughout the relevant range, the key is to increase the efficiency of utilization. One strategy, assuming there is excess office space, would be to recruit more producers, since this would not increase fixed costs, and all of the contribution margin contributed by the new producers would offset fixed costs. If recruiting is not possible but there is extra office space, then the doctor should consider subleasing it. The doctor should also closely examine whether fixed costs are truly in the relevant range for the current volume of work. Would it be possible to eliminate a clerical or support position? Are clerical workers being overpaid? Could leased or rented equipment be returned? These are the sorts of questions that should be asked.

Variable costs, on the other hand, are controlled through conservation. For example, the practice may try to reduce its variable costs by using the copier less, cutting back on paid business lunches, using supplies more judiciously, substituting no-cost promotion methods for paid advertising, and controlling long distance telephone calls. Most likely, the eventual solution will involve a combination of measures that attack both fixed and variable costs.

Exhibit 7-4 Break-Even Analysis

Gross Revenue	$270,229.47	
Variable Costs	$165,758.76	
Contribution Margin		$104,470.71
Fixed Costs	$115,283.91	
Net Income		($10,813.20)
Monthly Net Income (Net Income ÷ 12)		($901.10)

Obviously, you are not operating your practice with the objective of breaking even. You can also use a BEA to determine the volume of business necessary if you are to achieve a stated level of profit given your current fixed and variable cost conditions. For example, suppose that the owner of the practice in Exhibit 7-4 determines that she would like to have a practice annual net income of $20,000. Given the fixed and variable cost conditions, the contribution margin (38.66 percent) must exceed her fixed expenses ($115,283.91) by $20,000. This then becomes an algebra problem:

$$\frac{X}{.3866} = \$115,283.91 + \$20,000$$

$$x = \frac{(\$115,283.91 + \$20,000)}{.3866}$$

or

$$x = \$349,932.51$$

Table 7-13 shows what happens at various revenue levels for this same practice. The effect of the revenue level on the net income and contribution margin can be easily observed. The physician can then look at these figures and evaluate their desirability and feasibility. For example, is it a good assumption that fixed costs really would remain constant if revenue was increased to $400,000? Perhaps there would be adequate office space, but might the physician have to hire an additional clerical worker to handle the increased volume? If she discovers that in fact the $400,000 level would be out of the relevant range for current fixed costs, then she could estimate the new fixed costs, enter that figure into the BEA, and determine profitability given the new set of conditions. For example, the physician might conclude that she would have to hire one more employee at $13,200 (including FICA and benefits). Fixed costs would increase, therefore, to $128,483.91, result-

Table 7-13 Break-Even Analysis for Various Revenue Levels

Revenue	Fixed Costs	Variable Costs	Total Costs	Net Income	Contribution Margin
$260,000.00	$115,283.91	$159,484.00	$274,767.91	($14,767.91)	−5.68%
$270,229.47	$115,283.91	$165,758.76	$281,042.67	($10,813.20)	−4.00%
$280,000.00	$115,283.91	$171,752.00	$287,035.91	($7,035.91)	−2.51%
$300,000.00	$115,283.91	$184,020.00	$299,303.91	$696.09	0.23%
$320,000.00	$115,283.91	$196,288.00	$311,571.91	$8,428.09	2.63%
$340,000.00	$115,283.91	$208,556.00	$323,839.91	$16,160.09	4.75%
$360,000.00	$115,283.91	$220,824.00	$336,107.91	$23,892.09	6.64%
$380,000.00	$115,283.91	$233,092.00	$348,375.91	$31,624.09	8.32%
$400,000.00	$115,283.91	$245,360.00	$360,643.91	$39,356.09	9.84%

ing in total costs of $373,843.91. With a revenue level of $400,000.00, her net income would be $26,156.09 and the margin would be 6.5 percent.

Sometimes it is easier to grasp the relationship between variables by examining a graphic representation. Figure 7-2 displays the relationship between the fixed costs, variable costs, and the revenue and profit figures found in Table 7-13.

A BEA also can be used to examine the effect that an increase in fixed costs and revenues would have on profitability. For example, suppose you were considering enlarging your facility, hiring an additional secretary, and bringing on an associate. By adding the additional fixed costs to your current fixed costs, you would then be able to calculate how much revenue the new associate would have to produce in order to cover the additional costs. Correspondingly, you could evaluate your profitability by constructing a table with the new fixed costs and various practice income levels resulting from a range of revenue contributions made by the new associate.

Finally, a BEA can use any index of productivity in place of or in addition to income. For example, the practice in the example above could determine the relationship between the number of patients treated and revenue. This relationship could be estimated by dividing revenue by the number of patients treated over an extended period of time. This would indicate the average number of patient procedures needed to generate revenue. For example, if the $270,229.47 of revenue in Exhibit 7-4 was produced as a result of 4,620 procedures, this would equate to 385 procedures per month at an average fee of $58.49 per procedure. This procedure average of $58.49 can then be divided into each of the other revenue levels to generate the average number of sessions required to generate that level of revenue. These data are reported in Table 7-14. Once again, the physician can use these data to evaluate the feasibility of possible goals and make informed management deci-

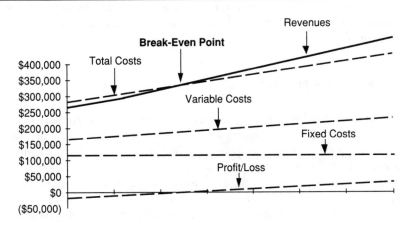

Figure 7-2 Break-Even Analysis Chart

Table 7-14 Break-Even Analysis Based on Average Number of Procedures

	Ave. Proc. per Month	Income	Fixed Costs	Variable Costs	Total Costs	Profit	Profit Margin
A	370.43	$260,000.00	$115,283.91	$159,484.00	$274,767.91	($14,767.91)	−5.68%
B	385.00	$270,229.47	$115,283.91	$165,758.76	$281,042.67	($10,813.20)	−4.00%
C	398.93	$280,000.00	$115,283.91	$171,752.00	$287,035.91	($7,035.91)	−2.51%
D	427.42	$300,000.00	$115,283.91	$184,020.00	$299,303.91	$696.09	0.23%
E	455.92	$320,000.00	$115,283.91	$196,288.00	$311,571.91	$8,428.09	2.63%
F	484.41	$340,000.00	$115,283.91	$208,556.00	$323,839.91	$16,160.09	4.75%
G	512.91	$360,000.00	$115,283.91	$220,824.00	$336,107.91	$23,892.09	6.64%
H	541.40	$380,000.00	$115,283.91	$233,092.00	$348,375.91	$31,624.09	8.32%
I	569.90	$400,000.00	$115,283.91	$245,360.00	$360,643.91	$39,356.09	9.84%

sions. Is it reasonable to expect a total of 570 procedures a month? If it is not, what are the additional fixed costs that would have to be incurred to support this volume of work? How would this then affect the profit picture? (This example assumes that the distribution of procedures offered by the practice, as well as collections and patients' ability and willingness to pay, would remain about the same. Since different procedures have different levels of profitability, this type of analysis can also be extended to look at the distribution and profitability of several procedures.)

If after conducting a BEA, the physician concluded that she did not want to do the volume of work necessary to generate the conditions in Row I of Table 7-14, then she could explore alternative ways of reaching a similar net income objective. This might include some combination of increased fees, reduced variable and fixed costs, and marketing aimed at generating higher fee patients.

If a practice encounters cash problems and it appears that examination of fixed costs or revenues may be appropriate, then conduct a BEA. In addition, a BEA can be run at any time as a planning tool, and one should always be run when you are considering practice expansion or contraction.

CAPITAL ASSET PLANNING

Capital asset planning is the process of evaluating the financial consequences of your investment decisions, including decisions whether to acquire new lab equipment, office space, furniture, computers, etc. Whenever you make an investment decision, you hope to see a return on your investment. The tools of capital asset planning will allow you to evaluate the potential financial consequences of alternative investment decisions. For example, suppose that you are considering the purchase of a new piece of lab equipment that costs $19,000. How do you know if this is a good investment? Should you lease the equipment instead?

In order to answer capital asset questions, it is important to appreciate the *time value of money*. A dollar you receive a year from now is worth less to you than a dollar in hand today, since the latter can earn interest for you. This concept is important to capital asset planning, because when you invest money in a piece of capital equipment, that money cannot be earning revenue for you through an alternative investment. You should evaluate the return, therefore, that you expect to receive from a capital investment, given the amount of time involved. To take this time component into account, you must consider the concepts of present value and future value.

Present value is the value today of an amount that will be received at some time in the future. Since you will be receiving the money in the future, you will not be able to generate revenue on it between now and then, so the present value of the sum will be less than the value of the same sum received today. The present value of an amount received in the future is a function of

1. the interest rate you could earn if you could invest the money
2. the length of time between now and the receipt of the money

Table 7-15 allows you to calculate the present value of an amount. A handheld calculator or computer spreadsheet program can be used to do the calculations that follow. The tables are presented to help you understand how the financial numbers are derived. The columns in Table 7-15 are for various interest rates and the rows are for various time periods. The entries in the table tell you the present value of $1.00 given the time period and the interest rate. For example, you receive an offer today of $48,000 for the lot you own adjacent to your office. You believe that the property will be worth $50,000 if you hold it for another year. What should you do? If you could earn 10 percent annual interest over the next year, then the

Table 7-15 Present Value of $1.00

Time Period	6%	7%	8%	9%	10%	11%	12%
1	0.9434	0.9346	0.9259	0.9174	0.9091	0.9009	0.8929
2	0.8900	0.8734	0.8573	0.8417	0.8264	0.8116	0.7972
3	0.8638	0.8163	0.7938	0.7722	0.7513	0.7312	0.7118
4	0.7921	0.7629	0.7350	0.7084	0.6830	0.6587	0.6355
5	0.7473	0.7130	0.6806	0.6499	0.6209	0.5935	0.5674
6	0.7050	0.6663	0.6302	0.5963	0.5645	0.5346	0.5066
7	0.6651	0.6227	0.5835	0.5470	0.5132	0.4817	0.4523
8	0.6274	0.5820	0.5403	0.5019	0.4665	0.4339	0.4039
9	0.5919	0.5439	0.5002	0.4604	0.4241	0.3909	0.3606
10	0.5584	0.5083	0.4632	0.4224	0.3855	0.3522	0.3220

present value of the $50,000 will be $45,455 ($50,000 × .9091). This indicates, therefore, that the value of the current $48,000 offer is worth more than the anticipated selling price in one year.

Future value is the value at some future time of an amount invested today. For example, suppose that you invested $10,000 today in a certificate of deposit that pays 10 percent annually for three years. The future value of the $10,000 is $13,310 (see Exhibit 7-5). A future value table, such as the one found in Table 7-16, can be used to make this calculation. Once again, the principal is multiplied by the factor found at the intersection of the appropriate interest rate column and time period row. The concept of future value is useful for evaluating the return from investing current funds in capital equipment.

The concept of annuity is also useful for evaluating capital investments. An annuity is a series of equal payments that are received periodically for a number of years. For example, if you received $1,000 cash each June 1 for three years and the interest rate is 10 percent, then the present value of the annuity is the present value of that stream of payments. Table 7-17 is a present value annuity table; it is used in a similar manner to the present and future value tables. The columns are for various interest rates and the rows are for the number of payments. In the example just stated, each dollar invested has a present value of $2.4869, so the $1,000 revenue stream for three years has a present value of $2,486.90. Stated another way, $2,486.90 invested today at 10 percent is equivalent to three annual payments of $1,000.

The concept of annuity is closely related to the concept of present value. In fact, you will notice that the entries for a single time period or payment (the top row) are the same in both the present value and annuity tables (Tables 7-15 and 7-17). In effect, the present value of an amount is equivalent to a one-period annuity. In addition, the annuity table entry for any given interest rate and number of payments is equal to the sum of the entries for an equivalent number of time periods in

Exhibit 7-5 Future Value Calculation

First Year Beginning Value	$10,000	
Annual Interest @ 10%	$1,000	
Total after 1 Year		$11,000
Second Year Beginning Value	$11,000	
Annual Interest @ 10%	$1,100	
Total after 2 Years		$12,100
Third Year Beginning Value	$12,100	
Annual Interest @ 10%	$1,210	
Total after 3 Years		$13,310

Table 7-16 Future Value of $1.00

Time Period	6%	7%	8%	9%	10%	11%	12%
1	1.0600	1.0700	1.0800	1.0900	1.1000	1.1100	1.1200
2	1.1236	1.1449	1.1664	1.1881	1.2100	1.2321	1.2544
3	1.1910	1.2250	1.2597	1.2950	1.3310	1.3676	1.4049
4	1.2625	1.3108	1.3605	1.4116	1.4641	1.5181	1.5735
5	1.3382	1.4026	1.4693	1.5386	1.6105	1.6851	1.7623
6	1.4185	1.5007	1.5969	1.6771	1.7716	1.8704	1.9738
7	1.5036	1.6058	1.7138	1.8280	1.9487	2.0762	2.2107
8	1.5938	1.7182	1.8509	1.9926	2.1436	2.3045	2.4760
9	1.6895	1.8385	1.9990	2.1719	2.3579	2.5580	2.7731
10	1.7908	1.9672	2.1589	2.3674	2.5937	2.8394	3.1058

the present value table. For example, the sum of the entries in the present value table for four periods at 10 percent is 3.1698 (.9091 + .8264 + .7513 + .6830), which is the same as the entry for a four-period annuity at 10 percent. (The difference, 3.1698 versus 3.1699, is due to rounding error.) In other words, an annuity calculation is a shorthand way of doing a series of present value calculations.

Let's now use these concepts to evaluate an investment in a new x-ray machine. This machine will require an initial investment of $30,000. You estimate that its useful life is five years and that you may then be able to resell it for $4,000. In addition, you must keep $5,000 worth of parts available in order to keep the machine in operation. These parts, however, can be easily resold, so when you sell the machine, you can recover your parts inventory costs. Finally, you estimate that if you purchase the machine, you will be able to generate an additional $12,000 in revenue each year as a result of providing additional services. Is this a desirable investment from a financial perspective?

Table 7-17 Present Value Annuity of $1.00

Number of Payments	6%	7%	8%	9%	10%	11%	12%
1	0.9434	0.9346	0.9259	0.9170	0.9091	0.9009	0.8929
2	1.8334	1.8080	1.7833	1.7590	1.7355	1.7125	1.6901
3	2.6730	2.6243	2.5771	2.5310	2.4869	2.4437	2.4018
4	3.4651	3.3872	3.3121	3.2397	3.1699	3.1024	3.0373
5	4.2124	4.1002	3.9927	3.8897	3.7908	3.6959	3.6048
6	4.9173	4.7665	4.6229	4.4860	4.3553	4.2305	4.1114
7	5.5824	5.3893	5.2064	5.0330	4.8684	4.7122	4.5638
8	6.2098	5.9713	5.7466	5.5350	5.3349	5.1461	4.9676
9	6.8017	6.5152	6.2469	5.9950	5.7590	5.5370	5.3282
10	7.3601	7.0236	6.7101	6.4180	6.1446	5.8892	5.6502

One way to analyze this situation is with a cost-benefit analysis. Table 7-18 lists the various elements of this problem as costs or benefits. Some of the elements, such as the $12,000 of revenue that the machine will generate each year, are currently stated in future value terms. Other elements, however, such as the initial capital investment of $30,000, are currently stated in present value terms. A simple analysis indicates that the equipment will generate $64,000 of revenue ($12,000 × 5 years plus $4,000 for the resale) and $35,000 of costs, for a net income of $29,000. This analysis, however, is misleading, because it does not take into account the time value of the funds involved. In order to evaluate the investment, all of the elements should first be converted into present value terms. This also has been done in Table 7-18 in the "Present Value Equivalent" columns. (The problem also could be approached by converting all of the numbers into future value terms; however, it is generally easier to reframe all of your thinking into current dollars.)

Let's examine the benefits first. The $12,000 annual revenue for five years has been treated as an annuity at an interest rate of 10 percent. This is the equivalent of $45,489.60 in today's dollars. The resale price of $4,000 will not be realized for five years, so this number is currently being expressed as a future value. It is necessary, therefore, to convert this into today's dollars, which is accomplished by calculating the present value of $4,000. At 10 percent interest, each dollar is worth .6209 of today's dollars, which equates to $2,483.60. The present value of the total benefits is therefore $47,973.20.

Examining the costs, the capital investment of $30,000 is already expressed as a present value, since you are paying that today for the equipment. The $5,000 parts

Table 7-18 Cost-Benefit Analysis

	Amount	Present Value Equivalent
Benefits		
Revenue ($12,000 per year)	$60,000.00	$45,489.60
Resale Price	$4,000.00	$2,483.60
Total Benefits	$64,000.00	$47,973.20
Costs		
Capital Investment	$30,000.00	$30,000.00
Parts Inventory	$5,000.00	$3,104.50
Total Costs	$35,000.00	$33,104.50
Present Value of Total Benefits	$47,973.20	
Present Value of Total Costs	$33,104.50	
Net Present Value	$14,868.70	

inventory, which will be sold in five years when the equipment is sold, has been expressed as a future value and must therefore be converted into present value terms. The present value of $5,000 in five years with 10 percent available interest is $3,104.50. The present value of the total costs is therefore $33,104.50.

The net present value of this investment, $14,868.70, is defined as the present value of the total benefits ($47,973.20) minus the present value of the total costs ($33,104.50). Since the net present value is positive, this indicates that the investment will make money. The effective value of the investment, however, is quite different from the value as derived by the original analysis, which did not take into account the time value of the funds involved. Since the net present value of this investment is a positive number, purchasing the x-ray machine is worthy of consideration. It should be evaluated, however, against competing investment proposals. For example, if expanding your facilities by making a similar present value investment resulted in a net present value of $30,000, it would be a superior alternative financially.

Finally, you should remember that the financial considerations are only one aspect, although a very important one, of your total decision-making process. For example, you might select the x-ray equipment option over expansion for ethical and professional reasons, even though the financial return is projected to be lower. You might also reject the expansion alternative because you don't want to go through the dislocations associated with construction, even though it may provide a superior financial return. The advantage of making these decisions *after* you have performed the appropriate financial analyses is that you will know what your ethics or convenience is costing you.

Another capital asset decision that you will encounter is whether to lease or purchase equipment. For example, suppose that you could buy a computer for $10,000 or lease it with the following terms:

1. an initial payment of $1,000
2. three annual payments of $2,500 at the end of each year
3. an option to buy the computer at the end of the lease for $3,500

In addition, you feel that the value of the computer in three years will be $4,000. Under both arrangements you will have to maintain the computer. The prevailing interest rate is 10 percent.

The real cost of the lease can be determined by looking at the present value of the three annual payments, which can be treated as an annuity. The present value of a three-year annuity at 10 percent with annual payments of $2,500 is $6,217.25 ($2,500 × 2.4869). Assuming that you want to keep the computer at the end of the lease, the present value of the $3,500 payment is $2,629.55 ($3,500 × .7513). Adding the initial $1,000 payment, the total present value for the lease comes to $9,846.80 ($6,217.25 + $2,629.55 + $1,000). The purchase alternative costs you $10,000, so that leasing the computer is $154 less expensive.

If you do not buy the computer at the end of the lease, the present value of the lease would be as follows:

Deposit	$1,000.00
Present Value of Three $2,500 Payments	$6,217.25
Total Present Value of Lease	$7,217.25

The value of the purchase alternative would be as follows:

Capital Investment	$10,000.00
Present Value of $4,000 Resale Price	($3,005.20)
Total Present Value of Purchase	$6,994.80

If you do not intend to keep the computer, the purchase is less expensive by $222.45. (This analysis has excluded the risk of obsolescence. It is possible that in three years the computer will be worth less than $4,000. The analysis could be repeated for any level of anticipated equipment value, and the physician could then make a decision to lease or buy based on the subjective probability of various resale values.)

Although the discussion so far has focused on the capital asset implications of the time value of money, the relevant concepts can also be applied to other areas of practice management. Suppose, for example, that Mrs. Smith is billed $1,000 for services provided today. Her bill-paying habits leave something to be desired, and it takes you one year to collect your fee. If you could have invested this money at 10 percent, then the $1,000 that she pays you in one year has a present value of $909.10. If your practice has a number of Mrs. Smiths, then the delinquencies could amount to a substantial transfer of wealth from yourself to your patients. Remember, the interest *is* being paid, it is simply being earned by the Mrs. Smiths of the world instead of yourself.

What does this imply regarding your patient fee policies? It certainly suggests that anything you can do to collect your fees sooner while at the same time not losing patients would be worthwhile. For example, some doctors do not bill patients for their copayment until after their insurance company has paid for the procedure. A better policy financially would be to have the patient pay the estimated copayment at the time of treatment and to reconcile the account when the insurance company pays its share. (This method has the added advantage of reducing mailing costs. Only patients who received inaccurate copayment estimates will receive mailed statements [or a refund]. This can reduce expenses attributable to postage, computer time, clerical time, supplies, and so on.) Obviously, if you are a nonparticipating provider, you are still better off. In this case, the patient pays for the service at the time of treatment and either you or the patient bills the insurance company. The payment then goes directly to the patient.

A similar problem occurs with your insurance receivables. The longer that the insurance company holds your money, the more you are effectively discounting your fees. If the normal turnaround for the receipt of payment is 13 weeks and you do $200,000 worth of business with an insurance company over the course of a year, then the company is holding on average $50,000 worth of your claims at any given time. The present value of this money, assuming 10 percent interest, is $48,863.75, for a net discount of $1,136.25 for one year. (The present value of $50,000 at 10 percent for one year is $45,455.00. Since the insurance company is holding your money on average for one quarter of a year, the discount is $4,545.00 ÷ 4, or $1,136.25.)

It should also be apparent that if you do a significant amount of insurance work, it is important to bill insurance companies as often as possible. If you are computerized, you may be able to file insurance daily. In addition, many insurance carriers will accept electronic submission of claims directly from your computer. In many cases, electronic submission of claims will cut several weeks off of the payment time. This *may* be to your advantage. Look closely, however, at the total costs for electronic claims, including access fees, on-line charges, and the cost of any additional equipment. Be certain to include in your analysis the expenses eliminated by not having to produce paper claims, such as the cost of postage, claim forms, envelopes, and clerical time used to review the paper claims and stuff envelopes.

BUDGETING

A budget is simply a formal statement of your financial plans for a specific time period. It is a plan stating what financial events *should* happen. If you have an expectation of the way that things should be, then you can gauge whether you are behind, matching, or exceeding your expectations. When preparing a budget, it can be useful to examine previous practice expenses and to consult published expense data to determine whether your expenses are in line with those of other medical practices. Survey data showing expenses as a percentage of cash collections are presented in Table 7-19.[2]

Budgets are very effective for communicating how you want your practice to operate. For example, when you budget for increased marketing expenditures, this communicates very graphically that you are serious about upgrading your marketing effectiveness. Similarly, when you budget for lower travel and entertainment expenditures, this conveys a far more serious message than simply stating, "Look, we really have to get this travel and entertainment thing under control!" Finally, budgets can be useful for creating discipline. For example, by stating, "This is all that we should spend for travel and entertainment," you create a limit and thereby direct yourself and others to adjust your actions in order to meet the objective.

Table 7-19 Mean Nonphysician Expenses as a Percentage of Cash Collections for Selected Single Specialty Groups

Nonphysician Expenses Category	Single Specialty Group Type							
	Anesthesiology	Cardiology	Dermatology	Family Practice	Internal Medicine	Neurology	Obstetrics/Gynecology	Ophthalmology
Nonphysician Salaries Subtotal	16.96%	13.71%	18.13%	23.68%	18.65%	18.60%	15.57%	19.63%
Executive Staff	*	1.81%	*	3.09%	2.09%	*	2.34%	1.81%
Business Office	2.88%	2.45%	*	3.91%	2.76%	*	2.16%	2.07%
Data Processing	*	.59%	*	1.42%	1.54%	*	*	*
Other Administrative	*	.97%	*	3.06%	1.01%	*	1.63%	*
Registered Nurses	*	3.44%	*	4.53%	4.37%	*	3.21%	*
Licensed Practical Nurses, Aides	*	1.84%	*	4.43%	3.61%	*	2.41%	*
Medical Receptionists	*	1.67%	*	3.55%	2.15%	*	2.15%	2.02%
Medical Secretaries/Transcribers	*	1.55%	*	1.54%	2.10%	*	.75%	*
Medical Records	*	.65%	*	1.14%	1.06%	*	.79%	.62%
Nonphysician Providers	*	*	*	2.93%	*	*	1.86%	*
Laboratory	*	*	*	2.46%	2.19%	*	*	*
Radiology	*	.92%	*	1.45%	1.16%	*	*	*
Physical Therapy	*	*	*	*	*	*	*	*
Optical	*	*	*	*	*	*	*	*
Housekeeping/Maintenance/Security	*	*	*	.88%	.40%	*	*	*
Certified Reg. Nurse Anesthetists	12.55%	*	*	*	*	*	*	*
Other Support	*	1.50%	*	2.77%	1.12%	*	2.23%	3.17%
Nonphysician Employee Benefits Subtotal	4.46%	3.52%	4.48%	4.40%	4.63%	4.21%	4.05%	4.23%
Taxes—FICA, Payroll, etc.	1.20%	1.34%	*	2.48%	2.04%	*	1.28%	2.03%
Insurance—Health/Disability/Life/etc.	1.19%	1.29%	*	1.48%	1.43%	*	1.27%	1.41%
Retirement and/or Profit Sharing	2.79%	1.06%	*	1.00%	1.48%	*	1.37%	1.64%
Other Employee Benefits	.63%	.64%	*	.54%	.28%	*	.38%	.39%
Data Processing Expenses Subtotal	1.95%	1.11%	.67%	1.69%	1.31%	1.60%	.74%	.86%
Service Bureau Fees	*	*	*	1.44%	1.01%	*	*	*
Equipment Rental/Depreciation	*	.84%	*	.92%	.52%	*	.40%	.44%

Equipment and Software Maintenance	*	.31%	*	.53%	.45%	*	.37%	.43%
Data Processing Supplies	.14%	.18%	*	.49%	.38%	*	.14%	.19%
Other Data Processing Expenses	*	*	*	*	.39%	1.08%	*	*
Laboratory Expenses Subtotal	*	1.21%	*	3.77%	4.32%	*	3.14%	*
Fees for Outside Laboratory Services	*	.66%	*	1.91%	2.79%	*	2.25%	*
Equipment Rental/Depreciation	*	*	*	.62%	.80%	*	*	*
Equipment Maintenance	*	*	*	.12%	.17%	*	*	*
Laboratory Supplies	*	.39%	*	1.71%	1.79%	*	*	*
Other Laboratory Expenses	*	*	*	*	.31%	*	1.24%	*
Radiology Expenses Subtotal	*	2.26%	*	1.35%	1.35%	*	*	*
Fees for Outside Radiology Services	*	*	*	1.61%	1.00%	*	*	*
Equipment Rental/Depreciation	*	*	*	.44%	.45%	*	*	*
Equipment Maintenance	*	.11%	*	.14%	.18%	*	*	*
Radiology Supplies	*	.56%	*	.66%	.74%	*	*	*
Other Radiology Expenses	*	*	*	*	.31%	*	*	*
Physical Therapy Expenses Subtotal	*	*	*	*	*	*	*	*
Equipment Rental/Depreciation	*	*	*	*	*	*	*	*
Equipment Maintenance	*	*	*	*	*	*	*	*
Physical therapy supplies	*	*	*	*	*	*	*	*
Other physical therapy expenses	*	*	*	*	*	*	*	4.06%
Optical Expenses Subtotal	*	*	*	*	*	*	*	4.06%
Equipment Rental/Depreciation	*	*	*	*	*	*	*	*
Equipment Maintenance	*	*	*	*	*	*	*	*
Optical Supplies	*	*	*	*	*	*	*	2.17%
Other Optical Expenses	*	*	*	*	*	*	*	*
Med./Surgical Supply Expenses Subtotal	*	1.34%	3.60%	3.62%	2.50%	.69%	2.48%	4.21%
Drugs and Medications	*	.09%	*	1.78%	2.03%	*	1.09%	3.62%
General Medical Supplies/Instruments	*	.95%	*	1.92%	1.24%	*	1.94%	1.96%
Laundry and Linens	*	.11%	*	.13%	.18%	*	.19%	*
Building and Occupancy Expenses Subtotal	.56%	4.30%	8.20%	7.93%	7.15%	7.13%	5.78%	7.82%
Rental/Depreciation/Occupancy	.51%	4.03%	*	6.16%	6.59%	*	5.16%	9.09%
Utilities	*	.48%	*	.93%	.58%	*	.47%	.59%

continues

Table 7-19 continued

<table>
<tr><th rowspan="2">Nonphysician Expenses Category</th><th colspan="8">Single Specialty Group Type</th></tr>
<tr><th>Anesthe-siology</th><th>Cardiology</th><th>Derma-tology</th><th>Family Practice</th><th>Internal Medicine</th><th>Neurology</th><th>Obstetrics/ Gynecology</th><th>Ophthal-mology</th></tr>
<tr><td>Housekeeping and Maintenance Supplies</td><td>*</td><td>*</td><td>*</td><td>.46%</td><td>.25%</td><td>*</td><td>.29%</td><td>.45%</td></tr>
<tr><td>Contracted Janitorial Services</td><td>*</td><td>.21%</td><td>*</td><td>.72%</td><td>.58%</td><td>*</td><td>.34%</td><td>*</td></tr>
<tr><td>Furniture/Equipment Expenses Subtotal</td><td>.47%</td><td>3.16%</td><td>*</td><td>1.49%</td><td>1.70%</td><td>1.93%</td><td>1.75%</td><td>3.71%</td></tr>
<tr><td>Rental and Depreciation</td><td>*</td><td>2.28%</td><td>*</td><td>1.24%</td><td>1.38%</td><td>*</td><td>1.23%</td><td>4.00%</td></tr>
<tr><td>Other Furniture/Equipment Expenses</td><td>*</td><td>.68%</td><td>*</td><td>.41%</td><td>.53%</td><td>*</td><td>.72%</td><td>.75%</td></tr>
<tr><td>Office Supplies/Serv. Expenses Subtotal</td><td>.41%</td><td>1.65%</td><td>3.27%</td><td>2.22%</td><td>1.63%</td><td>2.25%</td><td>1.51%</td><td>1.63%</td></tr>
<tr><td>Telephone Expenses Subtotal</td><td>.16%</td><td>1.18%</td><td>.90%</td><td>1.15%</td><td>1.17%</td><td>1.42%</td><td>1.11%</td><td>.92%</td></tr>
<tr><td>Insurance Premiums Subtotal</td><td>5.60%</td><td>2.92%</td><td>1.90%</td><td>4.03%</td><td>2.10%</td><td>3.08%</td><td>6.61%</td><td>1.80%</td></tr>
<tr><td>Professional Liability</td><td>5.95%</td><td>2.35%</td><td>*</td><td>4.02%</td><td>1.88%</td><td>*</td><td>6.72%</td><td>1.99%</td></tr>
<tr><td>Other Insurance</td><td>.11%</td><td>.20%</td><td>*</td><td>.42%</td><td>.19%</td><td>*</td><td>.26%</td><td>.35%</td></tr>
<tr><td>Outside Professional Fees Subtotal</td><td>1.32%</td><td>1.59%</td><td>1.73%</td><td>2.19%</td><td>1.52%</td><td>1.76%</td><td>1.44%</td><td>2.01%</td></tr>
<tr><td>Medical (Nonphysician) Professionals</td><td>*</td><td>.71%</td><td>*</td><td>.24%</td><td>.42%</td><td>*</td><td>*</td><td>*</td></tr>
<tr><td>Legal and Accounting</td><td>.70%</td><td>.60%</td><td>*</td><td>.67%</td><td>.66%</td><td>*</td><td>.75%</td><td>1.03%</td></tr>
<tr><td>Management Consultants</td><td>*</td><td>.70%</td><td>*</td><td>1.36%</td><td>.73%</td><td>*</td><td>*</td><td>*</td></tr>
<tr><td>Other Nonphysician Consultants</td><td>*</td><td>.37%</td><td>*</td><td>.94%</td><td>.62%</td><td>*</td><td>.71%</td><td>.32%</td></tr>
<tr><td>Promotion/Marketing Expenses Subtotal</td><td>.27%</td><td>.63%</td><td>.82%</td><td>.58%</td><td>.36%</td><td>.42%</td><td>.57%</td><td>1.42%</td></tr>
<tr><td>Group Interest Expenses Subtotal</td><td>.22%</td><td>.48%</td><td>*</td><td>.80%</td><td>.75%</td><td>.60%</td><td>.35%</td><td>.90%</td></tr>
<tr><td>Other Nonphysician Expenses Subtotal</td><td>1.34%</td><td>3.76%</td><td>*</td><td>2.97%</td><td>2.75%</td><td>5.56%</td><td>2.67%</td><td>3.32%</td></tr>
<tr><td>Total Nonphysician Expenses</td><td>31.95%</td><td>38.38%</td><td>46.63%</td><td>59.48%</td><td>49.53%</td><td>50.41%</td><td>45.85%</td><td>55.41%</td></tr>
</table>

Notes: An asterisk indicates that data are suppressed when the number of responding groups is less than six. Data for university and government affiliated medical groups are excluded from all tables. This table includes data for single specialty groups.

Source: MGMA *Cost and Production Survey Report, 1989 Report Based on 1988 Data,* reproduced with permission from the Medical Group Management Association, 104 Iverness Terrace East, Englewood, CO 80112-5306.

Budgets are not essential to the operation of a medical practice. They are a step above the minimum financial methods—such as cash accounting procedures—that are necessary to operate your practice. The sophistication that budgets can add to the process of identifying financial problems early enough to take effective action must be balanced against the time that they take to construct and utilize. Budgeting is very consistent, however, with the notion that as a physician you are a consumer of accounting information, who uses it to plan and make management decisions. Budgets do not replace your day-to-day involvement in the operation of your practice. Instead, they are tools that force you to think ahead, anticipate future conditions, prepare for them, and take action if things are not going according to plan.

Budgets can be established for virtually any quantifiable aspect of your practice, including cash receipts and disbursements, procedures, revenues, and expenses. Some practices may find the budgeting process to be useful for tackling very specific financial problems. For example, if an evaluation of office supply expenses indicates substantial waste, then budgeting for office supplies and closely following up on variances would be an effective cost control procedure. Similarly, other expense or revenue items can be selectively targeted and brought into line through the budgeting process.

Budget information can also be assembled into pro forma or forecasted financial statements, such as balance sheets and income statements. As you will recall, ratio analyses draw information from balance sheets and income statements. As a result, it is possible to construct forecasted ratios once you have constructed the underlying pro forma financial statements.

Let's examine how a budget could be used to help manage a group practice. We have previously examined some of Dr. Arnold Bennett's finances, including his balance sheet (Exhibit 7-2) and income statement (Exhibit 7-3). Dr. Bennett has two colleagues. He is undertaking the budgeting process because he expects that his practice will be growing and he wants to plan for the growth so that it takes place in an orderly, efficient manner. As a result, he has decided to construct a budget for the next three months.

Since many costs vary with the activity level of a business, the budgeting process often begins with the development of an index of "sales." Dr. Bennett asked his two colleagues to estimate the number of procedures that they would conduct and their revenues for each of the next three months. The physicians' revenue forecasts are found in Table 7-20. Since laboratory revenues historically had been at about 6 percent of clinical service revenues, he budgeted this amount for each of the three months.

Next, Dr. Bennett projected the following expenses:

1. Rent, interest, and insurance expenses were fixed, so he simply carried over the monthly amounts from the previous year.

Table 7-20 Pro Forma Balance Sheets for Dr. Bennett's Practice

	January	February	March
Revenues			
Clinical Services			
Dr. Bennett	$25,000.00	$25,000.00	$25,000.00
Dr. Warren	$19,000.00	$20,000.00	$20,500.00
Dr. Stewart	$18,000.00	$19,000.00	$20,000.00
Total	**$62,000.00**	**$64,000.00**	**$65,500.00**
Laboratory Services	$3,720.00	$3,840.00	$3,930.00
Total	**$65,720.00**	**$67,840.00**	**$69,430.00**
Expenses			
Clerical Salaries	$5,249.00	$5,406.47	$5,406.47
Professional Compensation	$40,920.00	$42,240.00	$43,230.00
Payroll Taxes	$4,155.21	$4,288.18	$4,377.28
Rent	$4,166.67	$4,166.67	$4,166.67
Advertising	$426.94	$426.94	$426.94
Office Supplies	$3,500.00	$3,500.00	$3,500.00
Medical Supplies	$1,971.60	$2,035.20	$2,082.90
Interest	$405.00	$405.00	$405.00
Local Taxes and Licenses	$775.50	$800.51	$819.27
Insurance	$1,580.00	$1,580.00	$1,580.00
Education	$500.00	$0.00	$1,200.00
Telephone	$304.00	$304.00	$304.00
Depreciation	$934.00	$934.00	$934.00
Total	**$64,887.91**	**$66,086.97**	**$68,432.53**
Pretax Income	$832.09	$1,753.03	$997.47
Income Tax Provision	$291.23	$613.56	$349.11
Net Income	$540.86	$1,139.47	$648.85

2. No capital expenditures were expected for the first three months, so he had his accountant determine the depreciation that the practice would incur based on previously purchased equipment.

3. Clerical salaries would remain the same for the first month and would probably increase 3 percent for the second and third months as a result of an anticipated employee pay raise.

4. Professional compensation would remain proportionally the same, but due to the projected increase in revenues it would probably rise each month.

5. Payroll taxes would rise in proportion to rises in clerical and professional compensation.

6. Dr. Bennett reviewed the expenditures for office supplies for the previous year with the practice business manager. He concluded that supplies were not being wasted. He assumed that supplies would be used at the same rate as last year, so he budgeted for one-twelfth of the previous annual supply expenditure. If he thought that there had been waste, he could have used the budget to try to reduce the utilization of supplies by budgeting at a level below the previous year's expenditures.

7. Medical supply expenses have historically been at about 3 percent of revenues. Since medical supply utilization would be correlated with practice activity, Dr. Bennett budgeted 3 percent of revenues for medical supplies.

8. Local taxes paid to the city based on the practice's gross receipts would be a function of the tax rate multiplied by the projected revenue for each month.

9. Education expenses were calculated by estimating the amount Dr. Bennett and his colleagues were likely to spend at the conferences they were planning to attend during the three-month period.

10. Telephone expenses were fairly consistent across the previous year, and Dr. Bennett saw no reason for there to be a change. In addition, he reviewed the long-distance charges and determined that they were reasonable. As a result, he budgeted one-twelfth of last year's telephone bill for each month.

11. Advertising consisted of two display ads each month in the "Science and Medicine" section of the daily newspaper. Dr. Bennett planned to continue this practice for the next three months.

Table 7-21 is a performance report, a comparison of January revenues and expenses with the budgeted amounts. Favorable variances occur when actual costs are less than budgeted costs, whereas unfavorable variances occur when actual costs exceed budgeted costs.

The data indicate that the practice had less net income than had been planned for January. An examination of the reasons for this shortfall indicated several causes. First, revenues were below projected levels. The primary problem areas were Dr. Stewart's revenue and the laboratory services revenue. Although total expenses approximated expected levels, some expense items greatly exceeded budgeted levels and others were below budget. Advertising and education had unfavorable variances; however, they were compensated for by favorable variances in professional compensation, office supplies, and medical supplies.

Dr. Bennett could now use the performance report to examine the causes of this situation. For example, was Dr. Stewart's revenue down because he made an unrealistic revenue projection? Was the shortfall due to illness? Or did the expected patients simply not materialize? After talking with Dr. Stewart, Dr. Bennett determined that the variance was due to a faulty revenue estimate. Examination of the

Table 7-21 Budget for January

	Budgeted	Actual	Variance
Revenues			
Clinical Services			
Dr. Bennett	$25,000.00	$24,785.00	$215.00 U
Dr. Warren	$19,000.00	$19,987.00	($987.00) F
Dr. Stewart	$18,000.00	$16,895.00	$1,105.00 U
Total	$62,000.00	$61,667.00	$333.00 U
Laboratory Services	$3,720.00	$2,897.00	$823.00 U
Total	**$65,720.00**	**$64,564.00**	**$1,156.00 U**
Expenses			
Clerical Salaries	$5,249.00	$5,249.00	$0.00
Professional Compensation	$40,920.00	$40,700.22	$219.78 F
Payroll Taxes	$4,155.21	$4,135.43	$19.78 F
Rent	$4,166.67	$4,166.67	$0.00
Advertising	$426.94	$587.26	($160.32) U
Office Supplies	$3,500.00	$3,215.72	$284.28 F
Medical Supplies	$1,971.60	$1,498.32	$473.28 F
Interest	$405.00	$405.00	$0.00
Local Taxes and Licenses	$775.50	$761.86	$13.64 F
Insurance	$1,580.00	$1,580.00	$0.00
Education	$500.00	$895.43	($395.43) U
Telephone	$304.00	$257.00	$47.00 F
Depreciation	$934.00	$934.00	$0.00
Total	**$64,887.91**	**$64,385.90**	**$502.01 F**
Pretax Income	$832.09	$178.10	$653.99 U
Income Tax Provision	$291.23	$62.33	$228.90 F
Net Income	$540.86	$115.76	$425.09 U

unfavorable variances in advertising and education both revealed acceptable but costly explanations. The advertising variance resulted from a display ad in a local newspaper during a local "high blood pressure awareness week." Dr. Bennett felt, after a review, that advertising in this edition of the paper was well justified. The education variance was explained by Dr. Warren's exceeding his budgeted education amount. This was due to a faulty estimate by Dr. Warren, and Dr. Bennett concluded that Dr. Warren's actual expenditures were reasonable.

Dr. Bennett may encounter some difficulties, however, in evaluating some of the other variances. For example, office supplies and medical supplies both showed favorable variances. The practice's activity level, however, was below expectations, so it really wasn't clear whether the lower utilization of office and medical supplies was due to treating fewer patients or to more efficient operations. Similarly, laboratory service revenue was down. Was this simply a function of lower than expected clinical service revenue? Unfortunately, such questions cannot be easily answered with the type of budget used by Dr. Bennett. They can be addressed, however, with a *flexible budget.*

A flexible budget utilizes a budget formula to express the relationship between those variables that fluctuate with the business activity level and an index of the activity level, such as revenue or number of procedures. Based on the previous year's data, Dr. Bennett expected that the following budget items would vary with physician revenues:

1. Laboratory services, since these services directly support clinical services.
2. Professional compensation, since Dr. Bennett and his colleagues pay themselves a percentage of the revenues.
3. Payroll taxes, since these are a function of professional and clerical compensation.
4. Office and medical supplies, since their consumption should vary with the practice's activity level.
5. Local taxes and licenses, since these are a direct function of the amount of revenues.

Dr. Bennett determined the flexible budget amounts by examining the relationship between these variables and clinical revenue for the previous year. Each dollar of clinical services revenue resulted in the generation of $0.06 of laboratory services revenue, $0.66 of professional compensation expense, $0.09 of payroll tax expense, $0.06 of office supply expense, and $0.01 of local tax expense. (Payroll taxes included FICA, which accounted for 7.51 percent of the first $48,000 in wages for each employee, and state unemployment taxes, which raised the overall tax rate to 9 percent at the wage levels used in the example.) In addition, each dollar of laboratory services revenue was associated with three cents of medical supply expense. These relationships are indicated in the "Budget Formula" column in Table 7-22. Items that do not have an amount in this column do not vary with the level of practice activity. The budgeted amounts for these items are the same as in the static budget (Table 7-21). Flexible budgets, therefore, adjust to changes in revenues and variable costs while allowing fixed costs to remain static over the relevant range.

Differences between flexible budgets and static budgets are due to variance in activity level and are therefore an index of effectiveness. Differences between flexible budgets and actual results are due to (1) efficiency, if the amount of inputs used for a given level of output varies from expectations, and (2) price variance, if the cost or price of a unit of service differs from that expressed in the flexible budget formula.

Table 7-22 Flexible Budget for January

	Budget Formula	Flexible Budget	Actual	Variance	
Revenues					
Clinical Services					
Dr. Bennett		$24,785.00	$24,785.00		
Dr. Warren		$19,987.00	$19,987.00		
Dr. Stewart		$16,895.00	$16,895.00		
Total	**$1.00**	**$61,667.00**	**$61,667.00**		
Laboratory Services	$0.06	$3,700.02	$2,897.00	$803.02	U
Total		**$65,367.02**	**$64,564.00**		
Expenses					
Clerical Salaries	Fixed	$5,249.00	$5,249.00	$0.00	
Professional Compensation	$0.66	$40,700.22	$40,700.22	$0.00	
Payroll Taxes	$0.09	$4,135.43	$4,135.43	$0.00	
Rent	Fixed	$4,166.67	$4,166.67	$0.00	
Advertising	Fixed	$426.94	$587.26	($160.32)	U
Office Supplies	$0.06	$3,700.02	$3,215.72	$484.30	F
Medical Supplies	$0.03	$1,936.92	$1,498.32	$438.60	F
Interest	Fixed	$405.00	$405.00	$0.00	
Local Taxes and Licenses	$0.01	$761.86	$761.86	$0.00	
Insurance	Fixed	$1,580.00	$1,580.00	$0.00	
Education	Fixed	$500.00	$895.43	($395.43)	U
Telephone	Fixed	$304.00	$257.00	$47.00	F
Depreciation	Fixed	$934.00	$934.00	$0.00	
Total		**$64,800.06**	**$64,385.91**	**$414.15**	**F**
Pretax Income		$566.96	$178.09	$388.87	U
Income Tax Provision		$198.44	$62.33		
Net Income		$368.53	$115.76	$252.77	U

The relationship between effectiveness and efficiency is important to understand. For example, you may have an objective of generating $30,000 in revenues in a month. You only generate $25,000, but you do this with the inputs specified in the flexible budget. Your production has been ineffective but it has also been efficient. Alternatively, you could have a $30,000 month but have unfavorable variances on several flexible budget items, in which case you have been effective but inefficient.

Examination of the flexible budget in Table 7-22 shows that office supplies and medical supplies were used very efficiently, since both were below budgeted amounts for the revenue levels even after taking into consideration the lower level of clinical services. The flexible budget also shows lower than expected laboratory service revenues, once again after taking into account the lower level of clinical services.

After examining the flexible budget and the static budget, several conclusions can be reached:

1. The unfavorable net income variance of $425.09 found in the static budget (Table 7-21) can be reduced to $252.77 (Table 7-22) as a result of lower than expected revenues. Therefore, $172.32 of the unfavorable variance was due to lower than expected practice activity (effectiveness), while the remaining $252.77 unfavorable variance is due to some combination of practice inefficiency or price variance.

2. Office supplies, medical supplies, advertising, and education had variances that were large enough to have a real impact on profitability if they continue at these levels over the course of a year. Dr. Bennett should pay particular attention to these variables.

3. Dr. Bennett should take a close look at laboratory services and determine the causes of the large variance.

4. Dr. Bennett needs to reevaluate the issue of discipline. Advertising and education had unfavorable variances because someone *chose* to exceed the budget. These choices could have been good decisions or wasteful decisions. A budget should not be viewed as inviolate, since situations change and organizations must have enough flexibility to respond effectively. On the other hand, a lack of discipline will almost always be clad in the armour of necessity. The effective manager will be able to determine when a variance is truly in the practice's best interest and when it is simply the result of extravagance.

In summary, the budgeting process can be used to help evaluate whether a practice is proceeding according to plan. However, it comes at a price in both effort and time. Someone, such as Dr. Bennett or his business manager, must construct the budget and watch out for and investigate variances. Only Dr. Bennett can determine whether this was or will be worthwhile in his particular situation. Some might believe that the variances that Dr. Bennett discovered hardly justify the effort expended. Dr. Bennett, however, may feel that the budget process is worthwhile if it gives him (1) some assurance that things are generally going according to plan, and (2) the capability of identifying specific variances as they grow, thereby providing the opportunity to control them before they reach critical levels.

THE INTERNAL CONTROL OF CASH

The object of internal cash control procedures is to prevent or detect theft. Cash, which includes currency and checks, is the asset most susceptible to theft. We have already discussed this topic from the perspective of job design. In Chapter 6, it was suggested that doctors should design front office jobs so that various responsibilities for handling cash are divided among the available positions. We now approach the same topic from a cash control perspective. To some degree, the size of your front office staff and your own possible unwillingness to involve yourself in some of the cash management responsibilities may require that you compromise on some of the standards that will be proposed. At a minimum, however, you will understand where your cash control procedures are weak, and hopefully you will be especially vigilant in those areas. The proposed standards are offered, therefore, as objectives, and the impracticality of implementing some of them in your practice should not preclude you from implementing as many others as are feasible.

The basic principle in controlling cash is to separate various functions and responsibilities so that they are performed by different persons. In this way you prevent theft by employees who also have the ability to hide their actions. Procedures that facilitate the internal control of cash include the following.

1. Keep the physical handling of cash separate from all phases of the accounting and recordkeeping function. The reason is obvious. If a person handling the cash also controls the function that can disclose a diversion, then hiding a theft becomes easy. This means, for example, that if your receptionist is collecting cash at the window, then he or she should not be involved in balancing your checkbook against the bank statement. If your business manager manages your checking account and also posts insurance payments, then the posting should be done from the insurance company remits and the manager should not have access to unendorsed checks. Similarly, the person posting payments to accounts should not open the incoming mail and thereby have access to check payments.

The practical reality in a small medical practice is that some cash handling and accounting functions must overlap due to staff size. In this case, you might want to institute procedures that create additional "trails." For example, you might inform patients and post a sign to the effect that anyone who pays in currency *must* receive a written receipt from a receipt book that leaves a copy. Require that all checks that come into the office must be immediately stamped "For Deposit Only to Account # . . ."

2. Separate the posting of procedures and payments to accounts from management of the checkbook. Since checkbook receipts and the receipts as recorded in your patient accounts must balance, these functions must be separate if each is to serve as a control for the other.

3. Make deposits to your checking account on a daily basis. If cash is not physically present, then it cannot be stolen.

4. Make all cash payments with prenumbered checks from one checking account. Using several checkbooks to make disbursements makes it more difficult for you to determine quickly where your cash is at any given moment. In addition, if all disbursements are made by check, then your checking account contains a complete record and there is no opportunity for funds to be lost in "petty cash."

5. *Establish a petty cash fund and petty cash account.* Petty cash is the cash that you need to provide change for patients. Keep this petty cash fund as small as possible, locate it in a lockable cash box, and always fund the petty cash box by cashing a company check. Do not use the petty cash fund for small expenses, such as stamps or a business lunch. Once the notion of making unrecorded withdrawals from petty cash has been established, it will be impossible to reconcile this account. An unreconcilable account is an invitation to exploitation. In addition, include the petty cash fund as an account in your cash receipts and disbursements journals.

6. *Keep check-signing authority in the hands of a practice owner.* Never give employees signature power on your checking account. Trustworthiness and loyalty are difficult to assess and liable to change. If an employee forges your signature, then you have possible recourse with the bank, since the bank is responsible for recognizing authorized signatures. If the employee has check-signing authority, then the question of whether an employee issued a check for an appropriate reason can be problematic (e.g., "I bought copier paper last February as a convenience to you, and you never did pay me back"). In any event, the bank is off the hook, and all your recovery options will probably be lengthy.

Larger practices may find the suggested restriction to be cumbersome, and they may have to resort to giving an employee check-signing authority.

7. *If you have more than one owner, separate the check approval process from the check-signing responsibility.* This separation of responsibilities will protect the interests of all owners. It provides each owner with a deterrent against inappropriate use of practice funds and an assurance that each will not be wrongly accused, since the actions of each will be routinely examined by a colleague.

The following cases illustrate the ease with which an employee can steal funds and cover it up if the proper controls are not in place:

- *Case A:* The business manager of a small practice posts all payments to patient accounts, manages the checkbook, and opens the mail. A cash payment is received for $100 on the Jones account. The business manager pockets the cash and writes off or credits $100 on the Jones account.

- *Case B:* The business manager has check-signing authority as well as the responsibility for paying all of the practice's bills. She issues a check to a fictitious creditor, such as an office supply store, and then cashes the check herself.

- *Case C:* A secretary posts all procedures to patient accounts and verifies his own work the next day by comparing postings to the appointment book. No one else validates his work. He fails to post some procedures and keeps the payments.

- *Case D:* A business manager posts all procedures and opens the mail. She posts a procedure, bills the insurance company, corrects the ledger to show a posting error, and then intercepts the insurance check when it arrives in the mail.

In all four of these cases, the faulty procedure fails to ensure that a record exists of the diverted funds.

All of the safeguards to theft that have been discussed can be overcome if employees act in collusion. However, the chances of collusion are obviously less than the chances of having one employee who is willing to steal if the opportunity presents itself.

THE DOCTOR'S ROLE

The doctor's role in the accounting and financial affairs of a practice is crucial. This role will vary somewhat with the size of the practice. In smaller practices, the doctor is regularly involved in cash control procedures. The doctor, for example, will be the only one with the authority to sign checks, although an employee should prepare the checks for signature. The solo practice doctor should also be ultimately responsible for managing the checkbook and reconciling it with the bank statement. Since balancing a checking account is almost certainly not a good use of a doctor's time, this task should probably be contracted out to a bookkeeper or an accountant. But even if the task is contracted out, the doctor retains the ultimate responsibility and should routinely review the consultant's work.

Doctors in all practices, irrespective of their size, should use financial, accounting, and production data extensively in their role as practice managers. The doctor is ultimately responsible for the financial health of the practice and has a duty both to himself *and to his employees* to use these data to ensure that the practice will survive and prosper. The following suggestions concern the appropriate role for the doctor:

1. The doctor should determine which financial tasks will be performed by the various front office personnel. If the practice has a business manager, the business manager may want to suggest appropriate roles, but the ultimate responsibility must reside with the doctor. This is essential to ensure financial control and reduce the possibility of collusion.
2. The daily receipts and adjustments and daily activity reports should be forwarded to the doctor each day after they have been reconciled. The degree to which the doctor should examine these reports on a daily basis can vary. The most important thing, as far as cash control is concerned, is that the doctor has the report and that employees know it. Spot checks by the doctor

on a random basis can be used to detect sloppy, misleading, or deceitful posting practices.

3. Cash receipt and disbursement reports and various other reports, including gross receipt, write-off, and aging reports, should be examined by the doctor. In larger practices, these reports would also be examined by the business manager; however, this is *never* a substitute for *close* review by the doctor. The business manager should be using these reports to direct day-to-day activities. Part of the doctor's job, however, is to ensure that the business manager is performing adequately, which requires that the doctor be personally familiar with the data in these reports. In addition, the doctor should be using these data to provide guidance regarding the growth and development of the practice. Personal familiarity with practice finances is essential in order for the doctor to make intelligent, rational choices. In this regard, it is always important to remember that the doctor is the best guardian of his or her own welfare.

4. Periodically—either every quarter or every six months—the doctor should set aside time to reflect on the implications of the financial data and consider plans for changes and improvements to practice procedures. Some amount of reflection should occur as a result of the daily, weekly, and monthly reviews of the data. It is important, however, to set aside time for developing a perspective on where the practice has been, where it is now, and various directions in which it might go.

5. The doctor and the practice's accountant should review the financial status of the practice annually. A logical time for this review is after the accountant has prepared the annual tax return. The accountant may be able to provide a perspective on the practice's performance and make helpful suggestions regarding, for example, modifying the practice's retirement plan, financing a proposed expansion, or leasing new equipment.

6. The doctor should determine which of the various accounting and financial tools will be useful for management purposes. The doctor then should direct employees to gather the appropriate information so that it will be available when it is needed.

Part of your responsibility as doctor is to manage the accounting, financial, and production data contained in the reports discussed in this chapter. Unfortunately, the task of managing data requires time, time that will be obtained by working more total hours or by sacrificing clinical hours. This is not to be avoided, however. Administrative responsibilities such as this are simply part of the baggage that goes along with *any* business organization. Furthermore, your work as an administrator will have an impact on your patients. It will assure them that you and your practice will be available when they need your services. Practices *do* fail as a result of mismanagement, fraud, and poor planning. Bankruptcy *can* occur even if you have first-rate clinical skills. Your role as a vigilant, involved administrator is *essential* if these problems are not to befall your practice.

A CASE APPLICATION

Chester Bramers, M.D., was an employed physician working for Dr. Smith, an orthopedist. Smith had visions of a large group practice, and so when he learned that Dr. Bramers was leaving the Navy, he agreed to take him on and help him to develop his practice. Dr. Bramers was still establishing his reputation in the community, but he had been relatively successful in his first year. His clinical skills were excellent, and he had gross receipts of almost $130,000.

Dr. Bramers' compensation was based on a fixed salary of $41,856 plus a bonus of 62 percent of his gross receipts in excess of $90,000. In addition, he also had a number of other benefits, including health insurance, a travel allowance, advertising, and what Dr. Smith felt was excessive utilization of a secretary. In addition, Dr. Smith had to lease an extra 1,000 square feet of space in order to provide an office for Dr. Bramers. Dr. Smith rented more space than he really needed for Dr. Bramers in anticipation of bringing on still more associates. Much of this space, however, was not currently being utilized. Dr. Smith had easily recruited Dr. Bramers and consequently had underestimated the difficulty of filling the additional office space.

Dr. Bramers' employment contract expired in 60 days, and he proposed that his compensation be changed to a flat 70 percent of his gross receipts, along with the elimination of most of the benefits (see Exhibit 7-6). Dr. Bramers commented to Dr. Smith, "Thirty percent should cover my share of the overhead." Dr. Smith realized that Dr. Bramers' practice was growing, and he estimated that Dr. Bramers would gross about $150,000 next year. He based his subsequent analyses on that assumption.

Dr. Smith used break even analysis concepts to evaluate Dr. Bramers' contract proposal and to look at the consequences for the practice if they were not able to reach an agreement. Dr. Smith's first observation was that Dr. Bramers' proposal shifted a considerable amount of risk from the practice to Dr. Bramers, since fixed expenses decreased from $68,143.95 to $21,013.95. This was primarily due to the elimination of the guaranteed salary component in favor of compensation completely based upon bonus. Next, he observed that the practice's net income attributable to Dr. Bramers would decrease by $23,813.43, from $42,694.68 to $18,881.25.

Dr. Smith then tried to put the practice's net income under Dr. Bramers' proposal into context. Dr. Bramers had a disproportionate number of Medicare and Medicaid patients, and he attracted clients that for one reason or another were not particularly responsible regarding their financial obligations. All of this required

Exhibit 7-6 Effects of Current and Proposed Contract Terms on the Projected Contribution to Practice Net Income for Dr. Chester Bramers

---

Current Contract Terms

Estimated Revenue		$150,000.00
Variable Expenses		
Salary (bonus)	$37,200.00	
FICA	$461.37	
Additional Supplies, etc.	$1,500.00	
Total Variable Expenses		$39,161.37
Contribution Margin		$110,838.63
Fixed Expenses		
Health Insurance	$1,200.00	
Gross Fixed Salary	$41,856.57	
FICA	$3,143.43	
Unemployment Insurance	$105.00	
Liability Insurance	$313.00	
Workers' Compensation	$250.00	
Pager ($27.50 per month)	$330.00	
Travel	$600.00	
Yellow and White Pages	$426.00	
Excess Secretarial	$4,992.00	
Office Space	$14,927.95	
Total Fixed Expenses		$68,143.95
Contribution to Practice Net Income			$42,694.68
Departure Adjustment for Receivables			$8,925.00
Adjusted Est. Contribution to Practice Net Income			$33,769.68

Proposed Contract

Estimated Revenue		$150,000.00
Est. Variable Expenses		
Salary (bonus)	$105,000.00	
FICA	$3,604.80	
Additional Supplies, etc.	$1,500.00	
Total Est. Variable Expenses		$110,104.80
Est. Contribution Margin		$39,895.20
Fixed Expenses		
Health Insurance	$0.00	
Gross Fixed Salary	$0.00	
FICA	$0.00	
Unemployment Insurance	$105.00	

continues

Exhibit 7-6 continued

Liability Insurance	$313.00		
Workers' Compensation	$250.00		
Pager ($27.50 per month)	$0.00		
Travel	$0.00		
Yellow and White Pages	$426.00		
Excess Secretarial	$4,992.00		
Office Space	$14,927.95		
Total Fixed Expenses		$21,013.95	
Est. Contribution to Practice Net Income			$18,881.25
Departure Adjustment for Receivables			$8,925.00
Adjusted Est. Contribution to Practice Net Income			$9,956.25

considerable and constant attention from Dr. Smith's business manager as well as a disproportionate amount of clerical support. In addition, Dr. Smith found Dr. Bramers to be a difficult person to work with. He was very self-centered and demanding. Finally, Dr. Bramers tended to isolate himself, and he was unwilling to discuss or have input into practice decisions. His typical comment when asked to think about a management issue was, "Well, George, this is your practice." As a result of these considerations, Dr. Smith asked himself, "Is it worth continuing with Dr. Bramers for $18,881.25?"

As he pondered this question, he began to consider for the first time the financial consequences of Dr. Bramers' departure. What effect would the departure have on the financial condition of the practice? Since all of Dr. Bramers' variable expenses would be eliminated, his real business risk was in the fixed expenses. Dr. Smith concluded that he could eliminate the salary, FICA, workers' compensation, pager, Yellow Pages ad, and travel expenses associated with Dr. Bramers. What about the secretarial and office space expenses? After considering the workload in the office, he decided that a part-time secretarial position could be eliminated without reducing secretarial support for himself. He also concluded that if Dr. Bramers departed, he really would eliminate this position.

The office space that Dr. Bramers used was going to be a problem. Dr. Smith had leased this space when Dr. Bramers joined his practice, and he was committed by lease for another three years. After contacting the renting agent for the building, he determined that the space was large enough and configured in such a manner that it could be successfully sublet. The office building was in a high-demand area, and the agent felt that the space could be rented in 45–60 days.

In exchange for helping Dr. Bramers develop his practice and for referrals, Dr. Smith was to get the receivables if Dr. Bramers left the practice. Dr. Bramers had receivables of about $15,000, and, based on previous experience, $12,750 of that would probably be collectible. Since Dr. Smith's portion of this under the proposed contract would have been $3,825 ($12,750 × .30) if Dr. Bramers stayed, this would result in a net gain to Dr. Smith of $8,925.00 from the receivables. This amount would have to be subtracted, therefore, from Dr. Bramers' contribution to the practice net income in order to determine the effect of his departure. When Dr. Smith did this, it left a projected contribution to net practice income of $9,956.25 under Dr. Bramers' proposal. Finally, Dr. Smith also noted that the workload for some of the other secretaries would decrease, but since he could not actually eliminate these fixed costs, he knew that they should not enter into his calculations.

Dr. Smith concluded that if he accepted Dr. Bramers' proposal, he would have $18,881.25 of net income next year due to Dr. Bramers, which could be used to contribute to practice fixed expenses or profit, and if he terminated Bramers, he would have $33,769.68 less net income next year as compared to this year.

Certainly *any* increase in net income would be justifiable on a financial basis. When he examined the difficulties of working with Dr. Bramers, he concluded that the financial gain associated with keeping him more than compensated for them. Although Dr. Bramers would only contribute $9,956.25 beyond his receivables, Dr. Smith realized that he would get those receivables sooner or later, so he viewed Dr. Bramers' estimated contribution to net income to be $18,881.25. (Dr. Smith could have guessed how long he intended to retain Dr. Bramers and discounted the value of the estimated receivables by their present value.) If he kept Dr. Bramers, it would allow him to retain his expanded facilities while looking for additional colleagues and would provide someone to share on-call and vacation coverage. Finally, it would end any worry that the rental agent might not be able to sublet the office space.

Dr. Smith felt, however, that he would be conceding too much at this point in the negotiations if he accepted Dr. Bramers' current offer. As a result, he made Dr. Bramers a counteroffer that split the difference between what Dr. Bramers proposed and the current contract terms. Dr. Smith also accepted the idea that if he could do no better, he would accept Dr. Bramers' current offer.

CONCLUSION

Routinely examining management accounting data is essential for maintaining a financially sound practice. The methods described in this chapter will give you the skills necessary to examine your practice's financial affairs in a proactive way so that you can address financial crises or take advantage of financial opportunities as quickly as possible.

Most of the management accounting data that you will need to make management decisions can be collected and reported upon on a routine basis by your medical office management software, your accountant, or accounting software. It is important for you to examine these data regularly and take firm control of the financial affairs of your practice. You should now understand the significance of various financial reports and should be able to structure your staff's activities to promote financial control. Deeper levels of inquiry, including the use of accrual data, break-even analysis, and budgets, are optional but in some cases desirable. If your practice is increasing or decreasing in size or undergoing other financial stresses, then these additional tools may help you steer an informed course.

Finally, this chapter should have provided you with a way of thinking about financial controls and how financial data can be used to manage your practice. If you are aware of how the available information can assist you, then you can make intelligent choices regarding what information you use and when you use it.

NOTES

1. Medical Group Management Association, 104 Inverness Terrace East, Englewood, CO 80112-5306.
2. See *The Cost and Production Survey Report* (Englewood, CO: Medical Group Management Association, 1989); H. Paxton, "Which Practice Expenses Are Out of Control?" *Medical Economics*, November 16, 1989, 104–13.

Chapter 8

Marketing

CHAPTER OBJECTIVES

This chapter will help you to develop an effective marketing program for your practice. You will learn how to evaluate your practice's competitive strengths and weaknesses. You will also learn how to identify and analyze potential problems and opportunities in your market. You will learn how to think about your market as a marketing professional would. This includes

- examining your potential patients by market segment
- using marketing research to understand your market and direct your planning
- using target marketing to position your practice to meet marketing objectives

Based on these marketing skills you will learn how to develop a marketing strategy, or overall marketing design, as well as specific marketing plans.

This chapter will also help you to develop promotional skills. Successful promotion depends on

- making personal contacts
- using the media for both paid and unpaid ads
- understanding the strengths and weaknesses of various media, such as TV, radio, and newspapers
- developing personal promotional methods

INTRODUCTION

The brief introduction to marketing in Chapter 1 emphasized the distinction between marketing and selling. To reiterate, doctors who market their services identify their patients' needs and provide the services they wish to offer in a form, at a price, and in a manner that make the patients desire to purchase them. These doctors, in effect, position their services before the patients so that the patients are likely to be aware of them and view them as valuable.

Many physicians believe that *marketing* and *advertising* are simply two different words to describe the same process. This is not true, and therein lies a fundamental misconception regarding marketing. Marketing, in fact, affects the quality and characteristics of the products or services being offered. As a result of your marketing efforts, therefore, your products and services will be changed so as to be more useful to your patients. When you market your services, you accept the reality that, no matter how excellent your clinical skills, you do no one any good if patients fail to use your services because (1) they are unaware of them; (2) your services are not as useful to them as someone else's services; (3) your services are offered at an inconvenient time or place or in an inconvenient manner, or (4) your services are not affordable or viewed as fairly priced.

Marketing professionals have traditionally talked about four types of decisions that must be made regarding the marketing of a product or service. Often referred to as the four Ps, these decisions concern

1. *product* or service characteristics
2. *place* or distribution of the product or service
3. *promotion* of the product or service
4. *pricing* of the product or service

The *marketing mix* is the specific combination of the four Ps that you develop for your practice as a whole or for particular services.

Product decisions concern the specific products and services you intend to offer. To make these decisions, you need to identify groups of potential patients, learn how they best can be served, and determine which products and services will attract them. The products you offer might well include more than your clinical services. For example, they might include the satisfaction and confidence felt by your patients. These products are affected by characteristics of your practice, including its physical attributes, such as the decor of your reception area and examination rooms and the exterior of the building. It also includes the dress and demeanor of you and your staff. Decisions regarding these issues should be reflected in the product plan.

Place (distribution) decisions concern where and when you offer your services. You want to choose a location and office hours that will contribute to your success. The use of satellite, storefront, and shopping center locations and of staggered and extended office hours are distribution options. In addition, convenient parking, easy access, and proximity to your patient base are fundamental considerations. Decisions regarding these issues should be contained in the distribution plan.

Promotion decisions concern the type and amount of promotion that you will conduct. Promotion can include various forms of paid advertising, speeches, seminars to likely patient referral sources, free or low-cost blood pressure or cholesterol checks, and any number of activities that will familiarize the public with your name and your professional abilities.

Pricing decisions concern the cost of your services. An important pricing consideration, for example, is whether to accept insurance company UCRs. With the increasing cost of health care, and with alternatives available, such as HMOs and PPOs, pricing can have a significant effect on a practice's ability to attract and retain patients. Doctors can adopt conscious pricing strategies to undercut, match, or lead the market. Each pricing strategy can be appropriate if it fits into a coherent marketing strategy.

Undercutting the market can result in a gain of market share at the expense of your competitors. Matching the market makes pricing a nonissue. If you adopt this approach, you will have to compete for patients on the basis of product, distribution, or promotion. Leading the market can be effective if your services are in great demand. Generally, consumers perceive higher priced products to be of superior quality, so a price leader position may promote the perception that your services are excellent.

Pricing can be based on costs. For example, it is possible to calculate the cost of an x-ray machine, including supplies, the amortized cost of equipment, labor, overhead, and so on, add a profit margin, and determine a fee. Very few doctors or people in other service industries use this strategy. Instead, pricing generally is based on guesswork and the market rate.

An effective marketing mix—the specific combination of product, distribution, promotion, and pricing—is the result of a carefully developed *marketing plan*. A formal, written marketing plan contains, therefore, a product plan, a distribution plan, a promotion plan, and a pricing plan. As indicated in Exhibit 8-1, the marketing plan is merely one part of the *marketing planning process*. The marketing planning process is intended to ensure that your marketing plan makes sense given the realities of the market that you operate in and your own personal objectives.

Medical practices do not operate in a vacuum. To some extent your marketing decisions will be governed by *external* factors, including the number, quality, and pricing of your competitors; local geography; the economy; state regulation of doctors and competing health care providers; and local ethics regarding acceptable forms of promotion. It is important for you to develop your marketing plan in the context of these external factors so that you can take into account problems they might create for you as well as take advantage of opportunities that they might offer.

Exhibit 8-1 The Marketing Planning Process

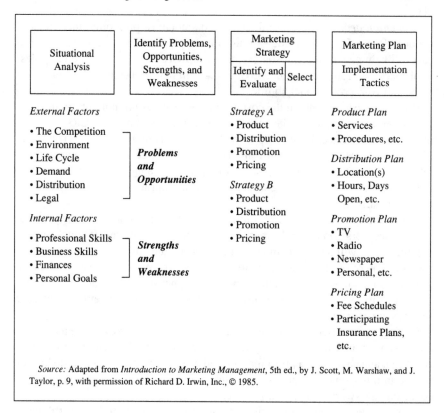

Source: Adapted from *Introduction to Marketing Management*, 5th ed., by J. Scott, M. Warshaw, and J. Taylor, p. 9, with permission of Richard D. Irwin, Inc., © 1985.

In addition, your marketing plan should take into account *internal* factors, such as your practice's financial position, the skills of your colleagues and staff, your equipment and facilities, and, most importantly, *your personal goals and desires.* Your marketing plan, therefore, should also be developed to build on the internal strengths of your practice and to compensate for its weaknesses.

An evaluation of external and internal factors is called a *situational analysis.* Exhibit 8-1 indicates that the situational analysis should lead to the uncovering of problems, opportunities, strengths and weaknesses, which in turn should define the boundaries for developing a specific marketing plan. Exhibit 8-1 also indicates that it is important to develop a *marketing strategy* before constructing a specific marketing plan. A marketing strategy is concerned with the long-range goals and general market orientation of your practice. It provides a context within which you can develop your marketing plan. The following are examples of types of statements that would appear in a document describing a practice's marketing strategy:

- My practice will seek middle- and upper-income patients. It will be based on patients with good insurance who will pay fair rates for superior, personalized care. It will offer state-of-the-art services in very comfortable surroundings. (Carriage Trade Strategy)
- My practice will be directed at lower paying patients who may not have good health insurance but who are most in need of care. My associates and I will provide our services in a "no frills" atmosphere so that prices will be affordable but we will still be able to operate at a profit. The practice will prosper by efficiently treating many patients at very competitive prices.[1] (McDonalds Strategy)

As you can see, once a marketing strategy is determined, a specific marketing plan will logically flow from it. Obviously, it would be counterproductive to develop a marketing plan with "McDonalds" product, place, promotion, and price characteristics if in fact your real intention is to be a carriage trade practice. If you do not precede the development of specific marketing plans with the identification of an overall market strategy, you may unintentionally back into a questionable market strategy as a result of a desire to undertake specific marketing activities. For example, if the McDonalds physician described above did not truly understand that she was a McDonalds physician, she might rent office space in a very expensive building not well located for her intended clientele. She might make this choice because she would personally like to be in the expensive office building. Similarly, she might decorate and furnish her waiting room in a manner consistent with her own personal taste, but once again this might be inconsistent with the McDonalds marketing plan she intends to follow.

The marketing planning process presented in Exhibit 8-1 indicates that doctors should obtain information for the situational analysis before they make decisions about marketing strategies and plans. They must understand the relevant external and internal factors, consider the practicality of various marketing strategy alternatives, and determine the likely effects of these alternatives. Marketing decisions should be made on the basis of informed speculation or market research. Both are legitimate sources of information for making marketing decisions. Market research methods will be discussed in detail later in this chapter. Fundamental to the whole marketing planning process, therefore, is the idea of making conscious, orderly, informed decisions on the basis of information as opposed to whimsy or impulse.

After reading about all the components of the marketing planning process, it would be easy to become intimidated. You may be tempted to say to yourself, "This is simply too much! All that I need to know is how to attract more patients. I don't need or want to spend all of the time or money that would be required to go through all of those additional steps and to develop all of those documents. I'll probably never really use them anyway."

Consider for a moment what the statement "All that I need to do is figure out how to attract more patients" really means. It means that you need to determine (1) what things will work given what you find acceptable, given what your competitors are doing, given the internal goals and limitations of your practice, and (2) what you can do given the constraints in your area. Determining these things *is* a situational analysis. In short, if you were left to your own devices and made more than a superficial effort at examining the problem, you would logically consider the issues listed in the first two columns of Exhibit 8-1.

By following the marketing planning process, you will force yourself to address marketing questions in a systematic and logical manner. If you confound your marketing strategy with immediate marketing plans, then you may go off on a tangent. The marketing planning process will give you a structure to ensure that your thinking and the resulting marketing plans are consistent. Remember, undertaking a thorough marketing planning process does not have to be a burdensome undertaking. There is no law that says that you must take three weeks to construct a 25-page written situational analysis document. A good hour spent thinking seriously about the issues, coupled with a few notes on a legal pad, may be sufficient. This is your practice, and you do not have to confuse formality with effectiveness. Ultimately, the only consideration is whether your marketing efforts are effective. Good ideas dashed on the back of an envelope can be quite useful if they are properly structured.

This chapter is organized around the marketing planning process found in Exhibit 8-1. In addition, a number of other topics essential for developing a marketing strategy and marketing plan are discussed. These other topics include marketing research, target marketing, and market segmentation.

MARKETING PLANNING PROCESS

Situational Analysis: External Factors

The object of doing a situational analysis is to discover all the external and internal factors that could affect your marketing plan. By taking these factors into account, your marketing plan will be able to benefit from some and avoid the pitfalls associated with others. First, let's examine the external factors listed in Exhibit 8-1.

The Competition

The place to begin is with the competition. In order to compete effectively, you must know who your competitors are and understand their competitive advantages and disadvantages. Questions to ask about your competitors include these:

- How many competitors do you have? Are you, for example, the only urologist in town, or is the market divided among many competitors?
- Who are your competitors and who are they likely to be in the future? Are they likely to be among the following?
  —old established practices
  —new physicians moving into the market
  —alternative providers, such as HMOs, PPOs, and EAPs
  —specialists who are broadening their spheres of practice
  —nonmedical competitors, such as chiropractors, psychologists, nurse practitioners, massage therapists, and health food stores
  —hospital emergency rooms
  —emergency care centers
- What are their competitive advantages and disadvantages? For example, do they have unique training, skills, or equipment that sets them apart? Do some have inside ties with hospitals and other potential referral sources? Do they have better or inferior locations? If you can understand the competitive advantages of your colleagues, then you may be able to
  —use similar strategies to your advantage
  —avoid head-to-head competition that you cannot win
  —devise strategies to circumvent your colleagues' competitive advantages
- What are their financial resources? Are they professionally well established?
- What promotional methods are used by your competitors and how well do they appear to work?
- Do you think that your competitors would respond to your promotional efforts? That is, would they react in a retaliatory manner? Might they try to neutralize your efforts or might they ignore you?

Environment

Environmental issues provide the scientific, professional, ethical, and social context for your practice. It is essential to take these environmental issues into account when designing a marketing plan. Some environmental issues come and go, whereas others are more or less permanent. From a marketing perspective, it is important to understand where we are in the life cycle of an issue. For example, as I write this book it is impossible to open a magazine, turn on a radio or TV set, go to a movie, or have an extended conversation with a friend without some mention of the "drug crisis." Our social and political environment is saturated with this issue. A marketing plan that takes into account the public's intense interest in the drug problem may benefit your practice as well as lead you to provide a needed public service.

In contrast, eating disorders, such as anorexia and bulimia, are no less real now than they were three years ago, but they no longer occupy the public spotlight. Does this mean that you shouldn't develop therapy programs or familiarize others with your ability to treat these disorders? Certainly not. However, your methods for promoting your treatment of eating disorders should take into account the current relative disinterest in the topic on the part of the media and the public as well as the large number of medical and nonmedical providers who are now competing for this market. These are all environmental considerations. As a result of the changing social environment, a marketing plan that you would design today for an anorexia or bulimia treatment program would probably look very different from one that you would have designed five years ago.

Changes in the scientific environment also have important marketing implications. For example, Doppler echocardiography appears to be changing the standard for assessing valvular heart disease.[2] Cardiologists might take this into account when they develop long-range marketing strategies and specific marketing plans. Increasingly, physicians are becoming aware of new treatments through unconventional means, such as press releases, direct mailings, and newspaper articles.[3] Monitoring the changing medical environment and then making clinical decisions as a result of the information obtained may be important for the successful marketing of services. For example, levamisole, in combination with 5-fluorouracil, was released as adjuvant chemotherapy for adenocarcinoma of the colon before experimental results were published in a medical journal. Similarly, the FDA and the manufacturer publicized aerosolized pentamidine prophylaxis for treatment of AIDS-related pneumonia before publishing the supporting clinical studies. In both cases, physicians who used nontraditional sources of environmental information had the opportunity to provide superior clinical treatment.

It is also important to take into account local environmental issues. For example, the Hampton Roads area in Virginia has a very large military population. This population is such a significant part of the market that it should be considered in the marketing plan of any local doctor. The implications of this market segment for a practice in the Hampton Roads area include the following:

- directing marketing efforts at young, low-income, temporary residents (Market segmentation)
- taking into account insurance coverage (CHAMPUS) and associated UCR rates (Pricing)
- accessing the CHAMPUS system and other referral sources that could selectively reach this market segment (Promotion)
- providing services that might be highly utilized by this segment, such as obstetrics and children's disease, alcoholism, trauma, and drug abuse treatment programs (Product)

- selecting a location that coincides with areas of heavy military housing, and providing practice hours to harmonize with military base commuting schedules and routes (Distribution)

Another environmental issue in the Hampton Roads area is the road system. The local highway system was poorly designed and does not have sufficient capacity. As a result, some parts of this area become virtually inaccessible between 7:00 AM and 9:00 AM and between 3:30 PM and 6:00 PM. Some creative engineers have managed to link Norfolk to Portsmouth (two dense urban areas) with a tunnel that opens onto a drawbridge. This means that at any given time a trip of a few miles can take half an hour or longer. These transportation problems have created a certain mindset on the part of residents: (1) They seek services in their immediate locality, (2) they avoid certain areas and roads except during midday, and (3) they plan commitments, such as medical appointments, so as to avoid the high-traffic times whenever possible.

These considerations should affect a local physician's choice of location. They should perhaps also affect when and where the physician offers certain services (e.g., public presentations or free blood pressure checks) and even the physician's hospital affiliations.

Another important environmental issue you should take into account when designing your marketing plan is local ethical standards regarding the use of promotion by health care professionals. For example, doctors in most parts of the country now feel comfortable placing a display ad in the daily newspaper describing their services. In addition, many doctors think that appearing on a local TV talk show is an appropriate public service. How do doctors in your area feel, however, about combining the TV medium with the newspaper message? For example, what would the reaction be to a 30-second paid commercial extolling your skills and services? Many doctors would feel that this goes beyond the bounds of good taste or is even unethical. What would the consequences be if you were one of the first in your area to use this promotional approach? How would your peers react to you, and might there be some form of subtle or not-so-subtle retaliation?

Another area of environmental concern is changing technology. For example, what new types of equipment or diagnostic procedures are becoming available, and to what extent will you need additional specialized training in order to utilize them? This issue, which obviously has educational, technical, and financial implications, also has significant marketing implications. How would new equipment allow you to provide new or better services to your patients? How can you let patients or referring professionals know about your capability to provide new services? To what extent will your colleagues follow suit, thereby limiting your competitive advantage to a window in time? Similarly, a technological change could be a major *threat* to your marketing plan if it eventually renders one of your services obsolescent.

Life Cycle

Another external consideration is the *life cycle* of each service or procedure you offer. It is easy to understand that a product such as a computer or a car can have a life cycle. It is introduced into the market, demand for it grows, the market eventually becomes mature and stabilizes, then the demand for the product declines as tastes change or as competing products enter the market, and finally there is little or no need for it. It is somewhat harder to apply the concept of a life cycle to medical services, but in *some* instances it is a useful concept to consider when making your marketing plans.

Some services and procedures and even some diseases do in fact go through a life cycle of birth, growth, maturity, decline, and death. In most cases, the underlying disease continues, but the services and procedures that doctors provide to treat the disease go through a life cycle. The change from one life cycle stage to another can be due to changing technology—such as new equipment or drugs, new clinical procedures—or changing public awareness and acceptance of the disease. For example, bulimia has reached maturity in terms of public interest, and the number of patients who seek services for this problem has leveled off. Most urban areas abound with a myriad of different types of treatment facilities and programs to deal with eating disorders. AIDS, on the other hand, is currently in the growth phase. By understanding where diseases, procedures, and services are in their life cycles, a doctor can plan to provide services that patients need and use the technology and methods that are most appropriate.

Marketing professionals have noted that products or services in a particular life cycle stage have characteristic attributes. For example, the introductory phase is characterized by low sales, technical and marketing problems, and high costs in relation to revenues. These characteristics are due to the startup costs and the costs of initial marketing. Doctors who decide to provide a service or procedure that is in the introductory stage should be future-oriented and be willing to assume some risk. Radial keratotomy, for example, is presently in this stage. Ophthalmologists who have invested their time and capital in acquiring the ability to perform this procedure face risks both in terms of its long-range effectiveness and the possibility that newer technologies, such as excimer laser procedures, may supersede it.

The growth phase is characterized by rapidly increasing demand for services by patients. Generally, the doctors who benefit most from the growth stage of a new service or procedure are those who first introduced it to an area. In the growth stage, it is not unusual for demand to exceed the ability to supply the service. The high revenues associated with the growth phase can also lead to a failure to control costs and create the temptation to overextend. Overextension can be manifested as risky growth, such as buying new equipment or acquiring new facilities that will only pay for themselves if the practice *continues* to grow. It can also be manifested as overwork. In short, the euphoria associated with the growth phase has inherent dangers. Husted, Varble, and Lowry, for example, report that high-technology home health care has profit margins as high as 25 percent, and that the industry's annual growth approaches 40 percent.[4] Industry analysts, however, have noted that there are not enough patients to support all of the companies that have moved into this market, and as a result many of them will fail.

The beginning of the mature phase is characterized by slowing growth. Eventually a peak is reached and patient demand may begin to decline. Most of your services and procedures will be in the mature stage, and some will remain there throughout your professional career. Practices that are well entrenched and well managed will prosper even when providing mainly mature services and procedures. Since growth is no longer occurring as a result of increased demand from patients, it must occur by increasing market share. In essence, a practice will grow to the extent that it takes business away from competitors, as opposed to growing because there are more patients asking for services. (Another source of practice growth is population growth. To the extent that the population is growing in your area, your practice can also grow without having to take patients away from your competition. In a mature market, you would experience this type of growth in any event, and it should not be confused with growth due to a procedure or disease that is in the growth phase of its life cycle.) Prospering on services and procedures that are in the mature stage can be achieved through controlling costs and increasing market share. Promotional efforts that differentiate you from your peers can be particularly effective in this stage. Effective choices in terms of location, hours, and pricing also are important for achieving success in this phase.

The decline stage of a procedure or service is characterized by a decrease in the use of a procedure or a decline in patient demand for it. This can be a slow and steady decline, such as would be characterized by changing social factors that might affect, for example, specific elective plastic surgery procedures. Declines resulting from technological change can, on the other hand, be precipitous. For example, the introduction of antibiotics in the 1940s and the polio vaccine in the 1950s created precipitous declines in the demand for services the need for which was eliminated by these new technologies. A current example may well be the introduction of Prozac and Clomipramine for the treatment of obsessive-compulsive disorder, which may result in a precipitous decline of alternative treatment regimens. Table 8-1 summarizes life cycle phases, along with associated characteristics and appropriate responses.

Demand

Demand is the extent to which current consumers seek the services or procedures you offer or intend to offer. In order to understand the demand for a given service or procedure, you must understand how potential patients currently buy similar services or procedures. Scott, Warshaw, and Taylor have listed a number

Table 8-1 Life Cycle Stages

	Introduction	Growth	Maturity	Decline
Characteristics				
Demand	Low	Fast growth	Slow growth	Declining
Profits	Negligible	Peak levels	Peak to declining	Low or zero
Patient Characteristics	Innovative	Mass market	Mass market	Laggards
Competitors	Few	Growing	Many rivals	Declining numbers
Responses				
Strategic Focus	Create/expand market	Penetrate market	Defend share	Productivity
Marketing Expenditures	High	High	Falling	Low
Marketing Emphasis	Patient awareness	Physician preference	Physician loyalty	Selective
Price	High	Lower	Lowest	Lowest
Service/Procedure	Quasi-experimental	Improved/developed	Differentiated	Rationalized

Source: Reprinted from *Principles of Modern Marketing* by S. Husted, D. Varble, and J. Lowry, p. 240, with permission of Allyn & Bacon, © 1989. Adapted from *Quarterly Review of Marketing*, p.5, Summer 1978, Marketing House Publishers Ltd.

of considerations related to the nature of patient demand for medical services.[5] These considerations include

- the number of physicians that patients consider when seeking medical care
- the extent to which patients seek information before selecting a physician
- the loyalty that patients have to physicians used in the past or referral sources, such as hospitals and other health care professionals
- the sources of information used by patients, such as the Yellow Pages, physician referral services, other health care professionals, and friends
- who makes the physician selection decision and who influences the decision, such as the husband, wife, father, or mother
- the degree of patient interest in the physician selection process (is the decision more like a decision to purchase hairpins or an automobile?)
- the perceived risk involved in making a bad physician selection decision
- attitudes regarding whether the illness or procedure is viewed as a necessity or a luxury (is the purchase of the medical service more like the purchase of food or a cocktail dress?)
- length of the anticipated time involvement with the physician (is the time involvement with the consequences of the purchase decision analogous to that of buying gum or dining room furniture?)

The object of asking these and other questions is to uncover implications for your services and procedures. By determining the answers, you may be able to design more effective marketing programs. One way to obtain an understanding of demand characteristics is to look at existing marketing research. Reviewing publications such as the *Journal of Health Care Marketing* and the *Journal of Medical Practice Management* can provide you with the latest research findings in medical practice marketing.[6] You can also obtain information by conducting your own marketing research. A later section of this chapter will describe how to conduct cost-effective, unobtrusive marketing research that will give you information specific to your practice and to your own particular marketing objectives.

Another issue related to demand is the concept of market segmentation. Market segments are groups of people who will respond in a similar manner to services and procedures. By understanding the different demands associated with the segments of your market, you can more precisely direct your marketing efforts. If, for example, a plastic surgeon determines that a significant number of his rhinoplasty patients are female, are between the ages of 25 and 35, and reside disproportionately in two of the seven local counties, then he can use this information to design a more effective marketing plan. Similarly, if the decision where to take a child with a cold for treatment is made by the mother in 75 percent of families, then this should also influence marketing decisions.

Legal Constraints

No matter what your peers may tolerate, legal limitations may restrict your marketing efforts. For example, your ability to supply and promote experimental services and drugs may be limited by state and federal law. Similarly, your ability to promote standard procedures or the use of specific drugs may be limited by state law or local ordinance.

Distribution Structure

How your competitors distribute or offer their services may affect your marketing strategy and marketing plans. Physicians should evaluate the distribution of competing services, such as traditional private practices, shopping center emergency care operations, and hospital emergency rooms. Market distribution factors can affect your distribution choices. For example, if your market is saturated with many private emergency care operations, your marketing strategy and plans should take into account that patients currently do not have to go very far to reach a competitor. You might then seek to differentiate your practice in such a way that patients will travel the extra distance.

Situational Analysis: Internal Factors

In addition to external factors, you must have a good understanding of your practice's characteristics before you can develop a marketing strategy and specific marketing plans. You should do a situational analysis of the internal factors to explore any intrapractice issues that could affect subsequent marketing decisions. Exhibit 8-1 lists some of these internal factors, including professional and business skill levels, finances, and personal goals.

Professional and Business Skills

In order to develop an effective marketing plan, you should assess both the professional skills and business skills of you, your associates, and your staff. Begin with an honest assessment of the depth and range of your own professional skills as well as those of any practice colleagues, including other doctors, nurses, and technicians. It makes no sense to market a service that cannot be delivered or to undersell a valuable or rare service. An additional perspective can be gained by comparing your skills and those of your associates with those of peers in other practices. Once again, self-deception is self-defeating. No one else need see your self-evaluation. Setting some practical goals, however, is obviously dependent upon a realistic determination of the relative quality of the professional skills available in your practice. In essence, you are trying to determine your distinctive competence.

You should also assess the business skills available in your practice. The business end of your practice provides the support necessary for the delivery of professional services. If your practice's business operations have weaknesses or strengths, then these must be understood, compensated for, taken advantage of, or changed. It is not advisable, however, to simply wish around weaknesses in office operations, or to fail to take advantage of a strength. How effectively is your practice managed? How much volume of work can your practice handle? In short, does your practice have the supporting structure necessary to provide your patients with the services you are skilled to deliver?

An assessment of your practice's business strengths and weaknesses is very important, because an effective marketing plan will put additional pressures on business operations. First, the marketing plan will hopefully result in an increase in patients treated, procedures performed, and so on. This of course will result in an increase in associated support work, such as laboratory testing, insurance filing, chart management, report writing, and telephoning. In addition, the marketing process per se may result in added pressures on a practice's business operations and financial resources. For example, marketing activities may include writing and typing news releases and speeches and arranging appointments with referral sources, all of which take time and energy. Do you have a business manager or another employee, for example, with enough skills to write a news release? Are your secretaries going to be able to take the additional load if you decide to produce a training and nutrition manual for the local Little League? Are you willing to commit time to do personal promotions, such as talking to civic groups?

Finally, you should evaluate your own promotional skills—and those of your colleagues if you are in a group practice. If you are terrorized by the thought of standing before an audience to give a lecture, then it is critical that you acknowledge this. You may choose to work on your fear or to avoid this type of promotion. Both are acceptable choices. What is not acceptable, however, is to base a marketing plan on something that you cannot or will not be able to undertake.

Finances

Any marketing plan you develop is going to have financial implications. Although some promotional methods may cost little or nothing, many others can be quite expensive. It is important to be realistic about the funds that are available for marketing. You do not have the time for pipe dreams, and your marketing budget may well eliminate ideas that in the abstract might sound very attractive.

Personal Goals

This is the single most important internal environmental issue. What do you *want* to do? What do you want your practice to be like? What kinds of patients (defined any way you like) do you want to treat, and what type of clinical work do you really want to undertake? There is nothing so frustrating as working hard to achieve success, only then to realize that what you accomplished was not what you really wanted.

In defining your goals, you should consider more than just your clinical work. If, for example, it is important for you to have significant amounts of time with your family, then this should be taken into account in your marketing plan. A plan, for example, that, if successful, would result in your conducting 45 clinical hours per week, not to mention marketing and administration duties, is obviously inconsistent with a significant home life. Other issues, such as your image in the community, your prestige, or your ability to help ameliorate social problems, may be important to you, and you will be happier and certainly more successful overall if your personal goals are reflected in how you run your practice. For example, the carriage trade practice and the McDonalds practice, which were described above, will have different degrees of attractiveness to different physicians. There is nothing inherently right or wrong with having either type of practice as an objective. The important point is for you to be honest with yourself regarding what you want your practice to be so that you can develop a marketing plan that will help you to get there.

Problems, Opportunities, Weaknesses, and Strengths

This next phase of the marketing planning process involves evaluating the information you have gathered in your situational analysis. In particular, you should try to determine your practice's problems, opportunities, weaknesses, and strengths.

Problems are external factors that result in a practice performing at lower levels than it would otherwise. Problems might include:

- numerous competitors in your specialty
- insurance carriers who have adopted less realistic UCRs and require more "hoops" to be jumped through as prerequisites for payment
- a new emergency care facility that has opened two blocks from your office
- a downturn in the local economy that makes preventive health care generally less affordable

Opportunities are openings in the external environment which your practice could take advantage of. Here are some examples:

- The local school system decides to contract with a physician to provide medical exams for all students in its special education program

- An older physician with a successful practice is retiring and is interested in working out an arrangement for the care of her patients.
- A major commuting route passes your office, which allows you to market treatment during commuting hours.

Weaknesses are internal factors that limit your practice's ability to compete for patients or provide them with services. Weaknesses might include

- a patient reception area that is too small to support practice growth
- a front office staff that is having difficulty coping with the current volume of patients
- a dislike on your part of talking before large groups
- a secretary who does not come to you with her work problems but instead takes them out on other employees
- computer software that is difficult for your clerical staff to learn to use effectively
- associates whom the office staff has difficulty working with

Strengths are internal factors that provide you with a competitive advantage over other practices. These might include

- your ability to use new procedures that have been mastered by only a few other local colleagues
- a staff that is well trained, effective, and courteous to your patients
- financial reserves that will allow you to deal with growth or any unforeseen circumstances expeditiously
- computer software that lets your staff identify delinquent accounts easily and study the demographic distribution of your patients so that you can evaluate marketing opportunities, bill insurance daily, and so on

It is important for you to examine the problems, opportunities, strengths and weaknesses realistically so that your marketing strategy and marketing plans will be more effective. Self-deception at this point may make you feel good, but it will ultimately result in wasting time and resources on developing marketing plans that are unrealistic or inappropriate.

Marketing Strategy

A marketing strategy is a statement of long-range marketing objectives. It should take into account the analysis of your practice's problems, opportunities, strengths, and weaknesses. Since the marketing strategy will be based on an evaluation of fundamental internal and external issues, it will serve as a useful guide for developing specific marketing plans. In particular, it will allow you to avoid fragmenting or misdirecting your efforts or developing specific marketing ideas that are inconsistent with your long-range plans and ultimate objectives.

Once you have evaluated your practice's problems, opportunities, strengths, and weaknesses, it is appropriate to evaluate alternative marketing strategies. Often, more than one strategy will be appropriate for achieving your objectives. At this point in the process, you want to be *creative*. You don't want to formulate just a passable strategy, you want to come up with a *great* one—one that will give you a sustainable competitive advantage. The reality may well be that you can't or don't come up with the "great creative breakthrough," but it is important for you to accept this challenge.

List the pros and cons associated with each strategy. Consider the implications of your situational analysis for each strategy. Carefully look at the risks that may be associated with a strategy and ask yourself whether they are reasonable and could be compensated for by a commensurate reward. There is no substitute for good, critical thinking. If you have confidants who are not competitors, share your potential marketing strategies with them. Sometimes simply expressing your thoughts will help you to clarify issues in your own mind and to recognize the importance of considerations you had not previously appreciated. However, when seeking the advice and commentary of others, keep in mind that this is your practice. Your confidants will have different degrees of risk averseness as well as their own personal goals, and these will influence their comments and recommendations. You must be the ultimate judge of the viability of a given marketing strategy.

As you evaluate various marketing strategy alternatives, pay attention to the various market segments and marketing mix implications. Consider, for example, the implications of each strategy for the decisions that must be made regarding product (e.g., services provided, procedures utilized), distribution decisions (e.g., location, time of service), promotion (e.g., paid and unpaid advertising, referrals from other health care professionals), and pricing (e.g., fee structure, accepting UCRs, being a PPO provider).

It is also important to remember that since a strategy should be based on the situational analysis, you must always be aware of changing environmental circumstances. Although your marketing strategy is ideally a long-term outline for how to proceed, it is important to appreciate that circumstances can change enough to merit a revision of a marketing strategy.

Exhibit 8-2 contains a marketing strategy statement for a family practice that wants to adopt a carriage trade approach. The statement provides a rough sketch of the physician's objectives. It provides enough detail in each area so that any fundamental inconsistencies with the subsequent marketing plan will be obvious. For

Exhibit 8-2 Marketing Strategy Statement for a "Carriage Trade" Practice

Overall Strategy Description

My practice will seek middle- and upper-income patients with good insurance who will pay fair but above average rates for superior, personalized care. It will offer state-of-the-art services in very comfortable surroundings.

Objectives

I want to be able to conduct about 35 clinical hours per week and manage the practice in an additional 5 hours per week. I want to earn income in excess of $200,000 annually. I want to minimize collection problems by working with patients who have "good" insurance and who will be more likely to meet their financial commitments. I want to collect the full fee at the time of service from a majority of my patients.

Target Market

The target market consists of people who are self-employed or work for private employers. This market can probably be addressed by segments, such as residential neighborhoods, employers, employment segments or industries, professional associations, and social organizations (e.g., churches, clubs, and interest groups).

The people in the target market want quality services but need to have them supplied in a timely manner. They do not want to waste time in waiting rooms or in getting an appointment. The key is to provide quality services in an efficient manner.

Marketing Mix Directions

The services and procedures that I currently provide will be adequate. Staying on the cutting edge, or at least being aware of state-of-the-art information, will be essential for working with these patients. I will try to be an innovator in this area, to become skilled in new procedures, and to introduce them as quickly as ethically and financially possible. Part of what I am offering is atmosphere and efficiency. The front office staff will always have to look professional, and I must remember this when I am hiring new personnel. My current location is ideal for attracting these patients, since I am located in one of the high-income areas of town. I probably need to rethink my hospital affiliations and make a move to Briarcliff. Promotional efforts should be directed both to my prospective patients and to potential patient referral sources. My overall pricing policy will be to set my fees at or somewhat above the median. I will participate with Blue Cross for the time being, and I will limit military patients by not participating with CHAMPUS.

Problems, Opportunities, Strengths, and Weaknesses

Problems: Other physicians in this area have very narrow standards for acceptable forms of promotion. This may greatly limit my ability to let prospective patients know about my practice's goals. Is the demand for this type of practice really there? My friends and associates all say that they would like to be able to go to a practice like this, and the income and education figures provided by the Chamber of Commerce indicate that the demand *should* be there. But will people really want it when it is available?

Opportunities: No other practice in the area seems to have adopted this strategy. If I can effectively dominate this market, I should have little direct competition for patients who are

continues

Exhibit 8-2 continued

---

sensitive to quality, exclusivity, and efficiency. I am already well located to attract these patients, and given the above average income and the high education level of the area, there should be a large, receptive market.

Strengths: My practice already operates effectively in terms of billing and the way that patients are treated. I have always kept professionally current and have invested in professional education for myself. I have also acquired excellent modern equipment. Financially, I am in excellent shape and can afford to adopt this strategy even if it results in a near-term decline in income. I belong to a country club and two social clubs, which could be good marketing sources.

Weaknesses: The front office staff doesn't always look as professional as they could. I don't really like to talk to groups of people. I know few other referring professionals, and I am not sure who to contact. About 20 percent of my current patients would probably tend to "mess up" a very nicely furnished waiting area. My associated physician, Floyd, may not have the personality or the "bedside manner" to develop a word-of-mouth referral network with more sophisticated patients.

---

example, the physician is uncertain whether her patients will be willing to pay a premium for more personalized service and whether target market patients exist in sufficient numbers to support her practice. Clearly, these are questions that need additional research. It should also be clear that it did not take the physician an excessive amount of time to construct this marketing strategy statement. Finally, by serving as a template against which all specific marketing plans must be assessed, the marketing strategy statement can prevent the physician from developing specific marketing plans that would not get her where she wants to go.

Marketing Plan

The marketing plan contains the operational details of how you will implement your marketing strategy. If the marketing strategy is somewhat analogous to the statement, "We will open a second front in France in 1944," then the marketing plan will indicate which divisions will land where, what their objectives are, and what equipment and supplies they will need. The four elements of the marketing plan must fit together into a synergistic whole, and there must be a logical tie back to the marketing strategy. The marketing plan should provide concrete guidance regarding products and services, distribution, promotion, and pricing, and it must be consistent with and reflect the knowledge obtained in the preceding phases of the marketing planning process. Exhibit 8-3 provides an example of a marketing plan for a psychiatrist.

A marketing plan is subject to constant revision. For example, suppose that the first of the quarterly workshops referred to in Exhibit 8-3 is a great success. Many people attend, and within a week, several have become patients. This would cer-

Exhibit 8-3 Marketing Plan for a Psychiatrist

Product Plan

My objective is to spend 60 percent of my time doing medication work and hospital rounds. I do not want to be involved in much short-term psychotherapy, so I will select my psychotherapy cases to be longer term, chronic cases. I will seek to refer out short-term psychotherapy cases while retaining the medical component of these cases.

I want to develop an eating disorders program. Once again, however, my primary interest is in the medication and hospitalization components. I will try to find a psychology practice with which to jointly develop and market this program. They will handle the psychotherapy and I will handle the medical component. If I can't find the right psychology practice, I will consider hiring a psychologist or clinical social worker and expanding my facilities so that I can provide these services.

Distribution Plan

My practice is currently well situated to serve my patients. I will not expand my hours. There is no room in our suite for growth. With the population explosion in the Churchland area, I must consider opening a satellite office there if growth is desired. One objective would be to have the allied practice be in Churchland. The eating disorders program will have to be based in the allied practice. If I can't find an allied practice in Churchland, then it should be in the eastern part of town, no more than 5 or so minutes from an expressway exit and no more than 15 minutes from my practice.

Promotion Plan

Paid Display Advertising

I will plan to spend $13,500 in paid print advertising. Based on market research provided to me by the publishers, I will spend $6,500 on biweekly display ads in the local entertainment newspaper and an additional $7,000 on a smaller display ad in the daily newspaper. The ads will stress
1. the personalized nature of my services
2. the comprehensiveness of psychiatry compared with psychology and other related disciplines

I am willing to devote an additional $5,000 to the eating disorder program and would expect that the allied practice would contribute an equal amount. The specific nature of these ads will be determined with the allied practice, but it is necessary that they reflect a high-quality, scientific, professional image, not a "pop psych" image.

Referral Source Development

1. I will refer out a significant proportion of psychotherapy patients to well-qualified and professionally competent allied providers, such as other psychiatrists, psychologists and clinical social workers with the object of receiving medication referrals. Once a provider has begun to supply me with medication referrals, I will continue to supply him or her with psychotherapy referrals.
2. I will develop a one-day training program for family practice physicians to acquaint them with ways of determining when child behavior problems should be referred to a psychiatrist. This program will be offered quarterly.

continues

Exhibit 8-3 continued

Television and Radio

I will have my secretary obtain a list of the names and addresses of all local talk show hosts. I will write each one a letter describing timely topics that I can talk about on his or her show. In addition, I will mail each one a press release on specific issues at least once every two months.

Free Media

1. I will write at least one news release each month. These releases will be on the latest developments in mental health. Sources of information will be my professional journals. The news releases will be mailed to reporters and to local TV and radio news departments.
2. I will conduct four free one-and-a-half-hour workshops each year, which will be held in a nearby church auditorium. The workshops will cover such issues as smoking, eating disorders, phobias, problem children, and so on. The workshops will emphasize the unique role of psychiatry in treating problems and disorders.
3. Six weeks before each free workshop, I will distribute a press release to all local newspapers and other media (for inclusion in their "Community Announcements") and to local churches and civic groups (for inclusion in their newsletters).
4. I will try to find some source of free recurring media exposure, such as a weekly mental health segment on a TV news program or a weekly or monthly newspaper column.

Pricing Plan

I will participate with Blue Cross/Blue Shield until I feel that my patients are no longer particularly sensitive to the UCR or until I have more patients than I can personally treat. At that point I will no longer be a participating provider. I will set my fees at about what my peers charge, but if I am off, I will be on the high side. My fees for the eating disorder program will not be different from my regular fees.

tainly suggest that the psychiatrist should consider revising his plans and should also try to determine exactly what happened at the workshop to attract the patients. Similarly, if the paid display ads are producing no noticeable results after six weeks, he should evaluate the ad content as well as the appropriateness of the media.

PROMOTION

Promotion is probably what first comes to most people's minds whenever they hear the term *marketing*. Promotion is the process of presenting your services to prospective patients. Your promotional activities will be the most visible part of your marketing activities to those outside of your practice, and they will make a statement about your practice and who you are. The object of this section is to acquaint you with a number of specific promotional activities and indicate how and when to use them.

Personal Contact

Personal contact is one of the most effective ways of promoting a medical practice. Personal contact means talking to large or small groups of people. It also includes one-on-one contact with another person. In either case, the target of personal contact can be potential patients or referral sources. One reason that this form of promotion can be so effective is that it is often not perceived as promotion. Another reason is that potential patients and referral sources get to know you and begin to see you as a person, not merely as a name or a title.

Let's first discuss how to promote yourself to groups of potential patients or referral sources. It is important to draw a distinction between making one or two presentations to groups and developing an ongoing personal contact strategy. The former is dabbling, the latter is promotion, and the distinction between the two is important. A real promotional effort requires *commitment*. In particular, it requires time and energy spent developing good presentations and a willingness to make presentations over an extended period of time.

Any form of promotion, in order to be effective, demands repetition, and personal contact is no exception. You must have ways of repeatedly developing interesting and effective presentation materials. How do you do this? You create a special niche for yourself. Think about your specialties and interests. Select two or three treatment or disorder areas that you are particularly knowledgeable about or would like to be knowledgeable about. Don't necessarily limit yourself to areas of current expertise. Be willing to expand your knowledge base when that is necessary or personally desirable. For example, if an employee assistance program will be conducting a seminar on drug testing, give it a shot even if you aren't an expert on the subject. A few hours of paid library work on the part of a student, coupled with a computer search, will give you the specialized knowledge that, in combination with your experience and medical education, will allow you to make an informative and effective presentation. Remember, you don't have to present yourself as an expert on a subject or procedure in order to make an interesting and effective presentation. You do have to present yourself, however, as one who knows what is current regarding a subject or procedure.

Remember also that the value of the personal contact is largely in the *quality* of communication between you and your audience. The very fact that you are there has promotional value. Develop your presentation so that whenever possible it involves your audience. Asking your audience questions and giving them plenty of opportunities to ask you questions will help you to establish a two-way dialogue. The presentation should allow your audience to sample your behavior. If your objective is to let the audience know that you are competent, concerned, and approachable, then conduct your presentation in this way. Give them facts but also show them the type of person you are. Conduct the presentation so that they understand you care about their problems and are willing to listen to them. "But I don't have the time to do all of that preparation," you say. If you really don't have the time, then you probably don't need to do the promotion in the first place!

Once you have defined a few presentation subjects, the next problem is to find someone who will listen. Begin by asking yourself, "Who else works in these areas?" For example, suppose that you feel that you could make an effective presentation on sexual abuse. You might want to contact family service agencies, rape hotlines, ministries, women's groups, police departments, and others who come into contact with sexually abused individuals. There are a number of ways that you can make these contacts, including these:

- You can send a letter outlining the services that you can provide or your willingness to talk about a relevant subject.
- You can make a phone call. This can be particularly effective if you are not certain who to talk to at an agency.
- A personal visit following a letter or phone call can be very effective in getting a commitment from a group to let you talk to them.
- You can make a call or send a letter in which *you* ask for advice. For example, state that you are looking for services that your patients might need, such as legal assistance or counseling.

Personal contact can also take place at the individual level. One of the most effective ways to conduct one-on-one promotion is over lunch. Meeting a referral source over lunch is advantageous in that neither of you "wastes" an hour (unless of course you normally don't eat during the day). It also pairs your message and your presence with food, which can have all sorts of beneficial unconscious associations. Finally, it allows you to develop a series of similar time-limited promotional opportunities that can be easily arranged by you or your secretary. If you make it a point to hold three luncheon meetings a week for a month, you will have captured approximately 12 hours of referral development time at virtually no cost in clinical hours.

Using the Media

Paid Ads

Paid advertising, irrespective of which media you use, is probably the most expensive way to generate referrals. Table 8-2 contains an evaluation of the strengths and weaknesses of various major media. Many physicians use newspaper display ads in which they state their names and the services that they offer. If newspaper ads are to work, they require repetition, and given the high cost of space in daily newspapers this will invariably result in a large initial outlay of money before results are seen. If you are considering placing a display ad in a

Table 8-2 Strengths and Weaknesses of Major Media

Source	Advantages	Disadvantages
Newspapers	• Good coverage in local markets • Short time commitment • Easy availability • Tangible and believable	• Low demographic selectivity • Relatively short life • Low reproduction quality
Television	• Combines sight and sound • High attention • Conveys "big league" image • Entertaining, energetic, and forceful	• Low demographic selectivity • Very short message life • High production and presentation costs • Commercial clutter
Radio	• Low production and presentation costs • High demographic selectivity • Reaches mass markets	• Less attention-getting than visual messages • Very short message life • Commercial clutter
Billboards and Signs	• High repetition • Low cost • Visual	• No demographic selectivity • Very limited message
Magazines	• High message permanence • High demographic selectivity • High reproduction quality	• Long purchase lead time • No guarantee of position
Direct Mail	• Demographic selectivity • Personalized • No competition surrounding your message	• High cost per number of exposures • Junk mail image

newspaper, be certain to ask yourself what will differentiate you from other physicians running similar display ads.

You should also consider the geographical area from which you draw patients. Although a newspaper may be read by hundreds of thousands of readers, most of this exposure may be of little value if your patients largely come from within a few miles of your practice. For example, a family practice located near residential neighborhoods may draw 90 percent of its patients from within a ten-mile radius. An advertisement in a widely distributed daily newspaper may be largely a waste of money, since most readers would not travel long distances because (1) there are likely to be many competitors who are located nearer, and (2) patients generally seek treatment at family practices for what are perceived to be less serious problems, thereby precluding the need to take extraordinary measures when seeking treatment. On the other hand, a specialist in internal medicine may have a regional clientele, in which case the wide circulation of the daily newspaper could be useful for reaching potential patients.

An alternative to advertising in the daily newspaper is to use smaller newspapers and newsletters. These can be especially effective if the publication targets an audience that is more likely to want your services than the general population. In addition, the lower advertising rates will allow you to achieve greater repetition. For example, a display ad in a Norfolk, Virginia, gay newspaper, which publishes monthly, can be run for a year for less cost than a single display ad in the daily newspaper. The gay newspaper could be a very good place for a practice to advertise if the gay population would be particularly interested in the practice's services. If gays would not be more interested than the general population, then it would in fact be a very expensive advertising outlet, since its circulation is much smaller than that of the daily newspaper.

For example, if an ad in the daily newspaper costs $400 and is seen by 500,000 readers, then each dollar of advertising translates into 1,250 readers. By placing a similarly sized ad costing $30 in the 10,000-circulation gay newspaper, you reach 333.33 readers for each advertising dollar. Advertising in the gay newspaper would be reasonable if you had a service or a message that would result in a response rate from the gay newspaper ad that was 3.75 times greater than the response rate from the ad in the daily newspaper. Promoting AIDS services or advertising the fact that you have special skills associated with helping gay and lesbian patients might produce a favorable return.

Whenever you advertise in a specialty newspaper or bulletin, you should consider designing your ad to speak *directly* to the publication's audience. Customizing the ad may cost a little more, but it will allow you to convey your message in a manner that might be particularly attractive to that market. Another benefit of utilizing smaller newspapers and newsletters is that some organization within the specialty audience may ask you to present a workshop or give a presentation, thereby providing you with additional exposure.

Another place to advertise is the Yellow Pages. Buying an ad in the Yellow Pages is a relatively passive form of advertising, since it does not increase demand for your services. A newspaper or TV commercial can educate potential patients regarding the symptoms of a problem or the need for preventive care, thereby increasing demand. If prospective patients are to find you in the Yellow Pages, they must already know that they need your services. If they already know you and simply wish to find your telephone number, they will most likely use the White Pages.

Many Yellow Pages referrals are price shopping. The Yellow Pages is also one of the last places people look—Yellow Pages shoppers often have exhausted other potential referral sources, such as friends and health care professionals. As a result, Yellow Pages referrals are less likely to show up for the initial appointment. One practice reported an overall first appointment "show rate" of 74 percent, whereas the rate for Yellow Pages referrals was 51 percent.

Yellow Pages ad copy should be designed for the consumer who does not know you. The top line should stress the services that you provide, not your name. (An exception is when the practice name is descriptive of the services provided, such as "Ear, Nose, and Throat Specialists, P.C.") Listing the most common symptoms you work with and a few of the most common disorders you encounter will also help Yellow Pages readers to determine whether you can help. Other Yellow Pages ad design pointers are as follows:

- Use a large black border around your ad. A 1/4" border will set your ad off from others.
- Color is not cost-effective. In addition, as more advertisers resort to color, the color ad's ability to catch the eye is lost. Finally, many color ads look gaudy and do not promote a quality image.
- Strive to get the ad placed near the alphabetical listing. This will result in increased readership. The "dollar bill"–sized ad has a greater chance of being placed near the alphabetical listing. An alternative is to create a small display ad in the alphabetical listing by purchasing several lines.
- Being toward the beginning of the listing is not that important. Many readers will fan through the book from back to front and will therefore search the listing in reverse order.
- Copy should use upper- and lower-case letters to increase reading ability. Put your name near the telephone number. Don't use a map. It will waste space and your ad may be torn out of the book. A short quote in parentheses will attract attention.
- If you have been practicing for a while, note that in your ad. A group practice may be able to state, for example, "Over 40 Years of Professional Experience."

Finally, Yellow Pages spending should be a carefully coordinated part of your overall advertising budget. By tracking how referrals are generated, you can determine the cost per referral, and comparisons can be made to other forms of promotion. The Yellow Pages budget can then be increased or decreased depending upon the relative usefulness of your Yellow Pages advertising.

Telephone and radio can also be used for advertising. Both media present messages that are very transitory. A daily newspaper may sit on a table for a day, and a monthly newspaper or newsletter may have exposure for several weeks. A 30-second television or radio ad is gone in 30 seconds. These media, however, can be exceedingly effective. The question is whether they are appropriate for your practice. Radio and television ads require significant repetition if they are to have a significant impact. A rule of thumb is that the ad has to be seen or heard at least three times before the viewer or listener will fully comprehend the message and be able to recall the advertiser's name. In addition, the development, design, and production of the ad is critical, since you have such a short period of time to make your point. Development, design, and production, of course, cost money.

Production and air time costs will vary greatly depending upon the market that you are in. In the Norfolk–Virginia Beach market (ranked 31st nationally), a simple 30-second television commercial can be produced and taped for about $1,500. The cost of air time will vary based on the ratings of programs on which your ad appears. For example, the local 6:00 PM news in this market costs about $600 for a 30-second ad. On the other hand, 30 seconds on David Letterman is currently selling for $150. If you have a $10,000 ad budget, the 6:00 PM news will not give you the repetition you need to have a good chance of success. Production costs for radio are substantially lower. Some radio stations will produce ads at no cost in return for the purchase of advertising time.

Understanding the characteristics of your patients is critical to using the electronic media effectively. For example, suppose that you are promoting a service that will be used primarily by women, such as cosmetic surgery. There are specific hours and programs that attract a disproportionate number of female viewers. Often, the rates will be lower for hours or programs that are most attractive to a particular market segment, because *overall* viewership may be lower. A well-designed plan for running an ad during hours and on programs where lower viewership is coupled with disproportionate viewing by your target market segment can make the cost-effectiveness formula for television and radio very favorable.

Television and radio stations have considerable data on ratings for various programs and time periods. Radio can be a particularly effective medium for targeting specific market segments, because each station has a well-defined format that appeals to a different segment of the population. For example, talk radio stations tend to attract higher income, better educated listeners, while rock stations have a high proportion of teenage and young adult listeners. When talking to a station's advertising personnel, you should remember that their job is to sell advertising. Advertising that works is going to be in their long-term interest, since you will continue to run ads if they generate patients. As with any purchase, however, you must be aware of the unscrupulous salesperson or the salesperson with a short-term profit orientation. According to one television executive, "A ratings book is like the Bible. You can find whatever you are looking for in it. An ad salesman will know what to show you to tell his story."[7]

Given the 30- to 60-second length of electronic media ads, your ad must be well designed if it is going to be effective. This is one area in which you should heavily rely on professional advice. Television and radio professionals know how to take your ideas and convert them into visual and audio effects that will attract viewer attention and communicate your message. You should be involved in the ad development process but should also recognize your limitations. Concentrate on communicating to the professionals the visual and audio message that you want to convey, along with some thoughts on advertisement characteristics. For example, you might outline the content of the ad and propose whether the message should be presented by actors in dialogue, by one actor, or by you talking directly into the camera. If the professionals suggest that you are in error and can give you a reasonable argument for proceeding differently, you should defer to their judgment.

You should also involve yourself in the selection of actors and graphic displays and other decisions that will affect the appearance and placement of the message. However, you should rely very heavily on professional advice in these areas. You should also defer to professional judgment regarding specific use of language and technical production considerations, such as lighting, background, music, camera angles, dress, and makeup.

An alternative to this level of personal involvement is to hire a media consultant to act as an intermediary between you and the advertisement production personnel and the television or radio stations. The media consultant will also be able to tell you which programs on the local stations will provide the best mix of viewers and listeners to meet your marketing objectives. If you use a media consultant, it is critical to spend enough time together and to make known your objectives and the image you wish to present.

If you decide to use paid advertising, you must be especially cognizant of the local ethics regarding this issue. If you get too far out in front of your colleagues, you may be subject to retribution ranging in form from mild ostracism or criticism to official censure. On the other hand, being out in front of your colleagues can be a very valuable competitive advantage.

Finally, if you determine that your practice might benefit from paid advertising, it might be worthwhile to read about some of the approaches used by successful advertising executives. This may give you some ideas for developing your own ads and ad copy and also help you judge the ideas proposed by marketing and media consultants. For example, David Ogilvy, who developed a number of successful advertising campaigns, has described his formula for print layout.[8] He concluded that the most effective way to lay out a print ad is to

1. place an illustration at the top of the page with a caption below it
2. print the copy in a serif typeface
3. set the copy in three columns 35–45 characters wide
4. start the copy with drop initials
5. print the copy in black ink on white paper

An example of a service ad utilizing Ogilvy's format is found in Exhibit 8-4. This ad provides a significant amount of information and tells readers why they should consider the service. Contrast this with a typical private practice print ad

Exhibit 8-4 Example of a Service Ad Utilizing the "Ogilvy" Format

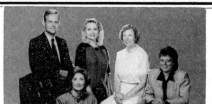

The Center For Anxiety & Stress Management: (L to R) Paul Clark, L.C.S.W., Gayle Cameron, L.C.S.W.
Bernadette Jones, L.C.S.W., Claire Goldhush, L.C.S.W., Kathleen Brehony, Ph.D.

"You don't have to be afraid"
Even if you are anxious, phobic, or stressed

We can help you overcome your fears, and put you back in control of your life. Panic episodes, fears of driving, being alone, speaking in public, crowds, heights, and others can be overcome.

How can we help

The Center for Anxiety and Stress Management's programs are based on intensive individual and group therapies, proven effective through clinical research.

We use cognitive, behavioral, and psychological methods based on an individual assessment of your problem.

You can learn how to manage your stress and anxiety, and how to confront rather than avoid your fears and phobias. Once you learn these skills, you will regain control over your life.

Make your butterflies fly in formation

We teach you specific skills and techniques that will help you gain control over your panic, or stop anxious feelings in their tracks. With phobias, we go with you as you slowly face your phobic situation...one step at a time. We'll be there to help you... 100% of the way.

Who can we help

We offer programs for people with stress or anxiety related disorders, including extreme levels

of anxiety, panic episodes, agoraphobia, and obsessive compulsive disorder.

What about medication

Medication, used judiciously, can sometimes be a helpful component of an overall treatment plan. Our programs, however, are not based on medication as the primary recovery method.

Why can we help you

We are licensed professionals who have worked for many years with these kinds of problems. Some of us have conducted and published research on these topics, and some of us have overcome our own battles with these issues. We know first hand what it takes to regain control.

Call for our Community Service Pamphlet, or a free confidential telephone consultation.

Norfolk   **671-2273**   Virginia Beach

In association with Greenwich Psychological Associates, P.C.

Source: Courtesy of Greenwich Psychological Associates, Virginia Beach, VA.

(Exhibit 8-5), which has more of the character of an announcement and does not try to sell the service directly. Ogilvy's aggressive approach to ad copy is certainly on the cutting edge in most areas of the country for private medical practices. Another example of aggressive and creative print advertising is the use of a testimonial ad (see Exhibit 8-6). In many areas, however, ads of this type for a hospital would not raise an eyebrow. Where hospitals and other health care providers pioneer, physicians often follow. The physician who is first in a market with aggressive ad copy may obtain a real competitive advantage—as well as the envy of and criticism from peers.

Kenneth Roman and Jane Maas have written a guide that concisely describes what they believe works best in print, direct mail, radio, and television.[9] In the case of television, they recommend attracting the viewer's attention in the first five seconds by presenting a single-minded, uncomplicated, short dramatic message featuring people instead of objects. In the case of radio, they suggest stretching the listener's imagination, presenting a memorable sound (e.g., an unusual voice), stating your name and your promise early, and target marketing by choosing sta-

Exhibit 8-5 Example of Typical Private Medical Practice Print Ad

The Staff of
Riverview Medical Center
Is Pleased To Announce
The Association Of
Franklin L. Herbert, M.D.
Otolaryngologist
(Ear, Nose, & Throat)   Audiology
February 1, 1991
Head & Neck Surgery   Laser Surgery   Cosmetic Surgery
By Appointment
(804) 555-7876
18768 Lexington Rd.
Hampton Roads, VA 34887

tions and timeslots to reach specific segments, such as teenagers or housewives. By doing a little bit of reading yourself, you may be able to differentiate your advertising from your competitors' even if you don't rely on professional consulting assistance.

Unpaid Ads

Some of the most effective promotions come in the form of "free" advertising. There are countless ways of getting free advertising, including

- writing letters to the editor
- placing announcements in community bulletins about new services that you will offer or workshops that you can or will conduct
- sending announcements to the local newspaper of honors that you have received or new associates who have joined your practice
- sending announcements to the local newspaper or appropriate community or church newsletters of "open houses," talks, blood pressure clinics, cholesterol clinics, and so on
- volunteering to write a column for a local newspaper or newsletter
- distributing a news release on a newsworthy subject
- appearing on a local television or radio program or obtaining your own program.[10] (Some radio and television stations will charge you for hosting a program, other stations will pay a salary for your services, while still others will neither pay a salary nor assess a fee. Generally, cable stations will charge a fee. Commercial stations may be more inclined to pay a salary. Some commercial stations may give you a program and pay you a salary if you advertise with them.)

Exhibit 8-6 Sample of a Testimonial Ad

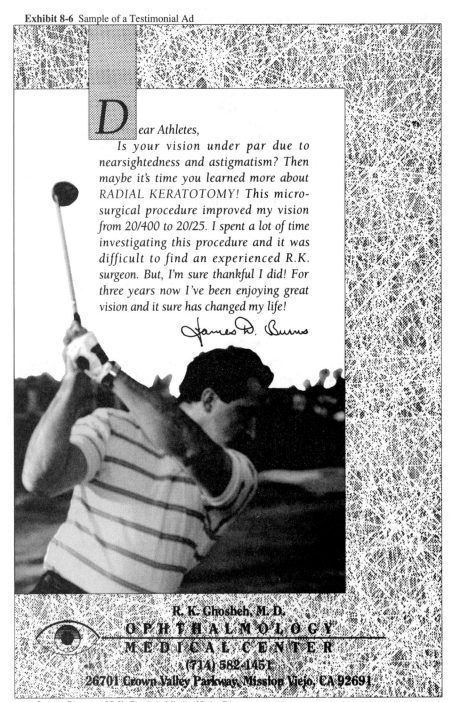

Dear Athletes,

Is your vision under par due to nearsightedness and astigmatism? Then maybe it's time you learned more about RADIAL KERATOTOMY! This micro-surgical procedure improved my vision from 20/400 to 20/25. I spent a lot of time investigating this procedure and it was difficult to find an experienced R.K. surgeon. But, I'm sure thankful I did! For three years now I've been enjoying great vision and it sure has changed my life!

R. K. Ghosheh, M. D.

OPHTHALMOLOGY
MEDICAL CENTER
(714) 582-1451
26701 Crown Valley Parkway, Mission Viejo, CA 92691

Source: Courtesy of R.K. Ghosheh, Mission Viejo, CA.

A few of these strategies deserve particular comment because of the exposure they can provide. News releases are a particular favorite in the free ad category. As you might imagine, TV ads during prime time can be very expensive. How much do you think that a two-minute advertisement would cost on the local six o'clock news? Writing effective news releases can get you the equivalent of several two-minute television ads per year as well as newspaper coverage that is equivalent to a large display ad.

The key to writing an effective news release is to remember who you are writing it for. Your target is a reporter who is in need of a story. A news release must tell the reporter that he or she can get an interesting, timely story by calling you. The format of a news release is important. It should cover the five Ws of newspaper reporting—who, when, what, where, and why—in a concise, clearly worded manner.

Exhibit 8-7 contains a news release. The *who* is of course you, but you want to indicate this in a clear and, if possible, visually exciting way. Next, you want to indicate the *when,* or the date of release. If you are releasing information that is not to be made public before a certain date, state "Not for Release before. . . . " The *what* should be summarized in your headline. The headline needs to be enticing, but it should not be sensationalistic. Reporters are bombarded with news releases, and if they sense that you are trying to overstate your case, you will quickly be filed in the wastepaper basket. The *why* should be in the body of the news release. You must demonstrate the validity of your release. Why should the reporter care? Why should his or her readers, listeners, or viewers care? Generally, a good tactic

Exhibit 8-7 Sample News Release

NEWS RELEASE FROM THE OFFICE OF
ROBERT BROWN, M.D.
JULY 18, 1991
FOR IMMEDIATE RELEASE

Driver Training Students Tour Bayview Hospital Emergency Room

Students in Riverview High School's Driver Education Program are being given a tour of Bayview's emergency room in an effort to educate them on the perils of reckless and drunk driving. Emergency room personnel familiarize the students with the typical injuries suffered by accident victims and the necessary medical procedures.

Dr. Robert Brown, who initiated the program, stated, "I hope that seeing the possible consequences of reckless behavior will act as a deterrent."

The program has been in effect for three weeks, and 47 students have toured the emergency room.

FOR ADDITIONAL INFORMATION CONTACT:
Robert Brown, M.D.
(804) 555-7639
or
5673 Anderson Rd., Virginia Beach, VA 23453

---

is to point out the personal importance of the information to the reporter's audience. If appropriate, state how it can affect their lives. Finally, you want to end the news release with a clear statement of *where* the reporter can go to get additional information. This can be a paper or workshop that you are presenting, your name and office telephone number, or both. News releases must be short and clearly written, and ideally they should include some numbers or catchy facts. You don't have to be a national expert to distribute a news release. The only requirements are that you are knowledgeable about the subject and possess a minimal amount of audacity.

Once you have developed a news release, the next task is to get it to the right people. Look in the local newspaper for reporters who are writing local articles. Don't limit yourself to the health, fitness, and science reporters. Your objective should be to gradually assemble a mailing list of local newspaper, television, and radio reporters. By reading the newspaper each day and by noting television and radio talk show hosts, you can establish a mailing list with virtually no effort. The same task can be given to your secretary or another employee.

Another tactic is to target a media outlet for concentrated attention. Since newspaper, television, and radio reporters receive dozens of news releases each day, 95 percent of them are thrown out immediately after or even before they are read. To be effective, you have to get enough distribution of your news release *within* the newspaper or station to overcome the natural propensity to throw it out. This can be accomplished by targeting a cross section of the organization. For example, you might target a television station by mailing releases to several reporters, the program director, the assignment director, and the public affairs director as well as the host and producer of each of the locally produced programs. A reporter may throw the release out, but perhaps it will appeal to the assignment director, who may then instruct a reporter to see if there is an interesting story there. Remember also that, in television, early morning news crews, noon news crews, and especially weekend news crews are often looking for program material. Be certain that your press releases get to these personnel. How do you obtain all of these names? Have your secretary call your targeted media outlets and ask for names and job titles. It is that simple.

Getting a mention in a newspaper article or TV story is often a function of timing. If you want to develop this aspect of marketing your practice, then you must be responsive to the needs of reporters. When a reporter calls, you must talk to him or her then or call back *very shortly* thereafter. Remember, reporters work under tight deadlines and they need answers quickly. A print reporter most likely will be in the process of writing the story at the time he or she telephones you. If you are not immediately available, the reporter will call the next physician down the list. The reporter will pass you by even if it was your news release that provided the initial idea for the story. Another advantage of consistently responding quickly to reporters is that they will come to rely upon you for medical information. Reporters will begin to call you and quote you in stories that they generate. For example, if there is testimony in a trial regarding a prescription drug, a reporter may contact you for information regarding the possible side effects of the drug. You may then be mentioned in the story: "Dr. Fred Wilson noted that the drug could cause the side effects claimed by the defense but that these side effects are rare." Another example of this type of promotion is found in Exhibit 8-8. In this article, several local physicians give their opinions about a national news item.

Don't overlook distributing news releases to appropriate church, community, and specialty newsletters. Although their readership may be small, your chances of scoring a hit may be significantly greater, if only because newsletters receive a lower volume of releases than newspapers and the media. Also, a church or community newsletter may give you exposure to a relatively high proportion of potential patients. Once again, sending your news release to multiple targets within each organization will increase your chances of scoring a hit.

A personal appearance on a local radio or television program is another favorite in the free media ad category. You need a "hook" to get on a program, and a news release is a good start. Another alternative is to call the talk show host and explain what you would like to talk about on the program. The reaction you will get to this approach will vary, with the probability of success being greater in smaller markets.

How should you conduct yourself when you appear on a local television or radio talk program? It is important to remember that in order to communicate effectively with the typical television audience, you must use a style of presentation appropriate for about an eighth-grade level. This means that you should use simple, direct language. If you use a technical term, you should immediately define it or explain it. Being very specific and using examples will also increase your communication effectiveness. Keep your discussion at the level of greatest general interest. It is important to remember that viewers will be less interested in your topic than your patients would be. Patients care about their bodies, so they tend to be interested in what you have to say. If a viewer does not feel that your discussion is directly pertinent, he or she will probably not care, and with remote control and 25 cable alternatives readily available, you may be quickly "deselected."

Finally, a word of caution. No matter what you say or how clearly you state it, reporters will make mistakes. You will be frustrated because they will miss a major point you were trying to make, misquote you, or present only part of the total picture. All of this "goes with the territory." As an example, take the story of a doctor who was trying to persuade the city council in a rural Virginia community to allocate more money for emergency treatment services. She told a local newspaper that the cost of 24-hour-a-day emergency services was about $1.50 per year for each county resident. In an attempt to put the cost of these services in perspec-

Exhibit 8-8 Newspaper Article Quoting Local Physicians

Henson's pneumonia treatable if diagnosed

Antibiotics could have saved him

By April Witt
Staff writer

The virulent strain of pneumonia that reportedly killed Muppets creator Jim Henson is common and usually curable if treated quickly with antibiotics, local doctors say.

"The streptococcus pneumonia is the most common kind of pneumonia to occur at home," Dr. William Edmondson, a Norfolk internist, said Thursday.

"It hits hard and once you have it you usually get sick enough to get help," he said. "It's something that drives you to the doctor quickly. It is the rare patient that toughs it out and does not get help."

Dr. Oscar E. Edwards, a Norfolk internist said: "Streptococcus pneumonia is tragic to die of. It is the most eminently treatable of them all. If he'd have just come in sooner, with a little bit of penicillin, and he'd probably have been well."

Henson, the creator of Kermit the Frog, Miss Piggy and a host of other beloved Muppets, died Wednesday in a New York Hospital of what his doctor said was "a massive bacterial infection, more specifically known as streptococcus pneumonia."

Dr. David M. Gelmont, director of intensive care at New York Hospital-Cornell Medical Center in New York, said the 53-year-old was healthy until coming down with flu-like symptoms Friday.

Asked why Henson failed to seek more aggressive treatment for his illness, Susan Berry, a spokeswoman for Jim Henson Productions, said: "My guess is he's totally absorbed. He couldn't be bothered. He was very cavalier with his health."

Henson worsened, returned to New York on Monday and checked into the hospital the next day. But by then the infection had spread through his body, damaging vital organs so severely that it could not be controlled by antibiotics, the usual treatment, Gelmont said.

Pneumonia, which strikes about 2 million Americans annually, is an inflammation of the lungs. Although a variety of bacteria and vi-

ruses can cause pneumonia, it is most commonly caused by streptococcus, the bacteria that reportedly killed Henson.

Once known as the "captain of the men of death," pneumonia has been much more easily treatable since the invention of antibiotics.

But pneumonia still kills more than 40,000 Americans annually. Most of those who do not survive pneumonia are either very young, elderly or debilitated by a serious disease such as cancer.

Among those at especially high risk of dying are people whose immune systems have been weakened by diseases such as AIDS or who are taking immune-suppressing medicines.

Asked Thursday whether Henson had AIDS, his doctor said: "Categorically, he did not have AIDS."

Dr. Scott A. Miller of Norfolk said no one needs to invoke AIDS to explain a pneumonia death in 1990. "If you get someone who comes in too late with this, you can't save them," said Miller, a Norfolk internist who specializes in infectious diseases. "It's upsetting, but it's the way of the world.

"A few years ago I took care of a 24-year-old woman — healthy, no AIDS — who came in with a little pneumonia and was dead in 24 hours. We don't have to invoke AIDS and we don't have to invoke alternative lifestyles to explain it. Mother Nature can do all of those things."

Streptococcal pneumonia is caused by a common bacteria. "Some people carry it in their mouths and are not affected by it," said Dr. Ignacia Ripoll of Norfolk, a specialist in pulmonary medicine.

People typically contract streptococcal pneumonia when "they have a little cold or a little virus," Ripoll said. "Then their body becomes more susceptible to this infection.

"Once they have this infection, they get sick very fast. Within a matter of hours, people are having chills and a fever and they feel quite ill."

Given a small dose of penicillin or another antibiotic, patients typically improve within 24 hours, Ripoll said.

Untreated, the infection can spread into the blood and damage vital organs, he said.

"We can still reverse it, but these people typically spend weeks in intensive care," he said. "When people develop multi-organ failure, 70 percent of them will die regardless of what you do."

Source: Reprinted with permission from *The Virginia Pilot-Ledger Star*, May 18, 1990, p. 2.

tive, she lightly dropped the comment that services were cheaper than a six-pack of beer. The next day a newspaper headline proclaimed, "Montgomery Emergency Services—Cheaper Than a Six-Pack!" To top it off, Montgomery was a dry county. Despite such possible pitfalls, it is important to remember that *all* exposure is valuable. Paraphrasing P.T. Barnum's adage, short of overtly negative statements, don't be concerned with what the media say about you as long as they spell your name correctly.

A letter to the editor is another useful variety of unpaid ad. Writing a letter to the editor will increase the chance that potential patients will hear your name or learn something about you. A good strategy for getting a letter published is to expand on an issue or topic already covered by an article printed in the newspaper. A sample letter to the editor is found in Exhibit 8-9.

But What Promotions Work?

At this point you may well be asking, "But what works? What will give me the most promotional effect for my time and money?" All of the ideas discussed can

Exhibit 8-9 Letter to the Editor

May 17, 1990

Editor
The Virginian-Examiner
150 W. Ambleton Ave.
Norfolk, VA 23510

Dear Editor:

I am writing in response to columnist William Johnson's article on "The Horrors of Child Abuse" (May 8, 1991).

As a practicing psychiatrist, I can testify that the horrors of physical and sexual abuse do not stop with the child and the child's parents. The scars and the pain follow the child into adulthood. As an adult, feelings of guilt, anger, and fear persist. Individuals abused as children feel different, and they struggle to trust others. Sexual problems are common. Alcoholism, compulsive eating, and violence are also frequent companions of the adult who was abused as a child.

Recently, the media has given much attention to the sexually abused child. We must not ignore the adult who carries his or her own pain into adult life and who may need help and encouragement in dealing with the wounds.

Respectfully,
George Gravely, M.D.

and do work *if you use them effectively and if you use them long enough.* A cornerstone of most successful medical promotion is personal contact with potential referral sources and patients, including one-on-one meetings, lunches, community services, and community presentations. Paid media can be useful if you can adequately finance the projects. The expression that "it takes money to make money" is particularly apt when it comes to advertising. Paid advertising, irrespective of the media, is most effective with repetition, and that costs money.

In general, the best way of generating referrals through the media is to get something to appear in print. People tend to cut out your name or your announcement or an article that you wrote or you are quoted in. They will often keep the clipping for weeks or months, and when they finally do need medical services, they will seek you out. In many ways, the ad, announcement, or article is like a business card with your name on it.

Television gives you outstanding visibility and name recognition. The fleeting nature of the medium, however, is a limitation, and you should not have great expectations based on a single appearance on a talk program. The cost of radio is substantially less than the cost of television. Once again, however, a few sporadic appearances will not constitute an effective radio campaign. Unless you devote substantial funds to advertising, the importance of these media lies in the part that they can play in your overall promotional effort, and this part should not be underestimated.

The final selection of a doctor is often the result of many events that occurred over an extended period of time. It may result from name recognition gained over months or years of published letters to the editor, appearances on radio and television programs, quotations in the newspaper, and a few personal encounters. Slowly a prospective patient or referral source becomes familiar with you and comes to believe that you are someone who may be able to help. When the prospective patient finally needs medical services, he or she is likely to call you because in a sense he or she has "known" you for an extended period of time. It should be clear from this that promotion is a long-term activity that must never cease but that may change in nature as your practice develops and matures.

Patients can come from anywhere, and virtually anyone can become a referral source. If you are cognizant of this essential truth, then any interpersonal contact has promotional potential. Whether you are visiting your dentist or lawyer, getting your car repaired or your plumbing fixed, or simply mingling at a party, you should always be open to the possibility that you are talking to a potential patient or referral source. When appropriate, manage to work a few comments into the discussion about your profession. The key word here is *appropriate*. Remember, if you do this in a clumsy manner or in a way that is inappropriate to the context of the conversation, you will be promoting yourself as a bore. Clearly, that is counterproductive. If you really are a bore, then you must learn when and how to drop a line or two about your work. It is not essential to list all of your accomplishments. It is far better to state your profession unobtrusively and then illustrate your good qualities by being an attentive listener and making appropriate additions to the conversation.

Finally, your own patients can be among your best referral sources. John Ernhardt, M.D., has offered several excellent suggestions for marketing to your own patients, including these:[11]

- Show regard for patient's time. This involves being punctual for your appointments and devoting sufficient time to each patient.
- Provide extra time for each patient who is hospitalized, and also make it a quality visit. Try to reduce the patient's anxiety. Also make courtesy calls, at no charge, to those of your patients who are under the care of another physician.
- Be available to talk on the telephone. In nonemergency situations, this could include having a staff person tell patients that you will return calls during a specified half-hour period.
- Provide patients with drug samples, thereby medicating them more quickly and relieving them of an expense if they cannot tolerate a new medication.
- Take the time to send appropriate letters and documents. This includes responding to patients who sent you greeting cards, forwarding medical records and test results to other physicians in a timely manner, and sending letters to family members of deceased patients.

It is important to approach these tasks with the proper mental attitude. They should not be undertaken as a way of manipulating patients. They should be done sincerely and considerately and should demonstrate that you are a professional who is concerned about your patients' welfare. If they are done with sincerity, then they will create patient good-will and will also set an example of appropriateness and courtesy for your staff to follow.

MARKETING RESEARCH

Marketing research is the process of obtaining marketing information that can then be used to make management decisions. Collecting marketing information can be done by using exceedingly complex, sophisticated, and costly methods or by simply asking patients for their opinions. Typically, the type of marketing research useful to the private medical practice is relatively simple and direct. The marketing research skills required to collect and interpret this information are well within the range and previous training of most doctors. However, if your time or interest precludes direct involvement in some or all phases of marketing research, you can contract out some or all of the technical tasks to a consultant.

Marketing research can be valuable to you for a number of reasons, including these:[12]

- It allows you to recognize, understand, and take advantage of opportunities in the marketing environment.
- It helps you identify competitive threats.
- It allows you to plan more effectively.
- It improves the quality of your marketing decisions.
- It reduces uncertainty and risk.
- It helps you evaluate patient reactions to new ideas, programs, services, and so on.

What should private medical practice market research typically involve? This question relates back to the marketing planning process that was presented in Exhibit 8-1. Marketing research is a tool you can use to better understand the external and internal environmental factors that confront your practice. For example, you can use marketing research to evaluate your competition; the feasibility of various practice locations; legal and ethical constraints; the life cycle of some of your more ephemeral services or procedures; patient demand, including demand for services that patients desire; and patient perceptions regarding your services and your practice. You can also use marketing research to test alternative marketing strategies and plans before you put proposed strategies and plans into operation.

The process of actually conducting marketing research can be broken into five phases:

1. defining the problem
2. designing the research study
3. collecting data
4. analyzing the data
5. interpreting the data

You must decide who should conduct this research. Some marketing research techniques, such as patient surveys, can be effectively implemented by doctors. This does not necessarily mean, however, that this would be a good use of your time or your staff's time. You may decide that hiring a marketing consultant will be the most cost-effective alternative.

Understanding how to conduct various forms of marketing research will help you to decide whether to undertake some of this work yourself or whether to retain a marketing consultant. If you do retain a consultant, knowing how marketing research is conducted will help you to understand and evaluate the work that the consultant will be performing for you. It is important for you to assess your own skills realistically in order to determine which research methods are reasonable options for you. If you have a strong statistical background—or if you have always wanted to learn more about statistics and have the time to obtain this knowledge— then quantitative research methods are a real option. If, on the other hand, you remember little more than how to calculate a mean, it would probably be best for you to limit yourself to qualitative research methods. The Sorcerer's Apprentice, you may recall, attempted to employ a seemingly easy-to-use but powerful tool without really having the appropriate knowledge or skill. The disaster that ensued should be food for thought. A modern equivalent of the Sorcerer's power is the personal computer coupled with statistics software. You could easily put yourself into the Apprentice's role, if you don't understand what you are doing, since many of these statistical packages can be operated so easily. Numbers will come out, but they may be totally meaningless if they are based on a faulty research design or if you have not met appropriate assumptions for the correct utilization of a statistic.

Creating a clear definition of the problem you intend to investigate is essential if the end product is to be meaningful. For example, suppose that you decide that you want to learn why your patients select and continue to use your practice. This question could be examined in a number of different ways. The answer could involve referral sources, advertising or other forms of promotion, the practice location, patient satisfaction with previous treatment, fee schedules, and so on. If you have not clarified in your own mind what you really want to learn, then you might easily design a study in which you waste time and effort collecting data that are not relevant to your real concern.

Designing the study is the next step in the process. At this point a decision must be made regarding how to collect the information. For example, will you use *quantitative* methods, such as a questionnaire, or *qualitative* methods, such as a focus group? If you are primarily interested in understanding concepts and issues, then a qualitative method will probably be appropriate. On the other hand, if you need statistical insight in order to answer your questions, then you will probably have to use a quantitative method. For example, if you want to know what the major patient satisfaction and dissatisfaction *issues* are regarding your billing, then you can obtain this information with qualitative methods. If you want to know what proportion of patients are satisfied and what proportion are dissatisfied, then you will have to use a quantitative method. If you decide to use quantitative methods, you should also decide which data analysis methods you will use. It is important to consider this question in the design stage so that the data that are collected will be appropriate for the data analysis methods.

The next stage involves collecting the data. Irrespective of whether you are using quantitative or qualitative methods, you will be confronted with the practical difficulties of conducting research in an ongoing business. Secretaries will not get questionnaires to patients because of ringing telephones or other job demands, patients will not respond because they don't have time, and sampling will be compromised when a questionnaire was given to Mrs. Smith instead of Mr. Jones because that was easier. Similarly, an interviewer may not ask the same questions of all interviewees. In short, the quality of your data will largely depend on how proficiently you and your staff conduct the study.

The next phase of marketing research is the analysis and interpretation of the data. Data analysis methods include examining simple descriptive statistics, such as means, standard deviations, percentages, and frequencies. Analysis of the relationship between two or more variables can be assessed by using, for example, correlation, regression, factor analysis, and cross-tabulation. Qualitative data must be analyzed by looking for common themes and ideas in subjects' responses. Consultants can be particularly useful in helping you with the mechanics of analyzing the data.

Once the data are analyzed, then the final task is to determine what it all means. Even if you conduct the research yourself, you may want to talk to a consultant regarding the interpretation, since a consultant will probably be less influenced by preconceived notions than you. The final interpretation, however, should never be totally left to a consultant. The study results are only useful to you if they directly pertain to the specifics of your practice. A consultant cannot know your practice as well as you do. It is essential, therefore, for you to subject any consultant's research conclusions to a thorough logical analysis based on what *you* know about your practice.

Marketing Research Methods

Secondary Sources

Secondary sources are sources of data that have already been collected for other purposes. One excellent secondary source consists of the records that already exist in your practice. For example, your medical office management database almost certainly contains important marketing research information. Data on patient demographics, referral sources, procedures conducted, diagnoses, and so on, may all be useful for answering marketing research questions. Internal sources of marketing data can be particularly attractive because you know something about their existence, thereby avoiding long, involved research. You also know something about their accuracy. You probably know, for example, if your secretary does a good job of determining referral sources before entering them in the computer. In addition, the data from internal sources have usually been collected and stored in a manner relevant to your practice, since you are probably already using this information for some purpose.

External secondary sources can provide you with a broad range of relevant information. In effect, the knowledge of the marketing world is available for you to utilize. One good place to start is at a university library. Computer searches of relevant topics, as well as reviewing selected periodicals, can provide doctors with significant marketing research information. Exhibit 8-10 contains a list of some periodicals that contain marketing research studies or summaries that may be of use to doctors. Other sources of marketing research findings include national and state professional associations; the American Marketing Association; the American Medical Association; state or regional offices on aging, adolescence, and so on; school boards; state hospital associations; state and regional economic development agencies; university bureaus of business research; and local chambers of commerce. Many of these groups publish marketing reports or studies containing data that can be used to evaluate various market segments. For example, the American Medical Association's Council on Long Range Planning and Development has assessed the changing demographics of internists' patient population.[13] They concluded that the increasing number of elderly patients will affect the nature of illnesses treated by internists. They also predict that there will be increasing competition between subspecialties within internal medicine.

The primary advantage of using secondary sources is that you can obtain market research data without having to collect it yourself. As a result, you may be able to answer market research questions without using your time or a consultant's time to construct a questionnaire, interview patients, and so on. You also will not have to ask your secretaries to distribute questionnaires or your patients to take time to answer interview questions or complete questionnaires. Assuming that there is nothing unusual about your market or your practice, that is, nothing that would make the study results inapplicable to your circumstances, use of published findings can be very cost- and time-effective. At a minimum, secondary source data will help you to more precisely define your research questions given the ex-

Exhibit 8-10 Publications Containing Health Care Marketing Papers and Research

American Demographics	*Journal of Pharmaceutical Marketing and*
Clinical Laboratory Management Review	*Management*
Guest Relations in Practice	*Market Focus*
Health Care Competition Week	*Marketing Showcase for Physicians*
Health Care Management Review	*Marketing to Doctors*
Health Care Strategic Management	*Mature Marketing Report*
Health Care Strategist	*Medical Care*
Health Marketing Quarterly	*Medical Economics*
Healthcare Advertising Review	*Medical Marketing and Media*
Healthcare Entrepreneur's Newsletter	*Physician's Marketing*
Healthcare Financing Review	*Professional Healthcare Marketing*
Healthcare Marketing Abstracts	*Selling to Seniors*
Journal of Ambulatory Care Marketing	*Senior Market Report*
Journal of Health Care Marketing	*Social Science and Medicine*
Journal of Medical Practice Management	*Strategic Health Care Marketing*

periences of other researchers. It can also give you ideas concerning questionnaire and interview question content, administration considerations, and data analysis methods.

Patient Surveys*

The patient survey is a cost-effective and practical market research method if you have some knowledge of or willingness to learn statistics and questionnaire construction. A patient survey can provide you with

1. a thorough understanding of your patients and why they came to you
2. data on your current referral sources
3. an evaluation of your practice's performance, including patient satisfaction, front office effectiveness, and so on
4. guidance for future marketing efforts

Since any marketing effort must be built on a thorough understanding of patient needs, patient satisfaction with current services, and the effects of current promotional efforts, the patient survey can be an excellent method for introducing marketing concepts into a practice.

Designing and conducting the study and analyzing the survey data involve going through a number of specific steps. Each step is essential to creating a survey that is minimally obtrusive to administer while also providing you with the information that you need.

Question Development. Asking the right questions is the most fundamental skill in constructing a patient survey. A good place to start is to organize your thinking around different groups of questions. For example, you might want to write a group of questions to assess patient satisfaction issues, another group to assess clinical need, and still another group to assess referral sources. Finally, you should also include a group of questions to assess the demographic characteristics of your patients. Demographic questions about age, sex, race, and so on, will allow you to break down your results by demographic categories. You may want to know, for example, if newspaper ads are generating significantly more female than male patients. A questionnaire coverage list used by a psychiatric practice that conducted an in-house patient marketing survey is found in Exhibit 8-11.

As you explore each question area, you will find that many specific issues arise. Each of these specific issues should be addressed in a separate survey question. For example, patients can express their satisfaction with your practice on a num-

---

*This section has been adapted from Robert Solomon, "Using a Patient Survey to Market Your Practice," *Journal of Medical Practice Management*, Vol. 6, No. 1, pp. 51–54, with permission of Williams and Wilkins, © 1990.

Exhibit 8-11 Questionnaire Item Coverage Used by a Psychiatric Practice

A. Demographic Questions		
Age	Sex	Education
Living Arrangements	Race	Employment
Income	Marital Status	Children
Legal Problems	Psych. History	Session Type
Insurance Company	A.A. Membership	
B. Clinical Question Coverage		
Anxiety	Depression	Alcohol//Drug
Self-Esteem	Marital Conflict	Eating/Weight
Child Problems	Sexual Concerns	Loneliness
Separation/Divorce	Violent Temper	Loss
Previous Treatment	Hospitalization	Medication
Homosexuality	Treatment Length	A.C.O.A.
C. Referral Sources		
Friend/Relative	Physician	Therapist
Clergy	CHAMPUS	Court/Legal
Attorney	Newspaper Ad	Yellow Pages
TV	Radio	Other Patient
D. Satisfaction Coverage		
Problem Now	Improvement	Quality
Location	Fees	Clerical Staff
Policies/Procedures	Recommend to Others	
Today's Session	Answering	

Source: Reprinted from Robert Solomon, "Using a Patient Survey to Market Your Practice," *Journal of Medical Practice Management*, Vol. 6, No. 1, pp. 51–54, with permission of Williams & Wilkins, © 1990.

ber of different dimensions, including the quality of your service, the reasonableness of your fees, the convenience of your location, and the friendliness and efficiency of your front office personnel. By addressing these issues in separate questions, you will be able to identify practice strengths and weaknesses precisely.

It is important to involve all categories of practice employees in the survey design process. As a result of their different jobs, front office staff, nurses, and colleagues will interact with patients in somewhat different ways. This will generate some unique satisfaction, service, and clinical issues that will be specific to each of these different organizational functions. A brainstorming session is a good way to get all employee groups involved in thinking about what issues should be covered by the survey and to obtain specific questions. Finally, reviewing the published papers of other researchers and practitioners can be a valuable source of ideas for areas of survey coverage and specific item content. For example, Barnes and Mowatt and Christensen and Giese provide good examples of survey coverage and item content.[14]

Scaling. Scaling is the process of attaching response scales to questions. Some questions can best be answered with a yes or a no. When asking yes/no questions, instruct the patient to respond to each question. If you tell the patient to check only those answers that apply, you will not know whether the absence of a checkmark indicates no or a failure to respond.

Other questions may require a "continuous" scale. Several examples of continuous scales are found in Exhibit 8-12. When writing continuous scales, the object is to make the anchors appear to be equally spaced. Generally, this type of scale contains four to six anchor points.

On occasion you may want to ask a question that requires the patient to write an answer (e.g., "In a few words, describe the problem that brought you to us"). It is a good idea to ask as few questions of this type as possible. Narrative write-in responses take patients more time to answer, and they are more difficult for you to interpret.

Questionnaire Design. The questionnaire should be designed so that it has a logical flow of questions based on subject area. Put all of the satisfaction questions in one area, the demographic questions in another, and so on. It is very important that patients be able to complete the questionnaire in a reasonable amount of time. Twenty minutes should be considered a maximum time limit. You can evaluate the clarity of questions and instructions and get a good idea of how long it will take to complete the survey by pretesting it on you and your staff. Usually you will find

Exhibit 8-12 Continuous Response Scales

Excellent 1	Good 2	Fair 3	Poor 4	
Satisfied 1	Somewhat Satisfied 2	Somewhat Dissatisfied 3	Dissatisfied 4	
Strongly Agree 1	Agree 2	Disagree 3	Strongly Disagree 4	
Not at All 1	2	Moderately 3	4	Extremely 5
Extremely Helpful 1	Very Helpful 2	Moderately Helpful 3	Slightly Helpful 4	Not at All Helpful 5

Source: Reprinted from Robert Solomon, "Using a Patient Survey to Market Your Practice," *Journal of Medical Practice Management*, Vol. 6, No. 1, pp. 51–54, with permission of Williams & Wilkins, © 1990.

that the first version of a questionnaire is too long. You then have to make some hard choices between what is essential and what would be nice to know about.

The survey instructions are critical to success. They should give the patient a reason for completing the questionnaire. For example, you might state, "We are very interested in the quality of services that we provide to our patients. You can help us provide the best possible care by candidly answering the following questions." The instructions should emphasize that responses will remain confidential. If you decide to conduct an anonymous survey, your instructions should make this very clear, and you should use a questionnaire collection method that guarantees this anonymity.

Sampling. It is important that patients who complete the questionnaire be representative of all of your patients. This means that their demographic traits, diagnoses, and so on, should be typical. If they are representative, then you can make inferences from your sample of respondents to the rest of your clientele. Obtaining a representative sample is not very difficult to achieve. If your practice has a high proportion of patients who return several times, you can offer virtually all patients the questionnaire. If patients tend to come for a single visit, then you can ensure representativeness by extending the study over a period of time, such as a month. This may require distributing a questionnaire to every fourth or fifth patient. Think very carefully about the survey administration and distribution procedures and consider whether they in any way tend to systematically exclude any type of patient. If they do not, then your sampling will almost certainly be representative.

The number of patients to survey is also important. An arbitrary but useful rule of thumb is to get completed questionnaires from 100 patients, or 75 percent of your clientele, whichever number is smaller. The object is to obtain a sample large enough to represent all facets of your patient population. On the other hand, you don't want to collect more data than you really need. Remember, all the data that are collected will have to be recorded for analysis, and that will take time.

Administration Procedures. It is important for the survey administration procedure to guarantee patient anonymity. This will increase the patient response rate and patient truthfulness. A good way to achieve this is by having patients place the completed questionnaires in a box in the waiting room.

Survey distribution, recordkeeping, and collection will compete with ongoing business operations for clerical time. It is critical to survey success, therefore, to take into account current office routines when designing questionnaire administration and collection methods. The object is to make the survey fit into the normal office routine as unobtrusively as possible. If staff members begin to feel that the survey is a burden, then haphazard recordkeeping and distribution may threaten the legitimacy of your sampling. By including the front office personnel in the design of the survey and the distribution method, you will allow them to feel a sense of ownership in the whole process. As a result, they will be more interested in making the distribution procedure work.

Data Analysis. Data analysis should be performed on a computer. There are many software packages for personal computers that are able to analyze the data from this type of survey. SPSS, SYSTAT, and StatView are examples of programs that can perform the necessary data analysis tasks. The statistical training that is provided in most medical school programs is adequate to understand the output from these programs. You may wish to do additional reading on specific statistical topics, such as factor analysis, significance testing, and correlation, as they become relevant. You may also wish to retain a consultant to assist you with the interpretation of the data.

Data analysis does not have to be complex. Simply noting the proportion of respondents who express a particular response on an item is often informative. For example, if 85 percent of the respondents rate your billing procedures as "Excellent," then this indicates a high level of satisfaction. Similarly, looking at the average response for different demographic groups can be informative. For example, if women average 3.0 on the question, "How responsive is the front office to your needs?" whereas men average 4.0, this may point to a potential problem. (To determine whether this difference is statistically significant, the means should be tested using an appropriate significance test, such as a t-test or a chi-square test.)

Marketing research that you produce yourself will probably not be elegant or publishable, because the refinements of methodology and data analysis usually associated with publication in scholarly journals are likely to be missing. It should, however, provide answers to the marketing questions that you have about your practice. It should do it inexpensively, and in a relatively easy and unobtrusive manner.

Case Example. CCV was an outpatient psychiatric practice with four full-time and four part-time professionals. The practice conducted a patient survey to obtain immediate information regarding current marketing efforts and to provide guidance for future marketing efforts.

Based on discussions with therapists and front office staff, an 80-question survey was designed to assess the variables listed in Exhibit 8-11. Ninety percent of the practice's 142 patients were offered the survey. Eighty-five usable questionnaires were returned over a five-week period.

The data analysis indicated that patients came to the practice with five distinct clusters of symptoms:

1. self-esteem, depression, and anxiety problems
2. sexual concerns
3. family problems
4. personal loss
5. latent substance abuse

As a result, a television commercial was designed that emphasized these five clusters. In addition, the ad was directed toward those with demographic characteristics associated with patients who had better insurance coverage. The study indicated that paid print advertising, such as Yellow Pages and newspaper advertising, generated patients who had less satisfactory clinical outcomes and lower incomes. As a result, the advertising budget deemphasized Yellow Pages advertising and eliminated general newspaper advertising.

"Friends" was identified as a referral category that generated a disproportionate share of patients who had experienced a personal loss. A waiting room flyer on loss was designed to address this referral source specifically. Similarly, gays and more highly educated patients also experienced disproportionate problems with loss. As a result, a display ad in a gay newspaper emphasized this issue. Therapists providing public service seminars understood that better-educated audiences might be particularly interested in this topic.

The groups that were most satisfied with the practice's clinical services included those who were divorced, adult children of alcoholics, the more highly educated, and gays. Since personal referrals were found to be the single best source of referrals, the practice implemented a bootstrapping strategy based on selectively marketing to those groups with the best chance of clinical success. At the same time, efforts to attract alcohol and drug treatment patients were reduced or eliminated, because this group had lower levels of clinical success. Finally, a new patient intake form was designed to collect information from all new patients on those questions found to be most important in the study.

Focus Groups

A focus group is a marketing research method. A group of eight to ten people is assembled for an open-ended discussion regarding one or several issues or topics. The object is to obtain rich qualitative information from the subjects. The discussion should be led by a professionally trained moderator, and you may be present as an observer if you wish. One advantage of a focus group is that the group "process," or the interaction between group members, can often disclose more about a topic than would be revealed by conducting one-on-one in-depth interviews or quantitative research. A focus group contains a small sample of non–randomly selected participants who may be subject to the biases of an analyst who may have preconceived notions regarding what will be discovered. If a focus group is properly conducted, however, and if you are aware of its inherent weaknesses, the weaknesses need not interfere with its usefulness to you.

Focus groups can be used for a number of different purposes. They are excellent for stimulating your own thinking regarding your practice and how your practice is perceived by your patients. Ideas generated by this exploratory approach may or may not then be tested using quantitative research. Focus groups can also be used to obtain information that is not accessible through quantitative methods. For example, information obtained from a focus group regarding the difficulties of scheduling a first appointment to address the problem of rectal bleeding would be very difficult, if not impossible, to obtain using an anonymous patient survey. It simply is too personal a matter to be explored in depth in a questionnaire. Focus groups can provide an opportunity to explore your patients' decision-making processes. Why do patients decide to return to your practice? What are the aspects of your practice that first attracted them? What issues do your patients consider when they evaluate the quality of your care or your fees? Focus groups can also help determine how patients and prospective patients will respond to a new service or advertisement.

Axelrod graphically described a further reason for using a qualitative approach, such as a focus group, when he stated that it is "a chance to 'experience' a 'flesh and blood' consumer [patient]. It is the opportunity for the client [physician] to put himself in the position of the consumer [patient] and to be able to look at his product and his category from her vantage point."[15] To put it another way, a focus group can let you "hear your patients talk." As Donald J. Messmer, president of Mid-Atlantic Research, stated, "Clients will often say 'This is the first time that I have actually heard my customers talk about my product or service.' You can't wipe that image of their comments away. It can be a powerful tool to get management's attention—it can be a revelation."[16]

Charles Keown has suggested a framework for organizing a focus group.[17] The first step in the process is to hire a consultant to conduct the focus group research for you. The consultant will arrange for an appropriate meetingplace, possibly find group subjects, and provide the group moderator.

There are several reasons for having a consultant conduct the focus group research. First, an effective focus group moderator must be trained and experienced in using a focus group to be able to stimulate a group process from people who are total strangers. In order to do this, the moderator must be able to determine the conscious and unconscious causes of behavior, and use the group process to obtain information that is more insightful than normally could be obtained through simple discussions. Most doctors have not developed these skills.

Second, since your practice is such a close, personal issue to you, you may tend to become defensive, or react punitively to direct or implied criticism. These types of reactions will quickly stifle free discussion. Finally, your presence may inhibit the willingness of focus group participants to speak candidly about your practice.

A focus group consultant can be retained through a marketing consulting firm or by contacting the business school at a local university. You should personally meet the consultant and be certain that he or she understands the objectives of your research. If you are not comfortable with the consultant, then select another one. If you are working with a consulting firm and they will not or cannot replace the consultant, then go to another firm.

A list of characteristics to look for in a focus group moderator is found in Exhibit 8-13. The moderator is under considerable pressure during a focus group session. If the moderator does not perform effectively during the few hours of the

Exhibit 8-13 Characteristics to Look for in Focus Group Moderators

Focus group moderators
1. must be specially trained in group processes
2. must be confident and self-assured
3. must be able to interpret responses outside of their own value systems
4. must be able to establish rapport with a wide variety of people
5. must be "intuitive" and be able to quickly develop communion with others
6. must be able to understand and appreciate marketing issues from the perspective of their clients

Source: Adapted from Y. Brugaletta, "Guidelines to Set Up, Use, and Analyze Focus Groups" in *Marketing News*, October 1975, with permission of American Marketing Association, © 1975.

session, then you will have wasted your money. The moderator must be able to respond to totally unpredictable events as they occur. This includes being adept at dealing with (1) quiet, passive groups or group members, (2) overly excited groups or group members, (3) outspoken group members, (4) the "wise guy," (5) inconsistencies that develop in the group discussion, and (6) groups that go off on a tangent.

In order to be effective, the moderator will have to do some homework. He or she must understand the characteristics of your patients so as to choose clothing and a communication style that will allow group members to work together effectively. The moderator will require spontaneity, humor, self-awareness of personal biases, and the ability to express thoughts clearly. In addition, the moderator should construct a moderator guide, which is an outline used to ensure that all of the relevant topics are covered. An effective moderator will use this guide as an initial agenda but will let a conversation develop if it appears to be relevant.

After you select a consultant, you must define your research questions. The consultant should help you with this process. Research questions involving more complex and personal issues will be most suited to examination through the focus group method. As the group session proceeds, patients will tend to explore the reasons for their actions, and they will probably develop a greater level of comfort in discussing them, since there will be others present who have been in similar situations or have experienced similar feelings. In a sense, there has to be something that is complex enough or debatable enough over which to develop a group process. Whether your waiting room should be pinky beige or powder blue is hardly the kind of topic to excite interest.

Next, you must decide who should be in the focus group. Should it be current patients or people who are potential patients? Often the research questions will help you identify the appropriate group participants. For example, if you are investigating questions related to patient satisfaction, you would obviously have to use current patients. On the other hand, if you are trying to assess the impact of a proposed television commercial or newspaper display ad on people who are unfamiliar with your services and skills, then a group composed of potential patients will provide you with better information.

Since people generally feel more comfortable talking to others who are similar, several focus groups, with different participants in each, may be necessary. For example, one group might be composed of mothers with children, another group might be composed of working white-collar men, whereas a third might include working women with no children. Nonpatient groups can be recruited from church, social, and civic groups as well as through notices in community newsletters and daily newspapers. Obviously, when you are using a patient group, confidentiality must be a primary concern. All patients whom you ask to participate should sign a written release stating that they will be voluntarily participating in the project and that they understand that their status as one of your patients will be revealed to others.

Normally, a focus group will be composed of 5–15 participants. The number of participants will depend on the preferences of the moderator, what you hope to obtain from the group, the meetingplace, the length of the focus group agenda (longer agendas call for fewer participants), and your budget. The number of groups are a function of the number of market segments and the size of your budget. (A market segment is a distinct group from whom you seek specific information. Segments can be defined on the basis of age, sex, diagnosis, treatment, and so on. Market segmentation will be discussed in more detail in the next section of this chapter.)

Generally you should organize at least one focus group for each distinct market segment. On occasion, a focus group will contain participants from more than one segment, such as heart condition patients and trauma victims. Such a focus group can be used to explore whether the segments act as different segments by gauging whether the two sets of participants respond differently to the issues raised in the group. By combining participants of more than one segment in a single focus group, the total number of groups can be reduced, thereby saving you some expense. Whether this is a feasible strategy depends on the complexity of the issues being discussed and the ability of the moderator to facilitate a group process in which the participants of neither segment inhibit the participants of the other segment.

In order to derive the most benefit from focus groups, they must meet in an appropriate facility. Groups can be run either in your office or in a facility designed for the purpose. Although using your office may save you several hundred dollars, using a commercial facility will usually give you superior results. This is because group members will respond in a more typical fashion if they are on "neutral turf." This is especially true if you are using patient groups, since feelings connected with being a patient, including being in a subordinate, dependent position, will be associated with your office. These feelings may interfere with the development of a group process and with the honest expression of opinions. In addition, commercial facilities have equipment that will help you to obtain the most information. This equipment typically includes

- a one-way mirror, so that you or several other observers can unobtrusively observe the group process
- taping equipment (video or audio), so that you can record the session for future reference and interpretation
- overhead projectors, flip charts, and other aids to help the moderator work with the group

It is particularly important for you to observe the focus group, either by using a one-way mirror or by viewing a videotape. (Group members should always be informed if they will be observed or taped.) This will help you interpret the moderator's findings. You may also have an opinion on the conduct and composition of future groups based on your observations of the content and intensity of participants' comments. Finally, your insight regarding your own practice and the issues raised in the focus group will help the moderator provide you with the most useful conclusions.

A focus group session usually begins with a "warm-up" in which the participants are greeted and introduce themselves briefly. The moderator then reviews the purpose of the focus group and the scope of the issues to be covered. The moderator then lays down some basic ground rules, such as the following:[18]

- There are no right or wrong answers, only points of view.
- Participants with minority opinions are encouraged to speak out.
- The moderator has no vested interest in the participants' supporting or rejecting any particular viewpoint. It is the moderator's responsibility to learn about the participants' viewpoints.
- The session is being recorded so that it can be analyzed for research purposes.
- After the meeting, participants will remain anonymous and will not be held accountable for their comments.

The moderator can then run the group by using a number of different strategies. A moderator using a directive style keeps strict control over the group. When a nondirective style is being used, the moderator will only become involved when the group starts to stray from the topic. The moderator can also adopt a "one of the group" role and mainly pose questions and hypotheses. The moderator can also "play dumb" by implying that he or she really doesn't know much about the topic and is interested in learning more.

The fourth step in the focus group process is to interpret the information obtained from the groups. Since focus groups are not composed of participants randomly drawn from the population of patients or potential patients, it is inappropriate to quantitatively categorize or interpret comments. A participant's statement could be idiosyncratic or it could reflect the views of many other patients or potential patients. What is essential is to understand the reasons behind the participants' statements. A good moderator will be able to comment on the reasons behind the statements. (In contrast, a quantitative method, such as a survey, would be more useful for determining how many patients or potential patients might hold a particular view. It would be very difficult, if not impossible, to understand the motivations behind the opinions expressed on a questionnaire, especially if the motivations were unconscious.)

Yolanda Brugaletta, vice-president for a marketing research firm that specializes in focus groups, has provided some guidelines for interpreting focus group sessions:[19]

1. Summarize what was said and what took place.
2. Analyze the meaning and implications of what was said.
3. Analyze the nonverbal responses as well as the verbal ones. Often facial expressions and body movements communicate as much as words.
4. For each topic, analyze the energy of responses, the spontaneity, and the degree of participant involvement.

Finally, the focus group findings should be classified into three categories. This last step can be used for any marketing research findings. The "no action" category includes findings for which it would be infeasible or undesirable to take immediate action. For example, comments that your practice location is inconvenient may be impossible for you to address until your lease expires. The "immediate action" category includes findings that are already confirmed by other observations, that are compelling in their own right, or that are unlikely to be confirmed or disconfirmed by additional investigation. For example, a hostile receptionist or confusing fee policies would fit into this category. Finally, the "further research" category includes findings that are important enough to examine through additional research and are amenable to additional research. For example, comments regarding your "bedside manner," the effectiveness of your clinical skills, and your reputation in the community should be of intense concern. If the focus group is raising questions in these areas, then you should consider additional qualitative or quantitative investigation.

The cost of organizing a focus group starts at about $2,500 but varies somewhat with geography. The cost breaks down in the following manner:

1. *Facilities.* A $500–$700 rental fee will usually get you a conference room, a one-way viewing mirror, and videotaping equipment.

2. *Incentive Fees.* Each participant will receive a fee of about $35. You may be able to avoid the fee if you are using current patients and ask them to serve on your "Consumer Advisory Panel," one duty of which is to participate in a focus group.
3. *Professional Fees.* The consultant's fee will be in the $700–$800 range. The "per group" fee may be somewhat lower if you are organizing more than one focus group session.
4. *Evaluation Fees.* The consultant will charge an additional $700–$800 to evaluate the results of the focus group and to write a report.

The cost can often be reduced if, for example, you find the group subjects or use your own facilities. Carefully weigh the cost of a focus group against the potential utility of the findings. For example, if you are considering running a $400 newspaper display ad for ten runs, it makes little sense to spend $2,500 on a qualitative investigation of the ad's attributes. On the other hand, if you are considering spending $3,000 to produce a TV commercial and $20,000 for air time, then $2,500 devoted to marketing research would be money well spent. Similarly, if you are developing your practice's marketing plan and it is likely to provide guidance for several years, then an initial investment in a focus group could easily pay off.

TARGET MARKETING AND MARKET SEGMENTATION

Market segments are groups of people who tend to behave in a similar manner or who have similar characteristics. Different market segments may have special needs and preferences, and this may justify developing special programs and marketing plans. For example, if people with homes in a particular zip code area are especially likely to come to your practice, then they are behaving differently as a result of their geographical location. You may be able to use this information to direct your marketing efforts toward segments (geographical areas) which are more likely to be responsive to your practice. Similarly, if you know that an important component of your practice consists of patients with hypertension, then you can develop programs and promotional efforts that will be particularly appealing to this market segment.

Identifying market segments is part of a marketing strategy called *target marketing.* Target marketing involves identifying one or more market segments and directing marketing efforts toward them. When a doctor adopts a target marketing strategy, he or she does four things:

1. identifies important market segments
2. systematically evaluates the attractiveness of each of the segments

3. selects one or more of the segments for special attention
4. positions the practice and services to establish a competitive advantage in each of the selected segments

It is important to understand that identifying useful market segments is one part of an overall marketing strategy; the other essential elements include evaluating the value of these segments and designing services and communications to tap into them. It is also important to note that although you may identify one or a few market segments deserving of special attention, your practice may still be largely composed of patients drawn from outside of these particular segments.

Developing Market Segments

The first phase of target marketing is to identify potential market segments. Obviously, it would *not* be worthwhile to customize your services to meet the needs of every possible type of patient. You may find, however, that patients can be divided into a few broad categories on the basis of their needs or the way they respond to marketing messages. If that is the case, then it may be worthwhile to try to make use of these differences.

The potential bases of segments are only limited by your creativity. Kotler has listed a number of commonly used segmentation variables, which are found in Table 8-3.[20] These segmentation variables can be classified as geographic, demographic, psychographic, and behavioral variables.

Geographic Segmentation

Geographic variables divide a market on the basis of location. Even though you may draw all of your patients from one city, you may be able to divide this area into useful smaller units, such as zip code area or district. If the practice is obtaining a disproportionate number of patients from particular zip code areas, then this may be a useful segmentation variable, because it could tell you *where* to direct your marketing efforts. If the practice has more than one location, then understanding which patients go to each location may allow you to determine more precisely the services and promotion activities that are best suited for each location.

Demographic Segmentation

Demographic variables divide the market on the basis of patients' personal characteristics, such as age, sex, and race. Demographic variables are the most commonly used basis for defining market segments. This is because patient desires, attitudes, needs, and utilization rates are often correlated with demographic variables. Segmentation on a demographic basis is commonly used in the market-

Table 8-3 Segmentation Variables and Typical Breakdowns

Variable	*Typical Breakdowns*
Geographic	
Region	Pacific, Mountain, West North Central, West South Central, East North Central, East South Central, South Atlantic, Middle Atlantic, New England
County Size	A, B, C, D
City or SMSA Size	Under 5,000; 5,000 to 20,000; 20,000 to 50,000; 50,000 to 100,000; 100,000 to 250,000; 250,000 to 500,000; 500,000 to 1,000,000; 1,000,000 to 4,000,000; 4,000,000 or over
Density	Urban, suburban, rural
Climate	Northern, Southern
Demographic	
Age	Under 6, 6 to 11, 12 to 19, 20 to 34, 35 to 49, 50 to 64, 65+
Sex	Male, female
Family Size	1 to 2, 3 to 4, 5+
Family Life Cycle	Young, single; young, married, no children; young, married, youngest child under 6; young, married, youngest child 6 or over; older, married, with children; older, married, no children under 18; older, single; other
Income	Under $5,000; $5,000 to $10,000; $10,000 to $15,000; $15,000 to $20,000; $20,000 to $25,000; $25,000 to $30,000; $30,000 to $50,000; $50,000 and over
Occupation	Professional and technical; managers, officials, proprietors; clerical, sales; craftsmen, foremen; operatives; farmers; retired; students; housewives; unemployed
Education	Grade school or less; some high school; high school graduate; some college; college graduate
Religion	Catholic, Protestant, Jewish, other
Race	White, Black, Oriental
Nationality	American, British, French, German, Scandinavian, Italian, Latin American, Middle Eastern, Japanese
Psychographic	
Social class	Lower lowers, upper lowers, working class, middle class, upper middles, lower uppers, upper uppers
Lifestyle	Straights, swingers, longhairs
Personality	Compulsive, gregarious, authoritarian, ambitious
Behavioral	
Occasions	Regular occasion, special occasion
Benefits	Quality, service, economy
User Status	Nonuser, ex-user, potential user, first-time user, regular user
Usage Rate	Light user, medium user, heavy user
Loyalty Status	None, medium, strong, absolute
Readiness Stage	Unaware, aware, informed, interested, desirous, intending to buy
Attitude toward Product	Enthusiastic, positive, indifferent, negative, hostile

Source: Reprinted from *Marketing Management: Analysis, Planning, Implementation, and Control*, 6th ed., by P. Kotler, p. 287, with permission of Prentice-Hall, © 1988.

ing of consumer goods. By understanding the demographic characteristics of market segments, it is possible to utilize marketing messages and media that directly address the most promising segments. For example, it is much more likely that Mercedes-Benz ads will appear in *Architectural Digest* or *Vogue* than in *Wooden Boat Magazine* or *Easy Rider,* because the demographic characteristics of *Architectural Digest* and *Vogue* readers are more similar to the demographic characteristics of Mercedes-Benz buyers.

Demographic variables can be important segmentation variables for a medical practice. Age, sex, family life cycle, income, occupation, education, and race can be important variables, because patient service needs vary across the segments defined by these variables. Women, for example, have a different distribution of diseases and procedures than men. In addition, women probably have more decision-making power in regard to the treatment of children. Lower income groups may be less able to afford elective procedures, such as annual examinations, contact lenses, and cosmetic surgery. Higher education groups may be more receptive to messages delivered through informational seminars, whereas lower education groups may be more responsive to Yellow Pages ads. It is important to understand that using demographic variables to define market segments does not mean that you need to neglect men, for example, or low-income and low-education groups. If in fact you want to attract these groups, then you will simply have to offer a different mix of services, which your segmentation research will help you to identify.

Age is another useful demographic variable. For example, the medical problems associated with sports differ among various age groups. Middle-aged athletes experience different types of injuries and have different medical needs than teenagers. Members of these two segments can also be attracted to a practice in different ways. Middle-aged athletes may be accessed through athletic and golf clubs and softball leagues, whereas teenage athletes can be accessed through schools, parents, and coaches. Each segment also may be responsive to different messages and media.

Perhaps the most obvious and important demographic variable is disease or health problem. Not every disease, however, has to be taken as defining a separate market segment. The issue is whether you can develop additional specific services for or ways of communicating with a group defined by a disease or health problem. For example, developing a program to help the families of terminally ill patients deal with the eventual loss of their loved one would be a service that you could provide to this segment. The particular causes of death would not have to be taken into account. An ophthalmologist might consider all patients who require sight correction to be a segment irrespective of whether correction is through the use of glasses, corrective surgery, or contact lenses.

When a market segment can be approached with a new technology, this can result in a powerful combination. For example, a dermatologist might consider people with tattoos to be a market segment. Recent research on Q-switched ruby laser treatment may offer a new technology that could be marketed to this segment.[21]

Examining market segments defined by diseases or treatments can suggest new services to provide or new ways to communicate with potential patients. Table 8-4 contains some diagnostic market segments arranged by medical specialty. Each of these diagnostic segments can be divided into smaller segments. For example, a dermatologist may choose to focus on the *adolescent* chronic dermatitis segment, whereas an orthopedist may market to *adult* sports medicine patients.

Psychographic Segmentation

Psychographic segmentation divides patients on the basis of social class, lifestyle, or personality. Social class is strongly associated with preferences for consumer goods, habits, clothing, etc. There clearly are social class differences in the kinds of medical treatment desired and needed. People lower down on the socioeconomic scale have more chronic health problems and have less sophisticated medical knowledge. This implies that the services you offer and the way you promote them will vary based on the social class of your present patients and of the potential patients you wish to attract.

Personality assessment, as we saw in Chapter 2, involves time-consuming assessment procedures. You can certainly make guesses about a patient's personality, but it is obvious that these guesses are going to be less accurate than your assessment of the patient's age, geographical residence, and sex. The marketing research literature is ambivalent about the real-world usefulness of personality segmentation. You may be able to devise some reasonable hypotheses, however, regarding personality segments. For example, if you have an oncology practice, you may well have a disproportionate number of situationally depressed patients. This would be a patient segment that could benefit from treatment for this problem and might be very responsive to a practice that communicates a recognition of this problem.

Behavioral Segmentation

Behavioral segmentation is based on attitudes toward, use of, or response to medical services. Table 8-3 lists a number of behavioral variables. For medical practices, two of the most useful behavioral variables are occasions and benefits.

Occasion buyers are people who will need your services at a given point in life. (The occasion, of course, is the onset of disease.) Many of your patients will be occasion buyers; if you are a specialist, perhaps all will be. You may also have a group of patients who are not occasion buyers but who are seeking preventive medical services. The services you offer to these two segments, as well as the effectiveness of your promotional efforts, will obviously be improved if you devise specific ways of reaching each segment. Professional referral sources and accessibility in emergencies will be important for attracting occasion patients,

Table 8-4 Market Segments by Specialty

Specialty	Market Segment
Cardiology	Post myocardial infarction
	Coronary bypasses
	arrhythmias
	Chronic congestive heart failure
Dermatology	Chronic dermatitis
	Skin cancer
	Allergic dermatitis
Endocrinology	Diabetics
	Thyroid disorders
	Adrenal disorders
Family Practice	Hypertensives
	Diabetics
	Chronic obstructive pulmonary disease
	Sick children
	Upper respiratory infection
	Psychosomatic illnesses
Orthopedics	Knee problems
	Sports medicine
	Arthritis
	Joint injuries
	Joint replacement
Pediatrics	Well babies
	Chronic ear infections
	Allergic children
	Asthmatics
	Orthopedic problems
Psychiatry	Depression
	Anxiety/phobias
	Sexual dysfunction
	Obsessive compulsive disorder
	Rape/sexual assault
	Physical and emotional loss
Pulmonary	Chronic obstructive pulmonary disease
	Asthmatics
	Industrial lung diseases
	Pulmonary fibrosis
Surgery	Cholecystectomies
	Gastrectomies
	Colostomies
	Trauma
	Postop care
	Separation and divorce

Source: Adapted from *Marketing Strategies for Physicians* by S. Brown and A. Morley, pp. 181–182, with permission of Practice Management Information Corporation, © 1987.

whereas community education and company wellness programs will be important for reaching the nonoccasion segment.

Segmenting patients on the basis of benefits means constructing groups based on what the patients seek from treatment, that is, the benefits that they desire. Kotler and Clarke state that most health care consumers can be grouped into the following four benefit-seeking segments:[22]

1. *Quality buyers* want the best product and are unconcerned about cost.
2. *Service buyers* are primarily concerned with acquiring the most caring and personal service.
3. *Value buyers* examine the price-quality trade-off. A value buyer would go to a doctor who had a "reasonable" reputation and who had "reasonable" fees.
4. *Economy buyers* are most interested in the least expensive alternative.

You may find that your patients are homogeneous with respect to the benefits that they seek. If that is the case, then you are probably conveying a message to prospective patients about the benefits that you provide. This may or may not be desirable. For example, if you are trying to provide family practice services to a broad spectrum of the community, yet your patients are mostly quality buyers, then you may be excluding a significant number of potential patients. If that is the case, you would do well to consider the nature of your practice's reputation. For example, are you conveying an unintended message that dissuades service or value buyers?

Multiple Segments

It is often possible to find more than one basis upon which to segment your practice. For example, you may find that young women with children, older patients, and professionals either are or should be important practice segments. On occasion you may find it useful to combine two segments. For example, Woodside, Nielsen, Walters, and Muller examined how demographic variables interacted with benefit segments when choosing a hospital.[23] They found that benefit segments were closely associated with unique demographic profiles. Since demographic variables are easily determined, their findings could be used by hospitals to develop new products and marketing strategies for promoting products and services to specific demographic segments.

Evaluating and Choosing Market Segments

The second and third components of target marketing involve evaluating and choosing segments. Larger health care providers, such as hospitals and nursing homes, determine the usefulness of various market segments through marketing research. The research process typically involves many in-depth interviews and focus groups composed of patients and potential patients. The data are then evaluated and a profile is developed of a potential patient's demographic, psychographic, geographic, and behavioral characteristics and media consumption habits. This obviously can be a time-consuming and expensive process. A more feasible approach for a medical practice is to look at current patients and search for prominent segmentation patterns. Concentrate on large, obvious groups defined geographically, demographically, or behaviorally. Don't try to create myriad narrow, multivariable segments, since each segment will be too small to market to effectively. Large homogeneous segments will allow you to make marketing decisions that will affect a substantial number of patients. Be sure to look for segments based on sex, family life cycle, occupation, disease or health problem, residence, and age.

When evaluating whether a segment will be useful for target marketing, consider the size and growth potential of the segment, its attractiveness, and your practice's objectives and resources. The size of a segment is important, because you do not want to put time, effort, and resources into a market that is too small to obtain a reward commensurate with your efforts. Growth potential is important, because successfully marketing to a growing segment will result in practice growth. But remember that a growing segment will tend to attract attention, which translates into competition. Good examples of growth potential leading to increased competition include the overeating-bulimia-anorexia segment in the 1980s and the contact lens market of the 1970s.

Another aspect of the attractiveness of a segment is the degree of existing competition. If there are already a number of other medical practices competing for a segment, you should ask yourself the following

1. Is this market segment large enough to support another provider?
2. Do I have a competitive advantage such that I will be able to do better in this segment than my peers?

Evaluation of the current attractiveness of a segment can be particularly important if you will be competing against nonmedical organizations or hospitals. Nonmedical competitors may be used to lower fees, and this may foreshadow an erosion of the profit potential of a market. Nonmedical competition may be encountered in problem segments such as smoking, weight loss, anxiety, pain management, eye care, and foot care. Hospitals can be tough competitors, because their enormous resources allow them to undertake expensive promotional campaigns that saturate a market with highly visible television, radio, and newspaper ads. They also can offer a service at a loss or a break-even price as a way of attracting patients, who will then turn to them for more involved services at a later date. Segments that have attracted the serious attention of hospitals must be approached with caution.

Perhaps the most important consideration when evaluating the desirability of a segment is the degree to which it is consistent with your own personal and practice goals. If you derive little or no satisfaction from working with children, then you should give careful consideration before targeting this segment, even if you are likely to reap financial rewards.

Ultimately, the selection of segments is a qualitative, subjective decision. It may be based on either objective data from sophisticated marketing research or upon intuitions derived from your personal knowledge of your patients coupled with a healthy dose of speculation. In the final analysis it is a *management* decision, and it should take into account the benefit that you can add to your patients. Going back to the four Ps, can you provide some benefit in terms of product (service), place (location), promotion (communications) or price that will give you a competitive advantage? If you cannot provide something of special value to patients in a given segment, then you should probably not select it for special attention.

Positioning Your Practice

The final phase of target marketing is to position your practice so that you will market to the previously identified target segment or segments. The positioning should be determined by your evaluation of the particular competitive advantages that you have vis-à-vis the segments. This should then be reflected in the marketing strategy you develop for approaching these segments and in the specific marketing plans you construct. A psychiatrist, for example, might identify the "upscale, higher income, better-educated" segment as deserving of special attention. She determines that her competitive advantages are as follows:

1. She is a *medical doctor,* unlike a psychologist or clinical social worker.
2. She can prescribe medication, unlike many of her competitors.
3. She can diagnose physiological problems, unlike many of her nonmedical competitors.
4. She has more years of postgraduate training than competitors with other kinds of degrees.
5. She is a psychoanalyst.
6. All major insurance carriers will cover her services, unlike competitors in other professions, who are only covered by some carriers.
7. Since she employs a psychologist, she can provide a *complete* range of mental health services, unlike many of her competitors, who can only provide some of these services.

After talking with several of her patients who are in the upscale, higher income, better-educated segment, she determines that they are largely "quality buyers." Her marketing strategy, therefore, is to approach this segment by appealing to the desire to obtain the best services from the most qualified provider. Her marketing plan for this segment is different *only* in regard to the promotion component. (The services that she will provide are the *same* as those offered to all her other patients. She is not providing additional services [product], offering different hours or location [place], or charging different fees [price] to attract this segment.) She places print ads emphasizing her superior position in the provider "pecking order," including her ability to diagnose physiological causes of mental disorders, and uses this to emphasize the superior quality of her services. She places television and radio ads on talk programs with demographics that are heavily biased towards the better-educated and upper income segments. Finally, she makes presentations before business groups and employers with more highly educated work forces, where she emphasizes the medical aspects of mental health and the overall superiority of psychiatry among mental health care professions.

CONCLUSION

Success *may* give you the luxury of not having to market. If you are in a specialty that is in high demand or if there are relatively few competitors in your area, you may be able to successfully limit your marketing activities to announcing your presence, affiliating with a hospital, and associating with colleagues. Apart from these circumstances, however, marketing should be a regularly occurring function within your practice. The question then becomes whether you will do it well or poorly.

Doctors who must market their services in order to prosper or even survive should undertake the complete process, including performing a thorough situational analysis, developing a marketing strategy, and writing specific marketing plans, including media plans and budgeting decisions. Marketing research should be employed to understand patient needs and to identify special opportunities for servicing particular segments.

You should be aware that you can do your homework, invest considerable personal time and money, and still observe little if any *initial* response. This creates a dilemma. Does a disappointing market response indicate a faulty plan or unrealistic expectations? If you have done your homework, then you can persevere in the knowledge that you should observe an effect. Conducting a thorough marketing evaluation will give you the confidence to stay with a plan long enough to know if it is viable. It is important, therefore, to be patient as well as diligent.

If you eventually conclude that your initial plans are not as effective as you had wished, then try other approaches. You may have to examine several segments or try variations on your initial marketing plans before you discover a workable formula for your practice. Through all of this, you need to remember that over a period of time competently performed marketing efforts *will* produce patients at your door.

You should now understand how to develop a marketing plan based on your patient's strengths and the opportunities present in your market. You should have obtained specific marketing skills, including an understanding of how and when to conduct marketing research and an appreciation of the importance of market segments and target marketing. Finally, you should be able to plan your promotional efforts, taking into consideration the various promotional and media alternatives, including television, radio, print advertising, and personal promotion.

NOTES

1. See, for example, J. Norman, "Can a Practice Serving the Poor Avoid Financial Quicksand?" *Medical Economics,* February 5, 1990, 79–87.

2. R.T. Lee, J.S. Satinder, M.D. Bhatia, and M.G. Sutton, "Assessment of Valvular Heart Disease with Doppler Echocardiography," *JAMA* 262 (1989): 2131–35.

3. R. Steinbrook and B. Lo, "Informing Physicians about Promising New Treatments for Severe Illnesses," *JAMA* 263 (1990): 2078–82.

4. Steward Husted, Dale Varble, and James Lowry, *Principles of Modern Marketing* (Needham Heights, Mass.: Allyn and Bacon, 1989), 237.

5. James Scott, Martin Warshaw, and James Taylor, *Introduction to Marketing Management,* 5th ed. (Homewood, Ill.: Irwin, 1985), 11–12.

6. *Journal of Health Care Marketing,* American Marketing Association, 250 S. Wacker Dr., Chicago, IL 60606; *Journal of Medical Practice Management,* Williams and Wilkins, 428 E. Preston St., Baltimore, MD 21202.

7. Personal correspondence.

8. David Ogilvy, *Ogilvy on Advertising* (New York: Vintage, 1985). Ogilvy devised the slogan for Rolls-Royce "At 60 miles an hour the loudest noise in the new Rolls-Royce comes from the electric clock." He also developed campaigns for Volkswagen, Dove soap, Hathaway shirts, and Marlboro cigarettes.

9. K. Roman and J. Maas, *How to Advertise* (New York: St. Martin's Press, 1975).

10. For an example of how a physician took advantage of serendipity to obtain a radio talk program, see D. van Amerongen, "I was Chicago's Answer to Dr. Ruth," *Medical Economics,* March 19, 1990, 101–5.

11. J. Ernhardt, "Marketing? My Patients Do It for Me," *Medical Economics,* October 2, 1989, 58–64.

12. L. Ring, D. Newton, N. Borden, and P. Farris, *Decisions in Marketing: Text and Cases* (Homewood, Ill.: Irwin, 1989), 97.

13. "The Future of General Internal Medicine," *JAMA* 262 (1989): 2119–24.

14. N.G. Barnes and D. Mowatt, "An Examination of Patient Attitudes and Their Implications for Dental Service Marketing," *Journal of Health Care Marketing* 6 (1986): 60–63; D.E. Christensen and T.D. Giese, "Assessment and Application of Patient Satisfaction Variables in Marketing a Psychiatric Practice," *Journal of Health Care Marketing* 8 (1988): 47–49.

15. M.D. Axelrod, "Marketers Get an Eyeful When Focus Groups Expose Products, Ideas, Images, Ad Copy, etc., to Consumers," *Marketing News,* February 28, 1975, 6–7.

16. Personal correspondence.

17. C. Keown, "Focus Group Research: Tool for the Retailer," *Journal of Small Business Management,* April 1983, 59–65.

18. Donald J. Messmer, personal correspondence with author.

19. Y. Brugaletta, "Guidelines to Set up, Use and Analyze Focus Groups," *Marketing News,* October 24, 1975.

20. P. Kotler, *Marketing Management: Analysis, Planning, Implementation, and Control,* 6th ed. (Englewood Cliffs, N.J.: Prentice-Hall, 1988).

21. J. Dover and K. Arndt, "Dermatology," *JAMA* 263 (1990): 2633–35.

22. P. Kotler and R. Clarke, *Marketing for Health Care Organizations* (Englewood Cliffs, N.J.: Prentice-Hall, 1987), 244.

23. A.G. Woodside, R.L. Nielson, F. Walters, and G. Muller, "Preference Segmentation of Health Care Services: The Old-Fashioneds, Value Conscious, Affluents, and Professional Want-It-Alls," *Journal of Health Care Marketing* 8 (1988): 14–24.

Chapter 9

Business Law

CHAPTER OBJECTIVES

This chapter will provide you with an understanding of fundamental business law concepts. As a result, you will be able to

1. prevent disputes
2. avoid lawsuits
3. anticipate the legal consequences of your actions

The chapter is organized around the following potential sources of liability or conflict:

1. torts
2. contracts
3. employment issues, including equal employment opportunity, employee contracts, contractor agreements, and the Fair Labor Standards Act
4. malpractice, which is a particular type of tort

After reading this chapter, you will understand how the legal system approaches these potential sources of litigation. As a result, you will be able to conduct your daily affairs with due consideration given to possible legal consequences.

INTRODUCTION

We are living in an increasingly litigious society. Many explanations have been offered for this, including a declining respect for authority, an ever-increasing number of lawyers, a rise in consumerism, and an evolving interpretation of what constitutes negligence. As a doctor, your relationships with your patients expose you to the risk of malpractice litigation. In addition, your practice has many of the legal vulnerabilities of any other business. Your practice's arrangements and dealings with insurance companies, landlords, suppliers, employees, contractors, partners, and so on, all have potential legal ramifications.

Legal considerations are best handled in anticipation of events. If you are aware of the potential legal consequences of an action, then you can often avoid a legal confrontation or, at a minimum, place yourself in a more favorable legal position. This strategy is called *preventive law,* and it is analogous to preventive medicine. By eliminating or minimizing problems before they occur, you may avoid the courtroom and all of the expense and personal disruption that is associated with this ultimate form of decision making.

This chapter will help you to recognize when you are entering territory with legal implications. In addition, by understanding the legal aspects of your actions, you will be able to communicate more effectively with your attorney. You should of course consult your attorney regarding situations with obvious legal implications, such as a contract, lease, or employee dispute. There will be many unanticipated situations, however, in which understanding the principles of law will allow you to make good operational decisions as well as help you to determine when you should involve your attorney.

Legal problems can arise from a number of different sources. In this chapter, these sources are classified as general torts, general contracts, employment issues, and malpractice. When a wrong has been committed that harms a person, that person can seek to recover money damages from the wrongdoer. If the harm was committed through the breach of a contract, then the process is governed by contract law. For example, if you have a contract with a cleaning service and you feel that its performance is inadequate, then your recourse will be governed by the content of the contract and how contracts are interpreted under contract law. When there is no contract, then the wronged party may seek recovery under tort law. For example, if a patient or member of the general public happens to fall in your parking lot, he or she may seek to recover damages under tort law, since there is no contract between the two of you.

Employment and malpractice cases are, respectively, specific types of contract and tort cases. For example, firing an employee who has an employment contract will be governed by contract law. Malpractice cases are generally governed by tort law, although some cases are filed as a breach of contract between the patient and the doctor.

Figure 9-1 outlines the general structure of United States law. *Statutory law* is the result of statutes enacted by state legislatures, ordinances enacted by municipalities, and laws passed by Congress. *Common law* derives from the decisions of judges:

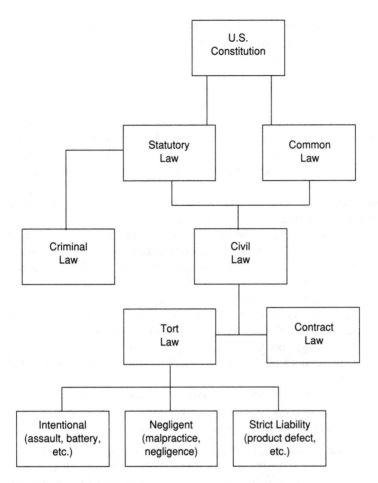

Figure 9-1 The U.S. System of Laws

Common law . . . makes itself up as it goes along; it sets precedents but they are never unalterable, because they are derived ultimately, not from a book of rules, but from a judge's intuitive feeling for equity and fair play. . . . Common law assumes a freely developing pattern which is nevertheless consistent with itself, like the development of a living language.[1]

Criminal law protects society's interest in order, safety, and the integrity of its institutions by defining and prohibiting unacceptable behavior. By definition, criminal law is statutory, since it derives from the actions of legislatures and Congress. *Civil law* also protects society's interests, but it does so by defining the rights and obligations of one person or business vis-à-vis another. Civil law can be either constitutional, statutory, or common (case or case-based).

TORTS

A tort is a civil wrong that has been committed against another party or another party's property but is not due to a breach of contract. A tort is distinct from a crime, which is an intentionally harmful act that is committed against society. As a result, tort actions are brought by individuals, whereas crimes are prosecuted by the state. Those responsible for a tort are referred to as *tortfeasors;* those responsible for a crime are referred to as *criminals.*

It is possible for an act to be prosecuted as both a tort and a crime. For example, an accident caused by a drunk driver could be prosecuted by the state under criminal law, and the injured party could independently seek remuneration under tort law. It is also possible for there to be a crime with no tort, such as the case of a physician who misrepresents his or her personal property assets to the local tax collector in an attempt to reduce tax liability. Since no individual has been harmed, there is no tort. Finally, there can be a tort with no crime. For example, if a patient inadvertently takes the wrong coat from a waiting room, this is the tort of conversion. This is not a crime, however, since the motivation necessary for theft is absent.

The simple fact that a person is harmed or injured does not in itself mean that a tort has occurred. In order for a tort to occur, there has to be a basis for liability. The following considerations can be used to establish a basis for liability:

1. *Voluntary Action.* The tortfeasor's voluntary actions or voluntary failure to act must have contributed to the harm. Actions resulting from immediate peril or fear are generally considered to be involuntary acts. For example, if you jump back at the sight of a snake, thereby inadvertently striking another person, the action would probably be considered involuntary.

2. *Intent.* Some torts require the demonstration of intent, whereas other torts do not. In tort law, the issue of intent relates to whether the tortfeasor intended to *commit the act, not whether harm was intended to the other party.* To prove intent, it is necessary to demonstrate that the actor either knew or believed that certain results were likely to follow his or her actions. This knowledge is determined on an objective basis, which is what a *reasonable* person would be expected to know or expect to occur under the circumstances.

   The following example illustrates the role of intent: "As a practical joke, Jack pulls a chair out from under Jill as she begins to sit, causing her to fall and sustain a hip fracture. Although Jack actually meant Jill no harm, a court could reasonably find that he knew with substantial certainty that Jill would attempt to sit down where the chair had been, and could fall and be injured. Hence, Jack had the knowledge required to support a finding of intent for tort liability. His intent was to do an act that he could have reasonably foreseen would cause injury to another."[2]

3. *Causation.* In order to sustain a tort, it must be demonstrated that there was a causal relationship between the wrongful act and the harm. State laws vary regarding how directly the act must be related to the harm in order for causation to be demonstrated.

The following example illustrates how the causal chain can become extended: "George Nesselrode was a passenger in an airplane made by Beechcraft Aircraft Corporation. A few minutes after taking off, the plane crashed and all occupants were killed. Action was brought by George's widow against Beechcraft on the theory that it was at fault to prevent the improper installation of certain parts in its airplanes, in consequence of which the parts could be installed in reverse or backwards, and this improper installation had caused the fatal crash. . . .

Judgement [was] against Beechcraft Aircraft Corp. Although no harm would have occurred if third persons had not made an improper installation, the fact remained that the prior failure of Beechcraft to give proper warning was a substantial factor in bringing about the harm. It therefore could not claim that the installation was an act that broke the causal chain. As a substantial contributing factor, the manufacturer was liable even though the wrong installation was the proximate cause and was the act of a third person."[3]

Notice that motivation is largely irrelevant to the above four considerations, other than perhaps as a way of demonstrating intent.

Torts can be classified into three basic groups:

1. *Intentional torts* result from intended acts, such as assault, battery, malicious prosecution, and defamation.
2. *Negligent torts* result from unintended acts, such as negligence and malpractice.
3. *Strict liability torts* result from a liability without fault. Examples include product liability cases in which the manufacturer is held strictly responsible for defective goods. For example, if a piece of glass was found in a can of soup, the manufacturer would be held strictly liable for any personal injuries suffered.

The following discussion will elaborate on some of the torts that a physician might reasonable encounter, either as the victim or the tortfeasor.

Intentional Torts

1. *Assault.* Assault is an act (more than words) that creates the apprehension of an immediate harmful contact. The important elements for demonstrating assault are the tortfeasor's action, his or her intent, the perception of fear or apprehension on the part of the assaulted person, and the causal relationship between the assaulted person's fear and the tortfeasor's actions. For example, Mr. Smith is dissatisfied with Dr. Jones' services. He confronts Jones and points an unloaded pistol at her while threatening to shoot. Assault has occurred, because Smith committed an act that a reasonable person would assume would create fear or apprehension whether or not the gun was actually loaded. Jones had those fears, and they were the proximate result of Smith's actions.

2. *Battery.* Battery is intentional, unjustified touching of another person's body. The contact does not have to actually cause physical harm. Battery has occurred even if the action is only offensive or insulting. For example, Dr. Brown intentionally and without consent unjustifiably kisses and fondles Ms. Arnold. Even though no physical harm is done to Ms. Arnold, a battery has taken place.

Defenses against assault and battery suits include *consent* and *privilege.* Consent exists if the allegedly wronged party implied or expressly stated that the actions were permissible. Privilege might exist if the alleged tortfeasor acted in self-defense or in the defense of others or of property. The level of force must be reasonable given the circumstances and cannot be retaliatory.

3. *Intentional Infliction of Emotional Distress.* This involves disturbing someone's peace of mind through outrageous behavior. The words or actions must be exceedingly severe; otherwise, torts could be claimed based on fictitious psychological damage. Doctors could be exposed to a suit through overly aggressive bill collecting procedures, which might include abusive or insulting language and threats of violence.

4. *Invasion of Privacy.* This is an infringement of the right to be left alone. Invasions of privacy fall into four categories. The first is intrusion into another's private affairs or solitude. The second is disclosure of private, embarrassing facts. The third is publication of information about someone that places the person in a false light. The fourth is the unauthorized use of someone's name or likeness for commercial purposes. A doctor can become exposed to an invasion of privacy suit by revealing confidential information about a patient to a third party (e.g., a social acquaintance at a party or even a professional colleague if a proper release has not been obtained from the patient).

5. *Abusive Discharge*. This tort occurs when an employee who does not have a written contract is discharged for a reason that violates public policy. For example, Dr. Wilson discharges Ms. Blakely because she has become pregnant and he fears that her attendance and job performance will deteriorate. This violation of public policy regarding sexual discrimination could be prosecuted under the equal employment laws and as a tort by Ms. Blakely.

6. *Disparagement or Trade Libel*. This occurs when there are false, injurious statements made about a competitor's reputation. This tort injures the business reputation of the victim, and often disparages the conduct of a competing commercial enterprise over time. For example, Dr. Wilson makes condescending and untruthful remarks about Benevolent Daughters Hospital.

7. *Interference with Contract*. This tort requires that (a) a contract exists between two parties, (b) a third party knows about the contract, and (c) the third party induces one of the other two parties to breach the contract or prevents one of the other parties from fulfilling the contract. For example, Fred Kane is a physical therapist with six months remaining on his employment contract with Dr. Jones. Dr. White is aware of this contract but mentions to Kane that he would be able to give Kane a higher salary if Kane would join his practice now. Kane leaves and works for Dr. White. Dr. Jones may sue Dr. White for interference and sue Kane for breach of contract. It is important to note that it is not necessary for Dr. Jones to prove that Dr. White intended to maliciously harm her. What is important is that White knew that there was a contract and that his actions interfered with the completion of that contract.

8. *Malicious Institution of Civil Proceedings or Malicious Prosecution*. This occurs when an individual initiates legal proceedings that are both unwarranted and unsuccessful. The plaintiff must show that the tortfeasor lacked probable cause to institute the legal proceedings. In essence, someone cannot instigate a frivolous legal action in an attempt to "even things out."

9. *Defamation*. This occurs when a reputation is injured due to false statements. If the statement is in writing, then this is called *libel*. If the defamation occurs verbally or by acts or gestures, then it is called *slander*. In most cases, the truth is a successful defense, even if the motivation was less than benevolent and even if the accused believed the statements to be false at the time they were made.

Defamation can be a particular concern when providing a reference to a former employee.[4] Stick to the facts regarding an employee's job performance. In that regard your performance appraisal records could be critical to a successful defense (see Chapter 3). It is generally okay to provide information about a former employee that might on its face appear to be defamatory if the information will help you protect an important interest. "Important interests" have been defined to include a legal or moral duty to speak, defend your own reputation, warn others of a prospective employee's misconduct or mismanagement, and protect the interests of a third party.

Conveying negative information is a privileged right that may be lost under some circumstances, including the following:

- You did not believe the reference you gave to be true.
- You had no reasonable grounds for your beliefs about the employee, even though you did hold your beliefs in good faith.
- The information you gave was not an appropriate response to the third party's inquiry.
- You gave information to a person who had no need for it.
- You gave information out of malice, which in a legal sense means recklessly, with an improper motive, with an absence of good faith, and with an intention to do harm.

Here are some guidelines to follow when providing references:

1. If the employee is being dismissed, explain why and let the employee review his or her personnel file.
2. Tell the employee that if he or she chooses to use the practice as a reference, you will respond truthfully.
3. Have the employee sign a form prepared by your attorney consenting to the release of information. (Have your attorney prepare a standard release form. Keep copies in your office so that it can be used as needed.) Do not release information if the employee refuses to sign the form. If the employee refuses to sign the form and subsequently uses you as a reference, tell the inquirer that you cannot supply information until the former employee signs a release.
4. Ask the inquirer if he or she has the applicant's permission to contact the practice and, if so, whether there were any restrictions placed on what could be discussed.
5. State that your evaluation of the former employee is your opinion and provide a full and accurate discussion of the facts supporting your opinion.
6. If you forward a written recommendation, be certain to mark the outside envelope "confidential" or "personal."
7. Do not volunteer information that has not been asked for.

8. Some employers will give employees who are discharged for inadequate job performance a generic written reference stating that the employee had been a "good employee." Never do this, since it could be used against you as evidence of wrongful discharge.

Negligence Torts

Negligence is the most common kind of tort. Negligence occurs when a person or company fails to act with reasonable care under the circumstances. In order for an injured person to be able to recover for negligence, the following five elements must be demonstrated:

1. *The Defendant Had a Duty to Exercise Reasonable Care.* What constitutes "reasonable" care is often a subject of debate in the litigation. Generally, the standard that is applied is what an imaginary reasonable person might do under the circumstances. Obviously, this type of standard is going to vary from one occasion to another, and ultimately the issue of reasonableness is only determined after the lawsuit has been resolved.

2. *The Defendant Breached the Duty to Behave Reasonably.* The standard of performance is not perfection. Instead, the standard is reasonable performance by the defendant under the circumstances. Generally, the more serious the hazard, the more care the defendant must exercise.

3. *Cause in Fact.* The plaintiff must demonstrate that the injury would not have happened but for the defendant's acts or omissions.

4. *Proximate Cause.* This concept deals with the foreseeability of the consequences of the defendant's act. (The term "proximate" is a lamentable choice of words, since the issue has nothing at all to do with closeness in time or place. The issue relates to how far courts will extend culpability in a chain of events.) Proximate cause exists when there is no intervening cause or chain of causes between the defendant's actions and the harm that occurred to the plaintiff. For example, Andrews is injured in an accident while a passenger in Hill's car. Hill removes Andrews from the car and lays him by the side of the road. Roberts, a passer-by, moves Andrews into the roadway, where he is struck by Thompson's car. Hill's alleged negligence is not the proximate cause of the injuries suffered by Andrews as a result of being struck by Thompson's car, although his actions are the proximate cause for the injuries suffered in the original accident.

5. *Injury, Damage, or Loss.* The plaintiff must demonstrate that personal injury, property damage, or economic loss actually occurred as a result of the act.

The following example will illustrate how the elements listed above can combine to form a tort. As a result of a snowstorm, the entrance to Dr. Framingham's office has become very slippery. Dr. Framingham has a contract with a cleaning service to provide snow removal. Dr. Framingham learned that the entrance was slippery when he arrived at his office. Before the cleaning service comes to clean the entrance, Mr. Newman slips on the icy entrance and breaks his leg.

Under these circumstances, it is likely that Dr. Framingham was negligent. Courts have generally held that it is a business's duty to provide a safe entrance. The fact that the cleaning service may or may not have responded does not relieve Dr. Framingham of this duty to the public to provide a safe entrance. Therefore, Dr. Framingham breached this duty. The snow at the entrance was the cause in fact of the accident, and the consequences of leaving the entrance covered with snow were foreseeable and known by Dr. Framingham. Finally, Mr. Newman did suffer an injury. As a separate issue, Dr. Framingham may be able to bring an action against the cleaning service based on the wording of the cleaning contract. For example, if the contract stated that snow would be removed before the office opened in the morning, then the cleaning service may have breached the contract.

Aside from negligent malpractice, which will be discussed separately below, a doctor's greatest exposure to negligence torts lies in the physical state of his or her office. People are very creative in their ability to misuse items and act without forethought. It is essential to examine how patients physically flow through your office and your physical facilities, and then rectify any potential hazards. The object is to prevent injuries, not simply provide a reasonable care defense. The following suggestions might be helpful:

1. Have all trash removed from your premises (not just your office) as quickly as possible.
2. Hallways and entrances should be routinely cleaned and maintained.
3. All office furniture should be routinely inspected for loose legs, loose backs, exposed wires, and so on.
4. Consider eliminating toys from your waiting room. Playing is correlated with activity, and activity is correlated with injury. If you must have toys, examine them for sharp edges, points, ingestibility, breakability, or any other potential danger.[5]
5. Be certain that the receptionist understands that he or she has a responsibility to keep order in the waiting room.
6. Be certain that all appropriate safety equipment is properly located and maintained. For example, have an adequate supply of properly placed fire extinguishers, be certain that exit signs are visible, and routinely check safety equipment such as ground fault interrupters, pressure relief valves, and locks.

Malpractice

The frequency of malpractice claims has generally increased from the late 1970s through the mid-1980s, although recent data indicate that the claims rate may be decreasing (Figure 9-2). In addition, the size of the average paid claim has risen steadily over the years (Figure 9-3). Malpractice claims vary by practice location and specialty, with specialties such as obstetrics, gynecology, and surgery having significantly higher claim rates than physicians in general, whereas psychiatrists experience significantly lower claim rates.[6]

Malpractice is the tort of negligence as it applies to a professional. In order for a patient to demonstrate malpractice, he or she must prove by a preponderance of the evidence that the five elements necessary for any tort are present:

1. *Duty.* There was a bona fide doctor-patient relationship, and the doctor owed the patient a duty to provide a certain standard of care.
2. *Breach of Duty, or Standard of Care.* The patient must demonstrate that the doctor did not provide a reasonable standard of care.

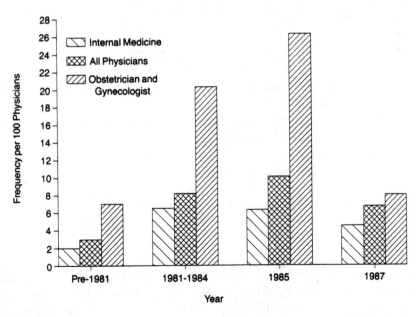

Figure 9-2 Frequency of Malpractice Claims. *Source:* Reprinted from *Journal of the American Medical Association*, Vol. 262, No. 23, p. 3321, with permission of the American Medical Association, © 1989.

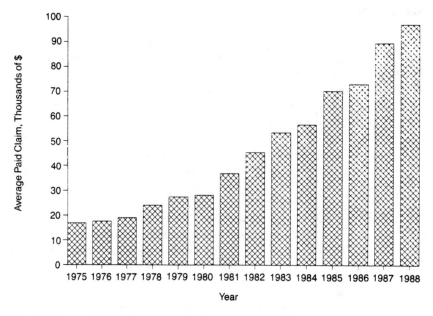

Figure 9-3 Average Malpractice Paid Claim by Year. *Source:* Reprinted from *Journal of the American Medical Association*, Vol. 262, No. 23, p. 3322, with permission of the American Medical Association, © 1989.

3. *Causation in Fact.* The injury would not have happened but for the actions of the doctor.
4. *Proximate Cause.* The consequences of the doctor's actions would be foreseeable by a reasonable, prudent person.
5. *Injury, Damage, or Loss.* The injuries caused by the doctor resulted in a physical, financial, or emotional loss.

These points will now be discussed in more detail.

Duty and Breach of Duty

Unless there is a doctor-patient relationship, there can be no malpractice liability. Once a doctor-patient relationship has been formed, however, the doctor has an obligation to care for the patient until treatment is completed or the relationship is terminated in a professionally appropriate manner. Failure to properly terminate a doctor-patient relationship can result in a charge of abandonment. Proper termination includes providing the patient with reasonable notice, assisting the patient in finding another doctor (when requested or when appropriate), and providing medical records when a signed patient release has been presented by the new doctor.

Obviously, the doctor must be particularly concerned about the abandonment issue if the patient is in an emergency or crisis situation. Special caution is called for if the patient has been diagnosed as suffering from a mental illness, since an abrupt termination of the case may exacerbate feelings of loss and abandonment and may precipitate suicidal or other irrational behaviors.

Once it has been established that there was a doctor-patient relationship, the *standard of care* then becomes an issue. The doctor owes the patient a certain quality of care, but at the same time the doctor is not required to guarantee a favorable outcome. Historically, the standard of care applied in a given malpractice case has usually been related to the standards of the local community and to the specialty and school of medicine practiced by the doctor. This standard, however, is usually established through the use of expert testimony. Historically, local experts testified to the standard of care provided in the community. Over the years, the "locality rule" has eroded, so that experts from outside of the defendant's practice area can be used as expert witnesses. As a result, the standard of care is now often regional or even national.

The demise of the locality rule has been due to a number of circumstances, including the hesitancy of local physicians to testify against one another; the adoption of national uniform standards for certification, residency, and training; and requirements for continuing education.[7] These latter two considerations have tended to homogenize and thereby raise the standard of care.

Within a specialty, a doctor is held to the standard of care of other specialists. A general practitioner, for example, is not required to provide the quality of care that would be provided by a specialist. The standard of care for a general practitioner, however, might well require a referral to or consultation with a specialist in a given set of circumstances. The standard of care is also related to the school of medical thought in which the doctor was trained. An osteopathic gynecologist is not held to the same standard as an allopathic gynecologist, and vice versa. There is a presumption that patients understand that different schools of medicine may practice differently and that they will take this into account when selecting providers.

Finally, the doctor has a duty to provide the patient with the opportunity to consent. If the patient did not consent to a treatment, the doctor could be liable for an intentional tort, such as assault or battery. Obviously, it is best to always obtain written consent from the patient, the spouse, or a legal guardian. Consent, however, may be implied in several circumstances, such as these:

- There are extensive discussions between the doctor and the patient, as demonstrated by the subsequent actions of both parties.
- An emergency arises and the doctor cannot obtain consent.

- Adjunct treatment is required because of a procedure to which the patient has consented.

If the doctor obtains the consent of the patient but the patient has not been properly informed of the potential consequences of the treatment, then the doctor has not obtained *informed consent*. Informed consent becomes an issue when the patient alleges that he or she was not provided with sufficient information to make a knowledgeable decision. Some courts have found that the degree of disclosure is determined by the standard of care generally applied by other doctors in similar circumstances. Some states, however, have adopted legislation requiring discussion of risks if a reasonable person in the patient's position would attach significance to the information. Finally, consent only becomes an issue if a reasonable person would have made a different decision as a result of the withheld information. Discuss the content of your state's consent laws with your attorney.

Consent can also be a question when the patient is a minor. Generally, it is best to obtain written consent from the parent of any patient who is under 18. Minors can provide consent under certain circumstances, including (1) emergency treatment, when the life of the patient is at risk, and (2) when the minor is emancipated, which can occur as a result of marriage, a court decree, or a failure of the parents to be legally responsible for the child.

Causation

The burden of causation requires that the plaintiff demonstrate by a preponderance of the evidence that the doctor's care was the cause in fact and the proximate cause of the damage done to the patient. The courts have tended to take two approaches to determining the question of cause in fact.[8] Using the "but for" standard, the question is whether the harm would not have occurred but for the actions of the physician. If the harm would not otherwise have occurred, cause in fact is taken to be demonstrated. A second standard that courts have applied concerns whether the doctor's actions were a "substantial factor" contributing to the patient's damage. If, for example, there were two causes of the patient's harm, then the substantial factor test would associate liability with the source of each cause. Generally, the burden of proof to demonstrate cause will be on the plaintiff. It can shift to a defendant, however, if one doctor is seeking to limit his or her liability with respect to a codefendant.

The issue of proximate cause is related to the "foreseeability" of the consequences of the doctor's actions. Negligence can only be found if the consequences were foreseeable by a reasonable, prudent person. If the consequences were not foreseeable, then the doctor did not have a duty to protect the patient from them, even though the doctor may have caused them to occur "in fact." The old parable—"for want of a nail, a shoe was lost; for want of a shoe, a soldier was lost; for want of a soldier, a battle was lost; for loss of a battle, a war was lost"—demonstrates the need for the concept of proximate cause. Still, a doctor can be negligent because he or she sets a chain of events into motion. The proximate cause standard, however, requires that the doctor be an *instrumental* cause of the injury in the chain of events, as opposed to simply creating conditions in which the harm was possible.

Another way in which cause can be demonstrated is through the doctrine of *res ipsa loquitur,* which is a Latin phrase meaning "the thing speaks for itself." Res ipsa loquitur allows a jury to reach a conclusion based on circumstantial evidence without the plaintiff having to demonstrate that the defendant actually caused the harm. This doctrine is often applied, for example, when a foreign object has been left inside a patient. The fact that the object is there is sufficient to demonstrate causation. Res ipsa loquitor has also been used to demonstrate cause for injuries outside of the area of treatment. For example, a patient receives burns during a procedure on a part of the body that is distant from the operation or a patient develops paralysis after receiving anesthesia. "It speaks for itself" that the harm was done while under the physician's care.

Courts have also applied this doctrine when many people have had control over a patient's unconscious body, such as during the preparation for, conduct of, and recovery from surgery. In this type of situation, it would be very difficult if not impossible for the patient to identify the *specific* person responsible for the harm. Res ipsa loquitur shifts the burden of proof to the defendant, who must then demonstrate by a preponderance of the evidence that he or she did *not* cause the harm.

In order for res ipsa loquitur to be applied by a court, the plaintiff must demonstrate that

1. the injury is of a type that ordinarily doesn't occur unless there is negligence
2. the injury was caused by something that was within the control of the defendant
3. the plaintiff did not contribute to the cause of the injury

Damages

In order for malpractice to be proven, the plaintiff must demonstrate that harm has occurred. The harm can be in the form of financial, emotional, or physical injuries. Compensation can be required for past and future medical costs, loss of income, funeral expenses, pain, mental suffering, and so on. The legal objective is to provide an award of money damages in recompense for the harm done to the plaintiff. In addition, courts occasionally assign punitive and exemplary awards over and above the plaintiff's actual losses, although these awards are usually limited to outrageous, malicious, or intentional acts.

Defenses

There are several defenses to a charge of malpractice. One strategy is to challenge the basis of the tort by claiming that the plaintiff failed to demonstrate that a duty existed, that the standard of care was not breached, that the doctor's actions were not causally related to the harm, or that the patient suffered no harm. In addition, the doctor can raise substantive defenses, which relate to the facts of the case, and procedural defenses, which relate to the legal basis of the complaint.

Substantive defenses include the contributory negligence and the comparative negligence defenses. Contributory negligence occurs when a patient contributes to the harm that occurred. For example, a patient who fails to follow the doctor's directions or provides false or incomplete information may be found to be contributorily negligent. Contributory negligence is a complete defense, in that if it prevails it will preclude *any* recovery by the plaintiff. Attorneys may hesitate to use this defense even if it is available, since a jury may resent an attempt to equate a minor indiscretion on the part of the patient with a major dereliction on the part of the doctor.

Comparative negligence defenses try to apportion the negligence between the plaintiff and the doctor. It is not a complete monetary defense, and the award of damages would be in proportion to the harm found to be done by the doctor. For example, if it was determined that the doctor was responsible for 80 percent of the damage, which was assessed at $100,000, then the doctor would be liable for $80,000.

Historically, case law has recognized the doctrine of contributory negligence; however, state legislatures have been replacing this doctrine with comparative negligence statues. The two doctrines are mutually exclusive and *only one will be in force in any given jurisdiction.*

A third substantive defense is called *assumption of risk.* This occurs when the plaintiff knows and appreciates the risk and voluntarily assumes the risk. Obviously, demonstrating that the patient gave informed consent is essential to this defense. Except where informed consent is present, this defense is usually not successful. Generally it is recognized that the doctor has superior knowledge of the risks involved and is better able to weigh information in making medical decisions.

One procedural defense is to claim that the statute of limitations has expired and that the doctor has thus been released from liability. A person who alleges injury must initiate legal action before the expiration of the time period referred to in that state's statute of limitations. Some states start the clock on the date when the alleged malpractice occurred. Since some injuries may not be observable for years, it is possible for patients to lose the right to sue before becoming aware of the problem. As a result, many states have adopted statutes that start the clock when the patient discovers or should have discovered the injury.

Some physicians have attempted to limit their liability by having patients sign forms releasing them from liability. These forms are generally worthless, since as a matter of public policy a person cannot contract away negligence. A release can be valid, however, in the case of experimental or inherently dangerous treatment. Under these circumstances, the release must be signed before the beginning of treatment, and it must pertain to the consequences of properly performed treatment. It will not constitute a defense for improperly or negligently performed experimental or inherently dangerous treatment.

In addition to legal malpractice defenses, you can implement financial defenses. One such defense is called *insolvency planning*.[9] The object is to make your assets as judgment-proof as possible. Since some aspects of insolvency planning may be inconsistent with prudent estate and financial planning, it is essential to consult your attorney and appropriate tax and financial planning consultants so that you can balance these competing interests.

Another financial defense is to maintain sufficient malpractice insurance and periodically reevaluate your level of coverage. Joint ownership of assets can also hamper creditors, especially in states that recognize the concept of *tenancy by entirety*. This requires that the asset be transferred to both a wife and husband, that the right of survivorship does not end with the death of one party, and that one party's interest cannot be transferred to a third party. Creditors of *both* the husband and the wife, however, can execute a judgment against this type of ownership. Some states have homestead laws that protect a portion of an owner's equity from a judgment. Retirement plans are also protected from creditors, although distributions from a plan can be subject to a judgment.

Finally, you can give away your assets. You may give up to $600,000 lifetime tax free to a spouse, or you may give assets to a reversionary trust (which is irrevocable for a period of time) or to an irrevocable trust. Life insurance that is placed in an irrevocable trust is also not subject to a judgment.

CONTRACTS

A contract is a legally binding agreement between two or more parties. Examples of contracts include agreements with your employees, your partners, your suppliers, the telephone company, and your bank. Contracts can be in written or verbal form. As a general rule, you should not enter into any significant contract without first having it reviewed by your attorney. However, you will likely have to enter into many contracts, and it would be time consuming, expensive, and cumbersome to have your attorney review all of them. For example, you engage a security service to install an alarm, a water company to supply bottled water, an employment agency to provide a temporary secretary for this afternoon, a store to supply a wingback chair, and a painter to repaint a chipped file cabinet. All of these transactions are contractual, yet probably none of them is of sufficient magnitude that it would warrant the inconvenience and cost of *routinely* forwarding it to your attorney for review. It is important, therefore, to appreciate how contracts are formed, interpreted, and enforced so that you can identify dubious or potentially disadvantageous situations and selectively use your attorney.

The objective of this section is to provide a basic understanding of how contracts are formed and interpreted by the courts. Whenever you are in doubt regarding the meaning of a contract or whenever a contract includes a substantial commitment of time, money, personnel, or other resources, you should have it reviewed by your attorney.

In order for a contract to exist, the parties must be competent, they must reach a mutual agreement, consideration must be provided, and what has been contracted for must be legal. *Competence* means that all parties are legally capable of entering into the agreement. Minors, the insane, and individuals who are intoxicated may be considered incompetent to enter into contracts. Entering into a contract with a minor is particularly dangerous, since the adult party may be held to the terms of the contract whereas the minor may withdraw at any time. For example, if you treat a minor without the consent of a legal guardian, you may not be able to hold the minor financially accountable, although the minor will be able to hold you to an acceptable standard of care. Although state law may hold the parent financially responsible, you then would have the problem of locating and collecting from the parent.

Mutual agreement means that there was both an offer and an acceptance. An offer means that you intend to be legally bound if the offer is accepted. Since offers may be preceded by preliminary negotiations, it is important to clearly indicate whether you are making an offer or merely expressing an intention to make an offer at some future time. For example, Dr. Kurth may state to Dr. Jackson, "I'm interested in selling my practice for $100,000. Would you be interested in buying it?" This is merely an inquiry, not an offer to sell. Dr. Jackson cannot force the sale for $100,000. If Dr. Jackson responded by promising to buy the practice for $100,000 or any other amount, that would constitute an offer. If Dr. Kurth then accepted the offer, a contract would then exist. Phrases such as "Would you be interested in," "I understand that you are looking for," and "How would you feel about" do not constitute offers. Since communications can become complex and the price of misunderstanding can be so great, it is always best to label an inquiry as such.

An offer can be terminated in several ways. The offeror can revoke it any time before it is accepted by the other party. For example, if Dr. Jackson offers Dr. Kurth $100,000 for his practice, he can revoke the offer at any point before Dr. Kurth accepts it. The revocation must be received before the offer is accepted in order for it to be valid.

An offer can be terminated by a lapse of time. For example, an offer can state when it will expire. If the offer contains no stated expiration time, a court will consider the offer valid for a "reasonable" length of time. What constitutes a reasonable length of time will depend on the facts and circumstances of the case.

An offer will terminate upon rejection or counteroffer. Once an offer is rejected, the person who rejected it cannot change his or her mind and then accept it. If an acceptance is conditional (e.g., "I will accept the offer if . . . ") or if the person to whom the offer is made changes some of the terms, the result is considered to be a counteroffer, not an acceptance. The original offeror, now the offeree, is free to accept the counteroffer, thereby binding the other party to a valid contract, or to reject it.

Once the person to whom the offer is made accepts the terms of the offer and conveys this acceptance to the offeror, the contract is binding. Communication of acceptance can take place in several ways. If the offer dictates the method of communication, such as by certified mail, then the acceptance must be communicated in that form. If the offer states that the acceptance must be made within a certain time, then once again the acceptance must occur within that time. Generally, an acceptance is considered valid after it is in the mail. In order to avoid problems with any offers that you make, you should always specify the manner of acceptance and when the offer expires.

Consideration is the exchange that takes place as a result of the contract. In order for a contract to be valid, something must be given and something received. For example, consideration exists if you agree to purchase bottled water at $7.50 per jug. Generally, the courts are not concerned with the adequacy of consideration. *If you strike a bad deal, you will be stuck with it!* Consideration does not exist if one party is not truly committed to provide something. For example, an agreement that states "If Dr. Sipos determines that he needs bottled water, he will purchase it for $7.50 per jug from the Gulch Water Company" would be considered an illusory promise. It would not demonstrate consideration, since Dr. Sipos is not promising to purchase water. In contrast, an agreement that stated "I promise to buy all the bottled water that I need from the Gulch Water Company at $7.50 per jug" would constitute a contract if it was accepted by the Gulch Water Company.

Finally, in order for a contract to exist, the subject matter must be legal. If a contract is in violation of any statutes or of public policy, it is not enforceable. For example, Dr. Saam contracts with Johnson Construction Company to enlarge his office. As part of the contract, he requires that Johnson Construction Company remove the fire doors after the project is completed, so that the building will no longer be in compliance with the building code. This is a violation of local ordinance and cannot be enforced under contract law.

Similarly, contractual terms requiring the violation of public policy will also be unenforceable. The term *public policy* is a loose one, but it generally means "protecting from that which tends to be injurious to the public or contrary to the public good, . . . or any established interest of society."[10] Contracts that obstruct justice; corrupt public officials; are immoral; are offensive to public decency; restrain trade; or discriminate on the basis of race, religion, sex, or national origin may violate public policy. For example, if the only two urologists in town contract to fix the price of urological services, this may be construed as a restraint of trade. If one of the urologists then violates the agreement, he or she could claim that there was no contractual relationship, because the content of the agreement violated public policy. In addition, *both* urologists might be prosecuted under federal or state antitrust legislation.

As you can see, the four requirements of a valid contract do not include the necessity of a written document. With certain notable exceptions, verbal contracts are generally enforceable if they are agreed to by competent parties and reflect mutual agreement, consideration, and legal content. Obviously, verbal contracts can be troublesome, since memories can become "selective." In order to protect your own interests, you should insist on a written contract whenever the worst possible outcome from a business arrangement is more burdensome than arranging for your attorney to prepare a contract.

Certain types of contracts must be in writing in order for them to be enforceable. These include

- The sale of land or an interest in land (in some states, a verbal lease of less than one year is enforceable).
- the sale of goods in excess of $500
- contracts that by their terms cannot be fulfilled within one year
- suretyship contracts (promises to pay for the debts of others)

When a written contract is drafted, it is critical that you or your attorney anticipate all possible consequences of the arrangement and ensure that the contract provides for adequate resolution. If a dispute should arise, a court will apply the "four corners" rule to resolve it. This means that the court will look first to *exactly* what is contained within the four corners of the contract. Irrespective of what you intended, the contract will be interpreted literally. (There can be exceptions to the four corners rule. For example, if the contract is ambiguous or contradictory, the court may look to "parole" evidence, evidence outside of the contract, to determine the intent of the parties.) Consider the following example:

Dr. Jones was working for Dr. Smith. Dr. Jones left Dr. Smith's practice, opened her own practice, and incorporated as Darla Jones, M.D., P.C. Dr. Jones' contract with Dr. Smith had stated that she, Jones, would pay Smith 15 percent of all fees received by her for any patients transferred from the practice for a period of six months. This was in consideration for Smith having provided referrals to Jones, and otherwise assisting in building Jones' practice. Jones' practice—Darla Jones, M.D., P.C.—paid Dr. Jones a salary of 60 percent of collected fees. Dr. Jones then paid Dr. Smith 15 percent of her salary from transferred patients, or 15 percent of 60 percent of transferred patient collections.

Dr. Smith objected on the basis that this was simply a subterfuge. Dr. Smith maintained that since Dr. Jones "was the corporation," the arrangement was simply a sham to avoid paying 15 percent on all fees collected from transferred patients. Dr. Jones refused to comply and Smith sued Jones.

Judgment for Dr. Jones. The contract clearly stated that the 15 percent payments were payable by *Jones* on fees collected by *Jones*. The fact that she interposed a corporation between herself and Dr. Smith did not change the clear language of the contract. The court reminded Dr. Smith that if his intention was to have Jones pay a fee on all collections for transferred patients, whether by her or by a corporation employing her, then this should have been so stated in the contract.

Attorneys are skilled at anticipating what can go wrong, drafting language to clarify what the resolution will be if something should go wrong, and positioning their client so that if a dispute does occur, the client will be in a strong position. Nevertheless, it is important, in any business arrangement, that your attorney fully understands your objectives, your exposure if the other party fails to fulfill the terms of the contract, and protections that you feel you need if the arrangement does not prove to be satisfactory.

As with an accountant, you are the ultimate consumer of your legal services. If an attorney does not fully appreciate your needs or drafts a document that does not fully meet your needs, you are the one who will ultimately live with the consequences.

EMPLOYMENT ISSUES

Many aspects of the employer-employee relationship have legal implications. The most basic legal consideration in the employer-employee relationship is the employment contract. Other legal considerations include employment discrimination, workers' compensation laws, and the Fair Labor Standards Act. Once again, it is important for you or your business manager to appreciate the legal issues involved so that you will know when to involve an attorney and be able to make daily decisions that are not legally risky.

Employment Contracts

As with other contracts, the employment contract can be written or verbal. A verbal arrangement is generally referred to as *employment at will*. It is important to appreciate the consequences of both types of employment arrangements so that you can choose the appropriate one for specific employees, jobs, or circumstances.

There are four major reasons why you might want to have a written employment contract with an employee. First, a written contract will decrease the chances that either party will misunderstand the mutual commitments. The process of negotiating the employment contract will require both parties to think about most aspects of the employment relationship, including compensation, vacation time, sick leave policy, work schedules, and termination. If disagreements are discovered in the contracting process, then they can be resolved before they lead to an employer-employee dispute.

Second, if you want a long-term commitment from an employee, it generally should be put in writing. To be enforceable, the contract must be put in writing if it is for a year or longer. For example, if you have a skilled radiology technician and you want to be certain the employee doesn't leave on the spur of the moment, you could negotiate an employment contract that states the employment would last for an agreed period of time, such as one year, or that required a notice period, such as three weeks or one month must be provided. (A long-term commitment of less than a year can be made verbally; however, if the contract has to be enforced there could be a disagreement regarding its terms. If your objective is to provide security, then the uncertainty created by the verbal contract defeats the purpose of seeking a long-term agreement.)

Third, you can include in the contract a noncompetition clause that will restrict the ability of the employee to compete with you after leaving your employment. Obviously, the issue of competition is only relevant for physicians or other skilled professionals. Generally, courts have found these clauses to be valid as long as they are limited to a reasonable time period and a reasonable geographical area. The standards of "reasonableness" vary with state law and local tradition. In the example above, the 15 percent fee on transferred patients that Dr. Jones was to pay Dr. Smith for six months might well be considered reasonable in many jurisdictions. A contract precluding practice in the same city for five years would generally be considered unreasonable. It is important to remember that the employee has a right to earn a living and that noncompetition clauses contradict the spirit of antitrust laws, which are based on the notion that open, robust competition is beneficial for society. As a result, courts will not enforce a noncompetition clause that unduly restricts this right. Some courts have struck down noncompetition clauses, whereas others have determined and then applied appropriate geographic and time restrictions. A local attorney's advice is essential in determining what might be a reasonable noncompetition restriction.

Fourth, an employment contract can increase a practice's financial security by committing revenue-generating employees to long-term employment. Practices that employ several doctors can coordinate the lengths of their contracts so that the expiration dates are staggered. This makes it more difficult for the employee physicians to conspire and decimate a group practice by leaving en masse. Other revenue-generating employees, such as nutritionists, physical therapists, and nurse practitioners, should also be considered for employment contracts.

The wording of the termination clause in an employment contract is very important. An improperly worded termination clause will restrict your ability to fire an employee. For example, the following termination clause was contained in an nurse's employment contract:

> This Agreement will be in effect for one year from the date upon which it was made and entered into. This Agreement can be terminated before the end of one year:
>
> A. At any time by the Employee with 30 days written notice;
>
> B. At any time by the Company for inadequate job performance.

During the term of the contract Nurse Roberts developed strong antiabortion attitudes. He did not allow them to interfere with his job performance, but his participation in public demonstrations and the extremeness of his attitudes caused Dr. Smith, his employer, to feel uncomfortable with Nurse Roberts. Dr. Smith no longer wished to employ him, but since his job performance had been adequate, Dr. Smith was committed to retaining him for the remainder of the contract.

From your perspective as an employer, the most favorable termination clause is one that states that the employee serves at your will and that you may terminate the employee (1) for any reason or for no reason and (2) at any time. Although this provision sounds harsh, it can be both legal and highly desirable from your perspective. There are few things as frustrating as not being able to immediately fire an employee when you feel that it is necessary and justified. There are also few things that are as destructive to the morale and effectiveness of an office as a dissatisfied and malevolent employee. Clever employees can be malevolent in passive-aggressive ways that are difficult to document, which can make it hard to show cause for terminating them. It is best to avoid having to show cause by retaining the prerogative to terminate an employee at your will whenever you want.

Since employees are interested in job security, they will naturally hesitate to sign contracts with strong at-will provisions. They will often seek to limit your ability to terminate them, or at a minimum they will seek severance benefits.

Kahn, Brown, and Zepke propose some provisions that attempt to balance the legitimate needs of doctors to terminate employees with the desires of employees for security:[11]

1. There should be a fixed length for the term of the agreement, such as one year, two years, and so on.
2. The employer should retain the right to terminate the employee in case of
   - the employee's death
   - a disability that prevents the employee from carrying out his or her duties
   - a failure of the employee to obey orders
3. The employer should retain the right to terminate the employee immediately for misconduct, with no severance benefits. Misconduct is to be defined at the sole and unrestricted discretion of the employer.
4. The employer should retain the right to terminate the employee for any reason, with notice (e.g., two weeks).
5. The employee should retain the right to resign at any time, with notice to the employer (e.g., two weeks).
6. The employee should agree not to work for a competing practice for a fixed period of time in a stated geographical area.

These termination provisions still give the doctor wide latitude to terminate the employee for inadequate job performance or any other reason, yet they provide some measure of job security and financial security for the employee. They also limit the ability of the employee to work for a competitor or to be stolen by a competitor for a higher salary during the term of the agreement.

An example of an employment contract is found in Exhibit 9-1. This contract has a number of typical features. First, it fulfills the minimal definition of a contract in that it provides for mutual agreement (Recitals and Paragraph 1) and consideration (Paragraphs 2, 3, and 4) and its contents are not in violation of statutes or public policy. The contract provides details regarding the employer's and employee's commitments, including the following:

1. salary and payment schedule (Paragraph 3)
2. vacation and sick leave (Paragraph 4)
3. the length of the contract and the reasons that it can be terminated by either party (Paragraph 6)
4. the manner in which one party should notify the other whenever notification is necessary (Paragraph 7)
5. a requirement that any modification of the contract must be made in writing (Paragraph 8)

Exhibit 9-1 Sample Employment Contract

EMPLOYMENT AGREEMENT

THIS EMPLOYMENT AGREEMENT is made and entered into this _____ day of _____, 1990, by and between Laura Smith, M.D., Ltd., a Virginia professional corporation, hereafter known as "Company," and _____, hereafter known as "Employee."

RECITALS

A. The Company has formed and developed a private practice providing medical services to the general public.

B. The Company desires the association and collaboration of the Employee.

C. The Employee is desirous of the benefits of affiliation and compensation provided in this Agreement.

NOW THEREFORE, for good and valuable consideration, the parties agree as follows:

1. *Mutuality of Interest.* The Company promises to pay such fees and compensation as set forth in Section 3 to the Employee for services provided under this Agreement, and the Employee promises to provide such services as set forth in Section 3 to the Company for the duration of this Agreement.

2. *Performance of Duties.* The Employee shall perform the duties of Radiologist Technician as determined by the practice Director. The Employee also shall comply in all regards with such policies and regulations as the Company may establish from time to time for the efficient operation of the Company's business.

3. *Compensation.* The Employee will be paid a salary of $_____ per year. This will be payable in 24 equal amounts paid on the 1st and 16th of each calendar month.

4. *Sick and Vacation Time.* The Employee will accumulate 1 day per month of personal time, which can be used as vacation leave or sick leave. Days may accumulate up to a total of 15 days, at which point, and at the sole discretion of the Director, a day must be used or the Company can provide compensation at a per day amount based on the following formula:

$$\text{Per Day Compensation} = (\text{Annual Salary} \div 2{,}080) \times 8$$

The Director will approve all vacation leave, and adequate notice of intention to take vacation leave must be given to the Director.

5. *Employee Status.* The Employee, for all purposes, including but not limited to federal income tax laws, state income tax laws, unemployment compensation laws, and workers' compensation laws, shall be an employee and agrees not to make any declaration or take any position for any matter to the contrary.

6. *Duration of Agreement.* This Agreement will be in effect for one year from the date upon which it is made and entered into. This Agreement can be terminated at any time by the Company for such acts of the Employee that the Company, in its sole and unrestricted discretion, may deem to be unethical, unprofessional, or illegal or for inadequate job performance. This Agreement can be terminated at any time by the Employee with 30 days written notice.

7. *Notification.* Any notices required or permitted to be given under this Agreement shall be sufficient if in writing and sent by certified mail to the Employee's last known address as reflected in the Company's records, and to the Company at its principal office.

continues

Exhibit 9-1 continued

8. *Waiver or Modification and Severance.* No waiver or modification of this Agreement shall be valid unless it is in writing and duly signed by both parties. Any part of this Agreement which is subsequently determined to be illegal may be severed from the remainder of the Agreement, leaving that remainder fully valid and in effect.

9. *Integration.* This Agreement contains the complete understanding concerning the arrangement between the parties and shall, effective as of the date hereof, supersede any and all other agreements between the parties. The parties stipulate that neither of them has made any representation with respect to the subject matter of this Agreement except such representations as are specifically set forth in this Agreement.

10. *Successors in Interest.* The rights and obligations of the parties under this Agreement shall inure to the benefit of and shall be binding upon the successors and assigns of the parties. The duties of the Employee are not delegable to any other person or entity.

IN WITNESS WHEREOF, the parties hereto have executed this Agreement on the day and date written above.

Laura Smith, M.D., Ltd.

By _____

Laura Smith, M.D.
President

_____

(Name)
Employee

6. a statement declaring that this contract is the total agreement between the parties and that nothing else is being implied or expected as a result of the agreement (Paragraph 9)

7. a statement that commits both parties to fulfill their obligations to their successors (Paragraph 10)

Regarding this last item, if the employee should die, for example, the employee's estate would be due any salary or benefits that had been accrued by the employee. Similarly, if Dr. Smith sold her practice, the employee would be committed to the new owner by this contract, and vice versa. This paragraph precludes the employee from meeting his or her obligation by hiring a replacement. He or she *personally* is committed to fulfilling the terms of the contract.

Finally, Dr. Smith signs the contract for the corporation. This makes the contract a corporate obligation, and Dr. Smith has no personal obligation to the employee. If, for example, Dr. Smith's practice went into bankruptcy, the employee would have to seek recovery for any unpaid wages from Dr. Smith's practice, not personally from her. Similarly, if the employee claimed that the contract was breached, he or she would have to seek recovery from the practice, not Dr. Smith.

Exhibit 9-2 contains a checklist of items that should be considered for inclusion in any employment contract. You can use this checklist to help ensure that you explore all relevant issues with the employee or applicant and with your attorney.

In general, you should only enter into employment contracts with very valued employees—and only after carefully considering the consequences and having the contracts drafted by an attorney. The difficulties and frustrations associated with *any* restrictions on your ability to terminate employees should not be underestimated. Generally, a written contract will be more restrictive than an unwritten agreement, simply because the employee will ask for restrictions that would not occur to him or her with an unwritten agreement.

The security offered by a long-term contract is often illusory. Even if you are able to convince an employee to stay contrary to his or her own true wishes, your victory is almost always merely Pyrrhic. Employees serving against their wishes

Exhibit 9-2 Employment Contract Checklist

1. Offer and acceptance of employment*
2. Description of duties, responsibilities, and so on
3. Provision that the employee devote full time and attention to the employer's business
4. Provision that the employee not engage in any other employment of any kind without disclosure and written permission
5. Duration of the contract*
6. Subsequent renewals (automatic or upon notice)
7. Compensation*
8. Discipline procedures
9. Other benefits, such as bonuses, insurance, and mileage
10. Severance benefits (allowed or not, earned or discretionary, accrued or forfeited)
11. Termination of employment (at will; for cause; whether employee is entitled to any compensation at termination and, if so, under what circumstances)*
12. Noncompetition covenants
13. Nondisclosure of confidential information, such as business plans and patient information
14. Provision for the employee in the event of sale, merger, and so on
15. "This is the whole of the agreement" clause ("zipper clause")
16. The procedure for amending the contract
17. Definition of what constitutes breach of the contract
18. Procedure for providing notice to the other party (e.g., by certified mail)
19. Governing law clause ("This contract shall be interpreted according to the laws of the state of _____ ")

*Item must be included in some form.

Source: Adapted from *Personnel Director's Legal Guide*, 1988 Cumulative Supplement, by S. Kahn, B. Brown, and B. Zepke, pp. S2-53–54, with permission of Warren, Gorham, and Lamont, © 1988.

will take their dissatisfaction out on you, your practice, and your patients, and a written contract will provide you with no effective defense against this form of retribution. It is better to replace employees who simply provide services, such as secretaries, business managers, and nurses, than to try to keep them against their will. Decisions regarding revenue-generating employees are more difficult. Following are three strategies for dealing with revenue-generating employees who are serving against their will:

1. Release them and consider the lost revenue to be the price for your own well-being and that of your employees and patients.
2. Negotiate a price for the employee to buy him- or herself out of the contract.
3. Enforce the contract and grit your teeth and bear it. If you pursue this alternative and the employee leaves, you may seek an injunction barring the employee from working for or becoming a competitor. Courts, however, generally recognize that slavery has been illegal for quite some time, so they are unlikely to force the employee to go back to work for you. Under these circumstances, you may seek monetary damages. You would have an obligation, however, to mitigate the damages by attempting to replace the employee. The damages that you may be able to recover would be the lost income less the damages that were mitigated.

    For example, Dr. Temple leaves Dr. Johnson's practice in violation of her employment agreement. Dr. Temple generated $200,000 in gross receipts and continues at this rate after leaving. Dr. Johnson hires a replacement, who generates $150,000 during the same time period. Dr. Johnson could seek damages of $50,000. If Dr. Johnson does not attempt to mitigate the damages, the court may decide that there would have been none and may choose to assign no damages. On the other hand, if Dr. Johnson made a good faith effort to find a replacement but none was available, Dr. Johnson may be awarded $200,000.

Your choice of strategy will depend on a number of issues, including the precedent that you want to set for other employees, the value of the employee's revenue to the financial health of the practice, and your own peace of mind.

Employment At Will

Employees with no written or stated verbal contract are employed "at will." An at-will arrangement, however, implies a contract. When a legally competent employee agrees to provide labor in exchange for compensation, there is consideration, mutual assent, and legal content, and therefore, a contract exists. Traditionally, at-will arrangements allowed employers to terminate employees for good cause, bad cause, or no cause at all. Over the years, however, courts and legislatures have placed limits on the employer's ability to dismiss employees.

Most states currently have laws that restrict the employer's ability to terminate at-will employees unless there is good cause. One type of restriction relates to *abusive or retaliatory discharge.* This occurs when the discharge is in retaliation for an employee's refusal to violate public policy. For example, many states do not allow dismissal for "whistle-blowing" or for failure to perform an illegal activity, such as refusing to commit perjury to protect the employer, refusing to commit bribery, failure to submit false insurance claims, and refusing to falsify records. Many states have made it illegal to dismiss an employee for filing a workers' compensation claim, for refusing to take a polygraph test, or for meeting military or jury duty obligations. In addition, federal and state antidiscrimination laws also limit the employer's ability to dismiss at-will employees without just cause.

An ex-employee's allegation that dismissal was in violation of public policy certainly doesn't mean that a court will uphold this allegation and assign damages. It does mean, however, that the employer may have to provide some evidence for dismissal that refutes the claimed violation of public policy. Documentation of inadequate job performance or insubordination, for example, is essential for a successful defense under these circumstances. The need to provide a defense in the first place exemplifies the erosion of the employer's traditional at-will prerogative to terminate an employee for "bad cause or no cause at all."

Another challenge to the employer's at-will termination prerogative arises from the concept of *implied terms* in the employment agreement. Courts have found that oral statements made to the employee, as well as written documents other than the employment contract, can become part of the employment agreement. This then makes dismissal conditional upon good cause. For example, some courts have held that an employee handbook can become part of the employee contract. In *Toussaint v. Blue Cross and Blue Shield of Michigan,* the court found that statements in the company's personnel manual indicating that employees would only be terminated for cause became part of the employment contract.[12] Other implied terms have been found in oral statements made at the time of hiring, such as "You'll always have a job here as long as you do as I say" and "I won't fire an employee until I give him three chances to improve."

Another attack on at-will employment is application of the doctrine that *good faith and fair dealing* is implied in any contract. Some courts have interpreted "good faith and fair dealing" to mean that the employer has an obligation to provide employees with due process and base terminations on just cause. If the employer has to justify the dismissal or provide an appeal process or a forum for the employee to contest the dismissal, then the at-will prerogative is obviously compromised. This doctrine has been used, for example, to invalidate terminations whose purpose was to avoid paying wages and a termination in which an employee was forced to write a resignation letter.

It should be noted, however, that there is wide variation in how far courts will go to find implied contracts. For example, a California court held that "merely exchanging pleasantries about the company during an interview did not imply a promise by the employer of job security."[13] Similarly, many courts have held that company handbooks and other written documents are simply unilateral statements. Since there is no "meeting of the minds," there is no contract.

There are several things that you, as an employer, can do to preserve your at-will prerogative to terminate employees in so far as your jurisdiction permits:

1. Make no statements in the employment process that could be construed as making an exception to at-will employment. For example, don't say, "You'll have a job here as long as you perform well" or "If your work isn't satisfactory, I'll give you a chance to improve."

2. Never give an applicant a policy manual or handbook during the employment process. If you do, it may be argued later that its contents were part of the reason that the applicant accepted the job, thereby making it part of the employment contract.

3. Tell the job applicant that the terms of employment are "at will" and explain what that means. Some companies will have new employees sign a document such as the one in Exhibit 9-3.

4. Always document reasons for discharge. Inadequate job performance, absenteeism, and insubordination are among the legitimate reasons for termi-

Exhibit 9-3 Statement Establishing At-Will Termination

I understand and agree that, if employed, my employment will not be covered by any contract for a specific term and that my relationship with the practice can, at any time, be terminated by the practice with or without cause, and with or without notice, and without prior notice or warning.

Frederick Jonson, M.D., P.C.

By _____   _____
    Frederick Jonson, M.D., President   Date

_____   _____
Applicant   Date

Source: Adapted from *Employee Discipline* by J.R. Redeker, p. 100, with permission of the Bureau of National Affairs, © 1989.

nation, and they can be used to refute allegations of abusive discharge or of an implied contract.

5. Have your attorney check state laws and court interpretations and inform you of illegal grounds for termination in your state.

6. Always review the facts of a termination with your attorney *before* you terminate the employee. Do this even if you feel the facts are very clear and your behavior is fully justified. Your attorney may have suggestions regarding how to document the facts and orchestrate the termination so as to provide you with maximum defensibility.

7. Review personnel manuals, employment applications, training materials, and so on, for any language that could be construed as limiting your at-will termination authority. These documents should contain a clear statement that employment is at will. In addition, each manual or handbook should contain a disclaimer stating that nothing in it is intended to create a contract with an employee.

8. If you create any documents specifying a code of conduct, always include a disclaimer in which you state that the document is illustrative. This will give you latitude, since it is impossible to anticipate all of the creative ways in which employees can violate the spirit of a policy without clearly breaching its specific content.

10. Review the suggestions for employee discipline and termination in Chapter 4. Using these ideas will strengthen your legal defensibility.

11. Apply your discipline and termination procedures with consistency.

12. Be honest with yourself regarding the real reasons why you are terminating an employee. Sometimes feelings of anger or betrayal may result in your doing something that isn't legally defensible. If you are honest with yourself, you will be able to avoid a questionable termination.

Equal Employment Opportunity

Federal and state legislation precludes employers from discriminating against employees on the basis of race, religion, sex, national origin, and age. This legislation encompasses all aspects of employment, including hiring, promotion, compensation, access to training, discipline, and termination. Employers covered by this legislation cannot use a person's race, religion, sex, national origin, or age (if over 40 years) to influence an employment decision. The primary federal equal employment opportunity (EEO) laws are the 1964 Civil Rights Act (in particular, Title VII), the Age Discrimination in Employment Act of 1967 (ADEA), and the Age Discrimination Act of 1975 (ADA). (Other relevant pieces of federal legislation include the First, Fifth, Thirteenth, and Fourteenth Amendments to the U.S.

Constitution, various executive orders issued by the President, and the Equal Pay Act of 1963.)

The Equal Employment Opportunity Commission (EEOC) was created as a result of the Civil Rights Act of 1964. Its mission is to administer Title VII of that act as well as federal age discrimination legislation. The EEOC interprets the meaning of civil rights legislation, provides guidance to employers, and enforces the legislation through prosecution in federal court. As a result of its central position in drafting, interpreting, and enforcing EEO legislation, the EEOC's interpretations, published in its guidelines to employers, are very important.

Most medical practices will *not* be subject to federal EEO regulation, because of their relatively small size. The Civil Rights Act of 1964 only covers employers who have 15 or more employees for each working day for 20 or more calendar weeks in the current or preceding year. The ADEA and ADA only apply to companies employing 20 or more employees for 20 or more calendar weeks in the current or preceding year. In addition, the ADEA and ADA only provide protection to employees who are 40 or more years old. Since most federal discrimination enforcement emanates from these acts, most medical practices are effectively exempt from federal EEO regulation.

Many practices, however, may be subject to state EEO laws. Since these laws vary considerably from state to state, it is essential that you contact your attorney to understand the compliance requirements in your particular state. In addition, some cities, such as New York City and San Francisco, have developed their own civil rights legislation, and once again you should seek guidance from your attorney.

The following discussion of federal civil rights legislation only applies *directly* to those medical practices that are covered by the Civil Rights Act of 1964, the ADEA, and the ADA. Smaller medical practices, nevertheless, may want to be familiar with federal guidelines. First, many state laws are based on the EEOC's interpretations of federal legislation. Understanding the EEOC's perspective may help doctors comply with state legislation. Second, the EEOC's perspective strikes a good balance between society's need for fair and equal treatment and the employer's need for competent, qualified personnel. Finally, the EEOC's thinking, as embodied in its recommendations to employers, is generally consistent with good personnel management and employment methods. Thus, understanding the EEOC's position may help doctors utilize better personnel management and employment methods.

The primary source of federal EEO enforcement is Title VII of the Civil Rights Act of 1964. Various EEOC publications provide the employer with specific guidance regarding how to hire, compensate, terminate, and otherwise deal with employees without discriminating. The following sections are designed to provide you with an overview of how to comply with the EEOC's recommendations.

Employment Methods

It is important to understand the technical definition of the word *discrimination* as it relates to employment. One form of discrimination is called *disparate treatment*, which occurs when the employer bases an employment decision on race, color, religion, sex, age, or national origin. In effect, disparate treatment occurs when the employer willfully discriminates. For example, not hiring males or females for certain positions, such as nurse or secretary, constitutes disparate treatment, and it is unlawful.

Another condition that may constitute discrimination is called *disparate impact*, which occurs when the employer's actions, even though apparently neutral, have the effect of disproportionately excluding one group. For example, during the interviewing process, while you do not consciously screen out females and the questions have no obvious gender bias, nevertheless you hire a substantially smaller proportion of females than males. This would constitute disparate impact, but it is not yet discrimination. At this point, the burden shifts to the employer to justify the disparity. A legal defense for disparate impact is business necessity. If the employment method (interviewing) assesses skills that are important and required by the job, then no discrimination has taken place. Persons in the affected groups simply do not possess the necessary skills in as high a proportion as members of other groups. In effect, *business necessity is a legal justification for disparate impact.*

An employer's ability to demonstrate business necessity will depend on the employment methods that are utilized. For example, suppose that you use an unstructured interview to fill a position. A female applicant who is denied the position claims that the real reason for the rejection was her sex. Your practice has previously rejected a number of female applicants. This fact would be documented by the completion of EEO Form 1, which is required of all employers covered by the 1964 Civil Rights Act. At this point there is strong evidence for disparate impact. You cannot show the job-relatedness of the unstructured interview questions because you don't have a record of them or of the applicant's responses. It is likely that the EEOC would determine that your employment procedures are discriminatory, since there is disparate impact with no documentation of business necessity.

If, on the other hand, you use a structured interview, you might be able to demonstrate that the content of the interview is closely related to job content, and this particular applicant's performance was inferior to the applicant who was hired. By establishing these two points, you would demonstrate business necessity and would probably be able to rebut the charge of discrimination.

Some race and sex groups do, in fact, perform differently on certain types of employment methods. For example, women have lower average scores than men on strength tests. Whites tend to have higher average scores than blacks on some standardized achievement tests.[14] Undoubtedly, many group differences are due to the effects of socialization, education, and previous discrimination, but rectifying past wrongs is not the employer's legal duty. The employer is fully justified in seeking the most qualified applicant, irrespective of race, sex, and so on. On the other hand, differences in group averages are not a justification for automatically rejecting all applicants from any group. Each applicant must be evaluated *as an individual*. If an employment method does have a disparate impact and the method is related to important job performance issues, then the employment method is justified and it is legally defensible.

The employer can demonstrate the job-relatedness of an employment method either quantitatively or qualitatively.[15] In a quantitative demonstration, the employer establishes that groups of employees who performed higher on the employment method also had better job performance than groups with lower employment method evaluations.[16] Most medical practices covered by Title VII will be too small to demonstrate the job-relatedness of their employment methods statistically. As a result, most demonstrations will be based on qualitative evidence.

A qualitative validation demonstrates that the content of the employment method is similar to the content of the job. For example, job analysis of a clerical position might show that the job requires considerable typing and that the typing is similar in nature to the content of the typing test that was used to screen applicants. It is important, therefore, to maintain accurate job descriptions and to use employment methods that can be shown to assess the job content. Another strategy is to use the results of studies conducted by employment test publishers. Employment tests put out by reputable publishers have been validated for various jobs. This research evidence, which is usually reported in the test manual, can also be used to argue that the test is job-relevant. In order to use this strategy, the employer must show that the job content is similar to jobs reported in the publisher's validation study. Once again, having an accurate job description is important for demonstrating this relationship.

If you use unstructured interviews that are unrelated to the job description, you may have a very difficult time demonstrating the job-relatedness of your employment method. More fundamentally, it should be obvious that relying on unstructured interviews is simply bad policy irrespective of its legality. Table 9-1 contains a guide on pre-employment inquiries. This will help you to think about the relevance of various interview questions that you might ask and how these questions might be viewed by the applicant.

Finally, the best and least expensive legal defense is always prevention. Even if an employment method *is* job-related, you always want to consider how it will appear to the applicant. An employment method that doesn't look job-related will raise questions in the applicant's mind. A litigious applicant may suspect that the test or interview is merely a subterfuge or an excuse to reject. It is a good idea,

Table 9-1 Preemployment Interview Guide

Subject	Unlawful Inquiry	Lawful Inquiry*
Name	If your name has been legally changed, what was your former name?	Have you ever worked for this company under a different name? What is your maiden name? *(May be asked of married female applicants, if necessary, to check educational or employment records.)* Have you ever been convicted of a crime under another name?
Age	[*Any question that tends to identify applicants aged 40 to 69.*]	Are you over eighteen years of age? If hired, can you furnish proof of age? [*Statement that employment is subject to verification that applicant's age meets legal requirements.*]
Citizenship	Are you a citizen of the United States (varies by state)?. Are your parents or spouse citizens of the United States? On what dates did you, your parents, or your spouse acquire U.S. citizenship? Are you, your parents, or spouse naturalized or native-born U.S. citizens?	If you are not a U.S. citizen, do you have the legal right to remain permanently in the United States? What is your visa status *(if No to above)*? Do you intend to remain permanently in the United States? [*Statement that employment is subject to verification of applicant's eligibility for employment under laws related to visa status.*]
National Origin/ Ancestry	What is your nationality/lineage/ancestry/national origin/ descent/parentage? How did you acquire the ability to speak, read, or write a foreign language? How did you acquire familiarity with a foreign country? What language is spoken in your home? What is your mother tongue?	What language do you speak, read, or write fluently? Do you have special familiarity with any foreign country? What is the nature of that familiarity *(if Yes to above)*?

continues

*Lawful only if job-related.

Table 9-1 continued

Subject	Unlawful Inquiry	Lawful Inquiry*
Race or Color	[Any question that directly or indirectly relates to race or color.]	[None.]
Religion	Do you attend religious services or a house of worship? What is your religious denomination or affiliation, church, parish, or pastor? What religious holidays do you observe?	[None.]
Sex	[Any inquiry as to sex, such as the following:] Do you wish to be addressed as Mr., Mrs., Miss, or Ms.? What are your plans regarding having children in the future? Do you have the capacity to reproduce?	[None.]
Relatives/Marital Status	What is your marital status? (If over 18) What is the name or address of relative/spouse/children? With whom do you reside? Do you live with your parents? What are the ages of your children?	What are the names of relatives already employed by the company?
Physical Condition	Do you have any physical disabilities? What is your handicap? What caused your handicap? What is the prognosis of your handicap? Have you had any recent serious illness?	Do you have any physical condition that may limit your ability to perform the job applied for? Do you need any special accommodations to perform the job applied for? Explain how you would go about doing the job applied for. How many days did you lose from work (or school) during the past year (or other period of time)? Do you have a temporary disability that will require absence from work for an extended period? [Statement that employment offer may be (is) made contingent on passing a medical evaluation.]

Subject		
Education	[Any question asking specifically the nationality, racial, or religious affiliation of a school.]	[Questions related to academic, vocational, or professional education of an applicant, including schools attended, degrees/diplomas received, dates of graduation, and courses of study.]
Experience	[Questions related to military experience in general.]	[Questions related to applicant's work history.] [Questions related to applicant's military experience in the armed forces of the United States or in a U.S. state militia.] Was your discharge dishonorable?
Organizations	To what organizations, clubs, societies, and lodges do you belong?	To what organizations, clubs, societies, and lodges do you belong? (Exclude those whose names or character indicates the race, religious creed, color, national origin, or ancestry of its members.)
Character	Have you ever been arrested?	Have you ever been convicted of any crime? If so, when, where, and disposition of case? Have you been convicted under any criminal law within the past five years (excluding minor traffic violations)?
Work Schedule/ Traveling	[Any question related to child care, ages of children, or other subject that is likely to be perceived by covered group members, especially women, as discriminatory.]	Do you have any family, business, health, or social obligations that would prevent you from working consistently/working overtime/traveling? Are there any reasons why you would not consistently arrive for work on time and work according to the company's (location's) work schedule?
Relocation	[Any question related to spouse's attitudes or other subject that is likely to be perceived by covered group members, especially women, as discriminatory.]	Do you have any family, business, health, or social obligations that would prevent you from relocating? Would you be willing to relocate?
Miscellaneous	[Any inquiry that is not job-related or necessary for determining an applicant's potential for employment.]	[Statement or notice to applicant that any misstatements or omissions of significant facts in written application forms or in an interview may be cause for dismissal.]

*Lawful only if job-related.

Source: Reprinted from Personnel Director's Legal Guide, by S. Kahn, B. Brown, and B. Zepke, pp 2-22–2-24, with permission of Warren, Gorham, and Lamont, © 1984.

therefore, to precede the use of any employment method that is not clearly job-relevant with a brief statement concerning why you are asking the applicant to perform this task. You might say, for example, "This questionnaire measures some job-related tendencies, such as your ability to get along with others and your desire to work."

Promotion

The same general issues that arise in the selection of employees also arise in the making of promotion decisions. For example, it is illegal to make a promotion decision based on an employee's race, religion, sex, national origin, or age. Documentation of adverse impact can arise from a number of sources, including (1) the words and actions of the supervisor, (2) a pattern of employees of a particular race or sex not being promoted into certain jobs, and (3) use of inconsistent promotion standards. Once the adverse impact has been demonstrated, the employer's task is to document the validity of the promotion decision. This can be done by producing performance appraisals and other evidence demonstrating that the promotion decision was based on job performance. Obviously, defenses based on a well-constructed and consistently applied performance appraisal process are more likely to be successful.

Sexual Discrimination

There are several additional points that need to be discussed regarding sexual discrimination. Obviously, there are some jobs in which a person's sex *is* relevant to job performance, for example, the preference for an actress for a female part in a play or the choice of a male as a guard in a male prison. In each of these exceptions, being of a certain sex is a *bona fide occupational qualification*. Because of the potential for abuse, bona fide occupational qualifications have been interpreted very narrowly by both the EEOC and the courts. For example, a bona fide occupational qualification would not be held to exist in either of the following circumstances:

- An employer refuses to hire an applicant based on the preferences of coworkers or patients. It is not permissible to reject a man for a nurse or receptionist position, for example, simply because staff or patients would feel uncomfortable.
- An employer refuses to hire an applicant based on assumptions about a certain sex (e.g., "Females are more likely to be sick or have higher turnover rates").

Discrimination on the basis of pregnancy is also prohibited under Title VII. You cannot terminate or refuse to hire or promote a woman solely because she is pregnant. In addition, it is illegal to set a mandatory pregnancy leave requirement. Pregnancy must be treated like any other short-term disability. Women who take a pregnancy leave have a right to reinstatement once they are able to perform the work if other employees who have been absent because of temporary disability have been allowed to return to work. Correspondingly, if you would terminate injured employees after they had used all of their sick leave, then you could treat the pregnancy "disability" in a similar manner. Finally, employers must treat pregnancy in the same way that they treat any other short-term disability in regard to fringe benefits, seniority, and so on. Practices not covered by Title VII may still have to comply with state regulations, so it is important to consult with your attorney on this matter.

Sexual harassment has increasingly been a source of litigation over the past decade. In addition to back pay and injunctive relief, plaintiffs often file tort claims in state court for assault, battery, and emotional distress. These tort claims create the possibility for both compensatory and punitive damages. The EEOC has defined sexual harassment as

> Unwelcome sexual advances, requests for sexual favors, and other verbal or physical conduct of a sexual nature . . . when:
>
> 1. Submission to such conduct is made either explicitly or implicitly a term or condition of an individual's employment;
>
> 2. Submission to or rejection of such conduct by an individual is used as the basis for employment decisions . . . or;
>
> 3. Such conduct has the purpose or effect of unreasonably interfering with an individual's work performance or creating an intimidating, hostile, or offensive working environment.[17]

As originally defined, claims for sexual harassment had to be related to the loss of a tangible benefit, such as the loss of a promotion, a salary increase, or employment. Under this "tangible benefits" doctrine, the employer was not subject to reprimand unless there was a clear job-related consequence of the harassing behavior. Subsequently, courts expanded the conditions under which sexual harassment could be found and included situations where the work atmosphere was hostile, intimidating, or offensive but where there was no tangible job loss as a result of the harassment. In these "atmosphere of discrimination" cases, the courts have issued injunctions to prevent the future occurrence of the harassing behavior. In many of these cases, employees have gone on to file tort claims for invasion of privacy, assault, battery, or infliction of emotional distress, and some have been awarded compensatory and punitive damages.

An important issue in determining whether sexual harassment has occurred is whether the sexual advances were welcome. If they were welcome, then they do not constitute discrimination. Obviously, the documentation necessary to demonstrate "welcomeness" may well be absent after a relationship sours. It should be understood that any sexual affair with an employee has the potential for being considered sexual harassment. Given the difference in power between doctors and employees, it may not always be clear whether a sexual relationship is truly welcome. It should also be noted that people vary in their sensibilities. Repeated sexual jokes and gestures can create an atmosphere of discrimination that may be very offensive to an employee, although this may not be perceived by the harassing individual. Finally, although males have historically been the harassers, sexual harassment is just as illegal and offensive when it is conducted by a female.

Age Discrimination

The general standards that have been discussed above also apply to age discrimination. Employers who are covered by the ADEA cannot discriminate against an employee who is 40 years or older on the basis of age. The standard defense to a charge of age discrimination is to document that the job action was based on job performance. If the charge relates to giving preference to a younger employee, then the defense is to document the superior performance of the younger employee in the employment selection process or on the job.

The ADEA also recognizes the concept of bona fide occupational qualifications. As with sexual discrimination, relatively few bona fide occupational qualifications are accepted as legitimate. Generally, these are related to public safety and to instances in which youth is essential to authenticity, such as a youthful part in a play or in an advertisement intended to promote the sale of a product to youthful consumers. Age-related bona fide occupational qualifications are largely irrelevant to medical practices.

A medical practice typically encounters the issue of age discrimination when an older person applies for a clerical or technical position. In these instances, utilization of the employment methods and strategies discussed in Chapter 2 will provide the basis for a sound defense based on business necessity if an age discrimination suit is brought. More importantly, using these methods will ensure that you will hire the best available applicant, who may well be older.

The Fair Labor Standards Act

This act is also known as the *wage and hour law*, and it was passed by Congress in 1938. Provisions of this act have been copied in so many state laws that the application of its provisions is nearly universal. Among other things, the act sets a national minimum wage, and it also requires the payment of time and a half for overtime in excess of 40 hours per week.

Not all employees are covered by the overtime provision of the act. Employees who are not covered by the overtime provision are referred to as *exempt employees*. Exempt employees are those who are employed in "a bona fide executive, administrative or professional capacity." Definitions of executive, administrative, and professional employees are found in Exhibit 9-4. Classification of a position as exempt can be difficult, and given that there may be significant financial implications, you should consult your attorney for the latest interpretations of exempt status. There are many positions in a medical practice that could be classified as exempt, including your business manager, office manager, and various nursing and technical positions.

Exhibit 9-4 Fair Labor Standards Act Definitions of Executive, Administrative, and Professional Employees

---

Executive Employee
1. Normally supervises two or more employees.
2. Has authority to hire and fire or has reason to expect recommendations regarding hiring and firing to be given serious consideration.
3. Primary duty involves managing the practice.
4. Regularly exercises discretionary powers.
5. Compensation at least $155 per week.

Also, any employee who receives $250 per week and manages a department or supervises two or more employees is considered to be an executive.

Administrative Employee
1. Primary duties consist of office or nonmanual work directly related to management policies or the general operation of the business.
2. Exercises discretion and independent judgment on a regular basis.
3. Regularly and directly assists executives, performs specialized work, or possesses specialized knowledge and exercises skills under general supervision only.
4. Receives a salary of at least $155 per week.

Professional Employee
1. Work requires advanced knowledge attained through a course of specialized intellectual instruction.
2. Work is original and is dependent upon the employee's imagination and talent.
3. Work requires the exercise of consistent discretion.
4. Work is predominantly intellectual and varied in character.
5. Receives compensation of at least $170 per week.

Source: Adapted from *Personnel Director's Legal Guide* by S. Kahn, B. Brown, and B. Zepke, with permission of Warren, Gorham, and Lamont, © 1984.

It is very important to document all time worked by nonexempt employees. Nonexempt employees can claim to have worked overtime, and if you do not have adequate documentation of their actual work hours, you may have to pay time and a half. The employer has a duty under the Fair Labor Standards Act to keep accurate work records. Exhibit 9-5 lists the data that should be kept for three years for each nonexempt employee. (Although the Department of Labor only requires that these records be kept for two years, an employee can bring an action for willful violation of the Fair Labor Standards Act for three years. It is safest, therefore, to retain these records for three years after employment ends.)

In order to maintain accurate records on the hours each employee works, time sheets should be completed by every nonexempt employee for each payroll period. Exhibit 9-6 is a sample time sheet for documenting data required by the Fair Labor Standards Act.

Nonexempt employees who work unauthorized overtime must be compensated for this time. In order to prevent unnecessary overtime, you should do the following:

1. Establish and distribute a policy stating that all work beyond normal work hours must be authorized.
2. Don't suggest, pressure, or condone coming in early, working late, or taking work home, unless you intend to pay for it.
3. Notice when employees arrive and leave. If they are coming in early or staying late, find out why.
4. Audit time sheets and be certain that they are being accurately kept.

Exhibit 9-5 Fair Labor Standards Act Recordkeeping Requirement

Full Name
Social Security Number
Address
Date of Birth
Sex
Job Title
Time and Day of the Beginning of the Employee's Workweek
Regular Hourly Rate
Hours Worked Each Day and Total Hours per Week
Total Daily or Weekly Straight-Time Earnings
Total Overtime Compensation for Workweek
Total Additions to or Deductions from Each Pay Period
Total Wages Paid Each Pay Period
Date of Payment and Pay Period Covered by the Payment

Source: Adapted from Sec. 211C of 29 U.S.C. §200 ETSEQ, 1938.

Exhibit 9-6 Employee Time Sheet

Name									Social Security #									
Week Ending									Week Ending									
EARNINGS TYPE	SAT	SUN	MON	TUE	WED	THU	FRI	FIRST WEEK TOTAL	SAT	SUN	MON	TUE	WED	THU	FRI	SECOND WEEK TOTAL	TIMESHEET TOTAL
Regular																	
Overtime																	
Vacation																	
Sick Leave																	
Personal/Business Leave																	
Holiday																	
Floating Holiday																	
Salary Continuation																	
Other (Specify)																	
LWOP																	
TOTALS																	
Employee's Signature									Supervisor's Signature									

5. Remember, it is ultimately *management's* responsibility to make certain that time sheets are accurate and that employees only work the hours that you intend.

Independent Contractor Agreements

An independent contractor is one who contracts to render personal services as well as provides the means to perform those services. Consulting physicians, psychologists, social workers, physical therapists, nurses, and a number of other types of workers are sometimes engaged as independent contractors by medical practices. The distinction between an independent contractor and an employee has important financial and tax considerations for the employer. For example, independent contractors are not covered under the Fair Labor Standards Act or workers' compensation laws. Employers also do not have to withhold federal and state taxes on wages, pay the employer's share of FICA, or pay federal and state unemployment taxes for independent contractors. Because of these financial considerations, federal agencies, including the IRS, may closely examine independent contractor agreements.

Often the distinction between an employee and an independent contractor is hard to ascertain. Federal agencies such as the Department of Labor and the IRS have an interest in classifying workers as employees, since that generates more taxes and creates more federal control. The costs associated with treating workers as independent contractors, if the IRS or the Department of Labor subsequently determines them to be employees, can be substantial. The IRS, for example, often seeks to collect FICA taxes not withheld, plus interest and penalties. As a result, whenever you are considering treating someone as an independent contractor, it is important to discuss this with your attorney. All written independent contractor agreements should be prepared by your attorney.

The overriding issue when determining whether a worker is a contractor or an employee is the degree of *control* exercised by the employer. There are a number of "tests" that have been established to determine contractor or employee status. Exhibit 9-7 contains some tests used by the IRS. Imagine that passing a test results in one checkmark on the employee or the contractor side of a ledger. The preponderance of the checks *may* determine the worker's status. The word *may* needs to be stressed because of the predisposition of federal agencies to decide in favor of employee status. Ultimately, both the courts and federal agencies look to the "reality of the relationship" as opposed to simply counting the number of characteristics associated with contractorship or employee status. (The IRS will issue a declaratory ruling for tax purposes. However, it also may view your inquiry as a red flag and target you for an investigation. If possible, have your tax attorney or accountant submit the factual information without revealing your identity.)

Exhibit 9-7 IRS Tests for Determining Contractor or Employee Status

---

FACTORS ASSOCIATED WITH EMPLOYEE STATUS

1. The employer has the right to direct and control the individual's performance, including the means, methods, and details of achieving the results. This control does not have to actually be exercised; it simply has to be available to the employer.
2. The employer can discharge the individual.
3. The employer furnishes tools and other equipment for performing the work.
4. The employer furnishes a place to work, and the individual regularly works there.

FACTORS ASSOCIATED WITH CONTRACTOR STATUS

1. The employer only determines the end to be accomplished, not the means to reach the end.
2. The individual furnishes his own tools and his own normal workplace.
3. The individual represents him- or herself to the public as available to perform similar duties for others, including working as a contractor for others in the same type of business.
4. The individual does not in fact spend most of his or her time working for one employer.

Source: Adapted from *Personnel Director's Legal Guide*, 1988 Cumulative Supplement, by S. Kahn, B. Brown, and B. Zepke, pp. S3-16–S3-17, with permission of Warren, Gorham, and Lamont, © 1988.

The use of independent contractor arrangements can also create some insulation from liability. Since an independent contractor operates outside the control of the employer, this can provide a defense for the employer in tort cases, such as malpractice. In order to assert this defense, however, the employer cannot lead a third party, such as a patient, to believe that the contractor is an employee. To ensure that the provider is perceived as an independent contractor, all letterheads, pamphlets, and publications should clearly indicate the provider's contractor status. In addition, request-for-treatment or financial forms signed by patients should clearly state that the provider is an independent contractor and not under the supervision or control of the practice.

SELECTING AN ATTORNEY

Since the law permeates all aspects of business, it is essential that your practice have an attorney who is readily available. The time to develop a relationship with an attorney is before you find yourself in a crisis.

You should consult your attorney whenever you are considering any action with legal implications or receive any document with legal implications. The following documents and actions, among others, require a consultation:

- written employment contracts or verbal employment agreements
- contracts with vendors, suppliers, or independent contractors
- participating agreements with insurance companies
- notification that a lawsuit has been or will be filed against you or your practice
- termination of an employee
- apparent violation of any employment contract or vendor, supplier, or contractor agreement
- injury to any patient, employee, contractor, or member of the general public on your premises
- all leases

Recommendations from other doctors or health care professionals can be helpful in the screening process when choosing an attorney. In addition, you should interview attorneys before making a decision. Many attorneys will not charge a fee for this type of consultation. Finally, once you select an attorney, you should continue to evaluate the quality and timeliness of his or her work. If you become dissatisfied, discuss this with the attorney; if there is no change, select another attorney.

It is not essential, for your general legal needs, to retain a lawyer or firm that specializes in medical practices. Larger firms have the advantage of being able to offer attorneys who specialize in various parts of the law, such as tax law and employment law. However, this can also work to your disadvantage. For example, if you call with a question that is about a contract but that also may have tax implications, the firm's contract lawyer may consult with the firm's tax lawyer, and you will be billed for both attorneys. Is this kind of intrafirm consultation really required? In some instances, it may be, whereas at other times it may be a strategy for "running the billing clock." In addition, you may find it more difficult to establish a personal relationship with an attorney in a larger firm. If you like to play golf or socialize with your attorney, then you may be more satisfied with a smaller firm that gives you personalized attention.

Keep in mind that you may be a medium or large account to a small firm, whereas you will probably be a small account to a large firm. A small firm or an attorney with a general business practice will generally possess adequate knowledge to handle your legal problems, and the firm or attorney can always refer you to a legal specialist when necessary. A potential disadvantage to using a solo attorney is that administrative tasks may consume enough time that he or she cannot be as responsive to your needs as an attorney in a large firm.

Fees should be discussed in your initial meeting with the attorney. Generally, the attorney will be your legal representative, file annual corporate papers, and do specified other tasks for a flat fee, which will vary with your geographical location. Additional tasks, such as providing an opinion on a contract, representing you in litigation, or giving advice on how to terminate an employee, are generally handled on an hourly basis. Hourly fees will vary with geography and with the experience of the attorney.

CONCLUSION

By reading this chapter, you should have gained an understanding of the legal responsibilities and implications associated with owning a private practice. You should have a basic understanding of contracts and torts, which you can use to identify potentially threatening or litigious situations. You should understand the theory of malpractice. You should be able to deal with employment and personnel matters in such a way that you do not implicitly forego your employer prerogatives, while at the same time complying with federal legislation, such as the Fair Labor Standards Act and the Civil Rights Act of 1964. You should understand the role of an attorney and be able to recognize situations in which you should seek legal counsel. Finally, you should have developed an awareness of how to avoid legal conflicts in the daily operation of your practice.

NOTES

1. Virginia Maurer, *Business Law: Text and Cases* (New York: Harcourt Brace Jovanovich, 1987), 5.

2. Ibid., 74.

3. R.A. Anderson, I. Fox, and D. Twomey, *Business Law* (Cincinnati: South-Western Publishing Co., 1987), 163; see also *Nesselrode v. Executive Beechcraft, Inc. and Beechcraft Aircraft Corp.* (Mo.) 707 S.W.2d 371 (1986).

4. S. Kahn, B. Brown, and B. Zepke, *Personnel Director's Legal Guide*, 1988 Cumulative Supplement (Boston: Warren, Gorham and Lamont, 1988), S2-27–S2-28.

5. Aside from the possibility of injury, children playing can be noisy and disruptive. The presence of toys tells children and parents that playing is appropriate. You may be doing the children and the parents a service by indicating that mature behavior is expected and that there are some places where playing is not appropriate. Stock your waiting room with children's books and encourage parents to read to their children or let them read.

6. J. Klein, J. Macbeth, and J. Onek, *Legal Issues in the Private Practice of Psychiatry* (Washington, D.C.: American Psychiatric Press, 1984), 62. The authors report a study estimating that for every five claims for physicians in general, there are one and a half claims for psychiatrists.

7. K. Fineberg, J. Peters, J. Willson, and D. Kroll, *Obstetrics/Gynecology and the Law* (Ann Arbor, MI: Health Administration Press, 1984), 21–22.

8. Ibid., 43–47.

9. See, for example, "Malpractice: Can You Really Protect Your Assets?" *Medical Economics*, October 30, 1989, 129–32.

10. Anderson, Fox, and Twomey, *Business Law*, 271.

11. Kahn, Brown, and Zepke, *Personnel Director's Legal Guide*, S2-42–S2-43.

12. *Toussaint v. Blue Cross and Blue Shield of Michigan*, 408 Mich. 579, 292 N.W.2d 880 (1980).

13. Kahn, Brown, and Zepke, *Personnel Director's Legal Guide*, S5-28.

14. *Wonderlic Personnel Test Manual* (Boston: E.F. Wonderlic and Associates, 1983), 17.

15. Specific technical requirements for demonstrating statistical adverse impact and job-relatedness can be found in "Uniform Guidelines on Employee Selection Procedures," *Federal Register* (1979) vol. 43, 38290–315. These guidelines are also available from the Equal Employment Opportunity Commission, which has offices in most large cities.

16. Current employees can be tested using the employment selection method and comparisons can then be made between their test performance and job performance. This approach is called *concurrent validation*. Alternatively, the employment selection method can be given to applicants and not used in the selection process. Several months or years later, their job performance can be compared to their test performance. This approach is called *predictive validation*.

17. Equal Employment Opportunity Commission, "Guidelines on Sexual Harassment in the Workplace," 29 C.F.R., Sec. 1604.11, *Federal Register* (1978) vol. 43, 74676–77.

Chapter 10

Collections

CHAPTER OBJECTIVES

This chapter will help you to increase collections from both patients and insurance companies. You also will learn

1. the appropriate role for the doctor in the collection process
2. what employees can do to increase collection effectiveness
3. strengths and weaknesses of alternative billing methods
4. why patients don't pay their bills
5. tactics for increasing patient payments, including education and collection methods
6. selecting and using a collection agent
7. using small claims court
8. how to manage insurance billing

In addition, you will learn how your medical office management software can guide collection activities so that you will obtain the greatest return from your efforts. Finally, you will learn how to construct a collection plan that will orchestrate the collection components into an effective, coordinated activity.

This chapter is not designed to teach you how to comply with the claim-filing procedures of specific insurance companies. These procedures vary by state and company, and they can change at any time. Staying current with particular claim-filing requirements is a daily task for your business manager.

INTRODUCTION

The following quotations have been drawn from *Strategies for the Harassed Bill Payer: The Bill Collector and How to Cope with Him,* by George Beldon.

This is a how-to manual designed to educate consumers on how to *avoid* collection. Hopefully, this will provide you with the motivation to improve your collection methods as well as a better understanding of the "rules of engagement":

> Doctors . . . are among the least effective collectors, yet they invite collections problems by loose credit practices. Professional etiquette discourages their working with patients on a pay-as-you-go basis . . . .
>
> COPING WITH DOCTORS . . . . In a pinch, pay your doctor last. There is not much he can do to you. The little dunning messages and stickers on the past-due bills are easily ignored.
>
> As in many collections situations, your worst enemy is your own potential for guilt and embarrassment . . . .
>
> When the doctor . . . . does try to collect in earnest, he will pass your account on to an agent, but not without reluctance because of the high fee. Usually, he does not do this until the sixth month of delinquency or later.[1]

Beldon also rates creditors according to how effectively they tend to collect. Doctors are assigned to the least effective category.

Effective revenue collection is neither an inevitable occurrence nor an accident. It only occurs as the result of hard, well-conceived work. There are many reasons why a practice may not collect a receivable. These include several factors related to your patients, such as

- economic hardship
- dissatisfaction with your services
- irresponsibility
- lack of information regarding the fee
- inadequate or inaccurate insurance coverage information

In addition, your practice can contribute to your collection problem by

- improperly educating patients regarding their financial responsibility and the likely size and nature of fees
- failing to obtain all necessary authorizations
- improperly completing insurance forms
- failing to process claims in a timely manner
- using deficient billing software
- using poor patient-billing procedures

Finally, insurance companies can contribute to the problem when they

- require overly complex filing procedures
- require unique forms or code numbers
- unreasonably deny or delay payment
- lose claims[2]
- improperly reimburse you by remitting an incorrect amount, which also delays the billing of the patient and secondary carriers

Effective revenue collection begins, therefore, by examining your practice's collection procedures and the reasons why fees remain uncollected. Generally, problems arising from multiple sources must be addressed by multiple solutions. There is no magic bullet for directly attacking all aspects of a collection problem, nor is there a single strategy for preventing the occurrence of one. Effective collection occurs when you successfully do a number of things, such as

1. systematically and consistently applying a well-designed collection strategy
2. motivating your employees to collect revenue effectively
3. educating your patients
4. fully utilizing the capabilities of your computer software and hardware

COLLECTION STRATEGY

A collection strategy will identify clear collection roles and responsibilities for your employees as well as state what collection procedures will be used and when they are appropriate. Since the sources of a collection problem can include patients, insurance companies, and the medical practice itself, each of these sources must be specifically addressed by the collection strategy. The collection strategy will be composed of the following elements:

1. the doctor's role
2. the employees' roles
3. billing strategy
4. patient collection methods
5. insurance company collection
6. the collection plan—a description of how accounts will be handled and the steps that will be taken when an account becomes delinquent.

Supporting your activities in these areas will be the reports and other pieces of information provided by your medical office management software. You will be able to use this information to direct and control your collection efforts.

THE DOCTOR'S ROLE

As a doctor, you will have little direct involvement in the collection process, although you may be directly involved in setting fees. Many doctors hinder the collection process by discussing payment arrangements with patients. Generally, any discussion of payments should take place between the collections administrator or business manager and the patient. (The term *collections administrator* will be used to refer to the front office employee primarily responsible for revenue collection. This employee may in fact be the business manager, office manager, accounts receivable manager, or some other employee.) Doctors should not discuss payments with patients, because

1. they usually aren't aware of all financial considerations regarding a given case
2. they often allow their feelings for a patient to interfere with what is essentially a business matter
3. their interference will frustrate the collections administrator, who, as a result, may hesitate to act for fear of being overruled

Doctors do have three important indirect roles in the collection process. The first role is to make certain that the practice has an effective collection process. The doctor must ascertain that collection procedures developed by the collections administrator make sense. Revenue collection is far too important to delegate to an employee without review by the practice's owner(s). This chapter will help you to evaluate whether your practice's collection procedures are comprehensive and effective.

The doctor's second role in the collection process is to motivate employees to collect fees. Many employees think that they and the doctor will be unaffected by "a few dollars that are not collected here and there." It is important that you tell your employees that this is not the case and that inattention to collection could jeopardize everyone's job. Many employees seem never to be aware of the link between their paychecks, their job security, and their role in collecting the fees that finance their paychecks. You can make employees understand this link through face-to-face meetings and practice documents, such as an employee handbook.

You can also affect employee motivation by evaluating collection efforts as an important part of employee performance evaluation. "Revenue collection" should be an evaluation factor for any employee with a role in the collection process. This includes the secretary who takes payments at the front desk as well as the collections administrator. In addition, an employee's evaluation on this factor should be tied to subsequent pay raises, rewards, discipline, or promotions.

Finally, the doctor has an important role as a control over the effectiveness of the collection process. By routinely examining management reports, you will be able to monitor your practice's collection effectiveness. Aging reports will tell you how long money has been outstanding on patient accounts. Examination of cash receipts and write-offs can reveal collection trends. A precipitous decline in cash receipts may indicate a collection problem, declining patient loads, or changing trends in treatment, among other things. An increase in write-offs might mean that (1) more insurance is being collected (most practices enter the contractual write-off at the time a claim is either paid or denied), (2) the volume of business is increasing, (3) more accounts are going bad, or (4) the collections administrator is manipulating the aging report by writing off accounts when they become old (this could occur for a variety of reasons, including bewilderment or indifference on the part of the administrator, who might simply be writing off insurance claims in an attempt to clear his or her desk of problems). It is essential to routinely review these and other financial reports, which will provide some indication of the quality of your revenue collection.

You may feel that this monitoring and control should be delegated to an employee. Consider the consequences, however, for a collections administrator who creates financial chaos. He or she will be fired and then will almost certainly find a job with another practice. The consequences for you, on the other hand, are not so easily resolved. A revenue collection crisis will strike at the heart of your practice's existence. A function this crucial to your livelihood must always be under constant review of a concerned, involved owner.

In summary, your personal collection responsibilities are based on your obligation to ensure that the personnel reporting to you perform in an effective manner. In point of fact, you will not personally use or implement most of the ideas discussed in this chapter. It is important, however, for you to be familiar with these ideas so that you can judge whether your subordinates are performing their collection roles competently.

THE EMPLOYEES' ROLES

The Collections Administrator

One employee, referred to as the *collections administrator*, should have overall responsibility for revenue collection. In small practices, the collections administrator may also be the business manager. (Throughout the remainder of this chapter, the term *business manager* is also used to refer to an employee whose job encompasses revenue collection tasks.) In this situation, the collection administration role is simply part of the business manager's job description. In a large practice, the collection administration tasks may be significant enough to justify a separate part-time or full-time position. This position should report to the business manager.

Some practices will be in a state of transition. Collection activities might begin to take too much time for the business manager to attend to all collection and noncollection responsibilities. If this happens, consider hiring a part-time employee who reports to the business manager. This part-time employee would perform the simpler collection tasks under the direct supervision of the business manager. You would then eliminate this part-time position if your practice grows sufficiently to justify a full-time collections administrator.

The collections administrator is responsible for developing specific collection methods, applying them to accounts, and supervising the activities of subordinates as they relate to collection activities. If the collections administrator is also the business manager, the supervision of subordinates on collection tasks will easily blend into the business manager's overall supervisory responsibilities. If, however, you have separate positions, the two employees will have to coordinate their activities. For example, a waiting room receptionist would report to the business manager and also to the collections administrator regarding collection issues such as collecting payments, deductibles, and so on, at the time of service.

You should review the suitability of the collections administrator's plans. The fees that will be collected or not collected are *your* fees, and the reputation that your collection methods will create for your practice in the community is *your* reputation. You should be satisfied, therefore, that the collection procedures are rational, appropriate, and effective.

Other Employees

Other employees may have an effect on revenue collection, such as the receptionist who collects fees at the window. *Each* employee with some collection responsibility must be held *accountable* for successfully completing these tasks. Accountability is achieved by ensuring there are undesirable consequences for failing to collect fees, as well as desirable ones when it is done effectively. Whenever there is a collection problem that can be traced back to a particular employee or job, it is important to analyze the reward contingencies. Does the employee benefit by a failure to collect? What happens when the collection does not take place?

Case Example

Nan was a receptionist for a group family practice that was having difficulty collecting copayments and deductibles. She reported to the business manager. Nan's collection responsibilities consisted of collecting payments, copayments, and deductibles at the time of service. Nan knew how to read a Blue Cross card to determine a deductible, and she was also told to refer cases to the business manager if she felt uncertain. In addition, she had been instructed to look up copayment arrangements in a database for patients who were returning for treatment.

On occasion, Nan simply did not collect payments and copayments. Her excuses included "I didn't see the patient leave" and "The patient told me he forgot his checkbook." The business manager routinely responded to these collection lapses by sending a bill to the patient or calling the patient and asking for payment by mail. The net effect, however, was that the business manager was devoting time to collection tasks that properly belonged to Nan. When the business manager was asked why Nan's behavior was tolerated, she stated, "Generally, Nan does a very good job. Revenue collection is an exception. Besides, once the patient leaves without paying, I can follow through faster than she can."

One problem was that Nan suffered no bad consequences when a patient avoided payment. On the contrary, if Nan didn't do her job, the business manager would do it for her. In effect, the business manager was rewarding Nan for not doing her job.

Once the business manager understood that she was rewarding unwanted behavior, she changed Nan's responsibilities. She told her that she was responsible for one effective collection attempt during each visit. If a patient managed to leave unnoticed or Nan dealt ineffectively with a patient's unacceptable excuse, she would be responsible for contacting the patient by telephone that day and asking the patient to put a check in the mail. Nan quickly learned that it was easier to collect from patients before they left the practice. This had two effects. First, Nan greatly improved her collection rate. Second, the business manager now had more time available to pursue other tasks.

The collections administrator must also consider the most appropriate use of practice personnel. Often, simple tasks such as calling or writing an insurance company, contacting a patient, or answering a patient's question can be handled by a cross-trained clerical employee. Why use a $10-an-hour management employee to perform a task that could be as effectively performed by a $6-an-hour receptionist? In addition, why use your most qualified collection employee to perform tasks that don't specifically draw upon higher level skills?

Ideally, the collections administrator should first devote time to those cases that can generate the most revenue and that require his or her unique skills. Tasks that require less skill or don't directly generate revenue should be assigned to other employees whenever possible.

BILLING STRATEGIES

A billing strategy is a plan for how and when to collect fees. There are two widely used strategies and several less frequently used strategies.

Insurance Pay–Patient Statement Summary

This strategy is characterized by the following sequence of events:

1. The patient receives services.
2. The physician bills the insurance company.
3. When the physician receives an insurance company payment or denial, the patient is mailed a statement.

This is one of the most commonly used billing strategies. The advantage of this strategy is that it results in uncomplicated patient billing. Since the patient is not billed until the insurance company's obligation is resolved, the balance owed by the patient is clarified before the patient receives a statement. The patient receives statements on a regular basis, such as each month or each time that an insurance claim reaches resolution. This system is particularly effective when the doctor's services are largely covered by insurance or when patients receive infrequent treatment.

This strategy becomes expensive and cumbersome when patients receive frequent treatment. When a doctor supplies patients with weekly services or with several services per week over a period of time, the doctor can wind up carrying large receivables on many patient accounts. This strategy also requires the mailing of a large number of statements. Since each mailing incurs postage, supply, and labor costs, this strategy becomes less efficient as the number of patients treated increases and as insurance coverage for typical services decreases. It also becomes complicated and time consuming when patients carry more than one insurance, since the doctor must then coordinate the payment of benefits between the two carriers before issuing a patient statement.

This strategy can become inefficient and ineffective in practices that perform many high-fee procedures, because a large fee can be under appeal with an insurance company for many months. As a result, the patient's first bill will be very old, thereby decreasing the likelihood of collecting the personal balance.

Finally, this strategy may inadvertently suggest to patients that it is the doctor's responsibility to collect from the insurance company and that if the insurance company fails to pay, this is the doctor's problem. Doctors who use the strategy should inform patients in writing that insurance is a contract between an insurance company and a patient and that each patient is ultimately responsible for any fees.

Patient Payment–File Insurance Strategy

When this strategy is used, the patient pays for the estimated share of the fee, or copayment, including any deductible, at the time of service, and the insurance company is billed simultaneously. This strategy is most appropriate when patients will receive continuing, frequent treatment. This approach is advantageous, because the physician collects the copayment at the time of service, thereby taking advantage of the time value of money (see Chapter 7). In addition, this strategy reduces the expenses associated with mailing statements, since statements are only mailed when (1) the insurance benefit for a procedure has been overestimated or underestimated; (2) a patient misses a copayment; or (3) upon termination of treatment, when the account closes with either a positive or negative balance.

In order to use this strategy, it is necessary to determine the patient's insurance benefits at or before the time of service. Exhibit 10-1 is a telephone referral information form. It can be used to collect the information necessary to verify insurance coverage. Benefits can then be confirmed by calling the insurance company before the first appointment. Some carriers may not reveal their UCR rates for fear of being accused of price fixing. These rates can be determined, however, by examining payments for previous claims for the same procedure.

This process of determining coverage at or before the onset of treatment works best in a practice that uses a fairly limited number of procedures and when most of a practice's patients use a small number of insurance carriers. Under these circumstances, it is relatively easy to determine UCRs. As insurance companies reduce coverage, require larger deductibles, and generally become increasingly difficult to collect from, this strategy becomes more attractive than the insurance pay–patient statement strategy to a wider range of doctors. As with the previous strategy, doctors who use this strategy should make patients fully aware that insurance coverage is based on a contractual agreement between an insurance company and a patient. If the insurance company does not pay, the patient will be expected to settle the account.

Modified Strategies

With both of the above strategies, the doctor assumes the risk that insurance companies will be slow to pay. My experience has been that insurance companies "lose" about 5 percent of filed claims. In some cases, insurance companies will

Exhibit 10-1 Telephone Referral Information Form

NEW PATIENT REFERRAL INFORMATION

Today's Date: _____   Physician: _____

Patient Name (and parent if applicable): _____

Home Telephone: _____ Work Telephone: _____

Referral Source: _____

Appointment Date: _____ Appointment Time: _____

Insurance Coverage: ___ Yes ___ No   Carrier: _____

If CHAMPUS, told patient to go through intake: ___ Yes   ___ No

Policy Number: _____   Carrier Telephone: _____

Insured's Name: _____

Insured's Employer: _____

Met Deductible: ___ Yes ___ No

Told Patient to Bring Form If Required: ___ Yes ___ No

Discussed Fee: ___ Yes ___ No   Told Patient to Bring Ins. or I.D. Card: ___ Yes ___ No

Gave Directions to Practice: ___ Yes ___ No

Detect Problems with Account: _____

Made Copy and Put Original on Board: ___ Yes ___ No

Person Who Handled This Intake: _____

Additional Comments: _____

To Physician:
DIAGNOSIS CODE: _____
We cannot bill the patient's insurance until you supply the Dx code!

---

classify a claim as "pending" for several months. As a result, a medical practice's business office must constantly monitor the status of claims, refile lost or improperly denied claims, and call or send interrogatories regarding claims. Available cash is reduced, since revenue is tied up in receivables. In addition, the eventual day of reckoning with the patient is delayed. Once again, the longer a debt is outstanding, the less likely you are to collect. Patients who do not receive a final statement for several months are less likely to pay and will consume more collection effort on the part of the practice.

Both of the first two strategies can become particularly burdensome to a practice when patients have more than one insurance carrier. When this occurs, all claims must be filed with the primary carrier, and copies of the explanation of benefits for each payment or denial from the primary carrier must accompany claims sent to the secondary carrier. Needless to say, this has the potential to become a protracted, paper-work-laden process. Unless the claims are large, doctors should not accept the responsibility of filing secondary insurance. This burden should be shifted to patients. When the primary carrier pays or denies a claim, the patient will also receive an explanation of benefits, at which time the patient can file the secondary claim.

Some practices have adopted a strategy in which they will try to collect from an insurance carrier for a stated period of time, such as 90 days. Delayed or denied claims are then billed to the patient irrespective of whether the practice could continue to pursue the claim with the insurance carrier. The patient is instructed to contact the insurance carrier if he or she has any questions. If the insurance company subsequently pays the claim to the practice, the doctor then sends a refund to the patient. An example of a letter that could be sent to a patient when a claim is delayed or denied is found in Exhibit 10-2.

Full Payment Strategy

With this strategy, the patient is expected to pay the full fee at the time of service. Insurance may be filed as a courtesy to the patient, with the payment going directly to the patient. (The practice, of course, can choose not to file insurance. Filing the claim, however, is a reasonable act of goodwill toward the patient.) This strategy has the advantage of increasing the immediate cash flow to the doctor and placing the burden of insurance company collection on the patient. It is consistent with the idea that insurance coverage is based on a contractual agreement between

Exhibit 10-2 Letter for Collecting Delinquent Insurance Claims from Patients

---

(Date)

(Guarantor Name)   Acct. #: (Account Number)
(Billing Address)   (Patient Name)
(Billing Address)

Dear (Guarantor):

An audit of your account indicates that you have a balance of $ (balance) that is more than 90 days past due. We have made every effort to collect from your insurance company, and we can no longer wait for its payment. Please forward payment in the amount of $ (balance) no later than (enter date two weeks from date of letter).

We file your insurance as a courtesy to you, and your insurance contract is an agreement between you and your insurance company. Any balance not paid by your insurance company is your responsibility. If you have any questions, please contact your insurance company regarding why it has not paid your claims.

Sincerely,

(Name of Business Manager)
Business Manager

---

a patient and an insurance carrier. It is also obviously the most advantageous strategy for the doctor and the least favorable one for the patient.

The full payment strategy is appropriate if there is more demand for services than a doctor can supply. The doctor can treat those patients who have the financial resources to wait for the insurance company's payment. Referrals who cannot afford this arrangement can be referred to colleagues who use one of the first two payment strategies. This strategy can be very efficient for well-established doctors who have associates in the practice without full caseloads. Under these circumstances, the referring doctor can keep the full payment patients while still retaining other patients in the practice.

A variation of this strategy is to use it for procedures below a certain amount, such as $300. Fees above this amount are billed using the patient–payment file insurance strategy.

Once again, as insurance companies become more difficult to work with and as coverage is reduced, this strategy will become increasingly more attractive to a wider range of doctors.

Patient Prepayment Strategy

In this strategy the patient prepays for services. The prepayment can take a number of forms. For doctors in very high demand, the prepayment can be for reserving an appointment. Patients who have ongoing but standard treatment plans can prepay according to a regular schedule. For example, a patient who receives a routine course of allergy desensitization injections can be billed prior to treatment on a quarterly basis, with insurance being filed as a courtesy to the patient at the time of treatment.

Summary

The most common billing strategy is to bill patients after resolution of the insurance claim. This is the least desirable method financially, since it delays cash flow and gives the patient the benefit of the time value of the fee. Its simplicity, however, may compensate for its disadvantages, especially in small practices.

Generally, it is not desirable to mix billing methods, although almost all practices do this to some degree. Mixing methods can create confusion among the front office staff, who may become uncertain when to ask the patient for nothing, a copayment, or the full fee. It can also result in statements being sent to patients who really don't need them.

There appears to be a trend for insurance coverage to provide fewer benefits with higher deductibles. It also seems that more carriers are developing unique filing requirements and taking more time to respond to claims. If these trends continue, doctors must seriously consider using billing strategies that place more of the collection burden on the patient.

THE PATIENT INTAKE PROCESS

Successful collections begin with the patient intake process. The patient intake process will vary to some degree depending on the patient billing strategy. The intake process will provide you with the legal authority to render treatment as well as the information and the legal standing necessary to pursue collection.

If you will be collecting a copayment at the time of service, insurance information may be taken over the telephone when the patient schedules the initial office visit. This task can be performed by a clerical employee after brief training by the collections administrator. (Practices with high "no-show" rates may find it a waste of time to verify coverage before the initial appointment. These practices should conduct the verification at the time of service.)

Upon arrival, the new patient should complete an intake form before receiving treatment, which solicits biographical information that could be useful for collection purposes and for initially evaluating the patient's creditworthiness. This form should also contain wording approved by your attorney that commits the patient to:

1. seek treatment
2. be responsible for the fee, including any deductibles or insurance denials
3. cooperate in the filing of insurance claims if the practice provides this service
4. be responsible for any collection fees, legal fees, or finance charges if the account becomes delinquent.

Normally, finance charges are not worth the bother to collect. They do have a deterrent value, however, and once again it is a way to convey the message that the practice is serious about collecting its fees. Note that state laws vary regarding provisions of this nature, so it is advisable to consult your attorney to obtain appropriate language for the assignment of collection fees and the assessment of finance charges.

If the patient is going to receive some form of extensive or ongoing care, such as repeated psychiatric visits or cancer treatment, it is also desirable to have the patient sign a method of payment form. Patients undergoing recurrent treatment have more potential to incur large balances, so the additional educational value of a method of payment form makes it worthwhile. The form contains detailed information about specific payment arrangements, what the practice expects of the patient, and other patient responsibilities. It also contains any specific payment plans, including time payment schedules and copayments (if known and applicable). A sample method of payment form is found in Exhibit 10-3. Placing provisions for legal and collection fees and finance charges in your method of payment form will achieve four objectives:

1. It puts the patient on notice that you have procedures for dealing with delinquent accounts.
2. It informs the patient that he or she will bear any costs of delinquency.
3. It creates a legal obligation that will allow you to pass delinquency costs on to the patient. (The language required will vary with state law. Consult your attorney for the most favorable language.)
4. It communicates this information in a tactful and socially appropriate manner. Most of your patients will not become collection problems, and they will view this wording as a necessary condition of doing business in the 1990s, not as specifically directed at them.

PATIENT EDUCATION

Educating patients regarding their financial commitment will allow them to make informed choices, avoid misconceptions, and reinforce your legal standing if you eventually must resort to collection proceedings. At a minimum, patient education should include information on the patient's insurance coverage and likely fees and terms of payment. You should also indicate what your expectations are regarding payment and emphasize that the ultimate responsibility for settlement of the account lies with the patient.

Patient education can proceed somewhat differently for patients who will be receiving long-term or repeated treatment as opposed to walk-ins or patients who will receive infrequent treatment. Both infrequent and recurrent treatment patients should receive written patient educational material. Patients who are identified as "infrequent" should receive a standard patient education pamphlet. This pamphlet should describe billing methods, emphasize the patient's responsibility for the account, outline expectations (e.g., the practice's appointment cancellation policy), indicate where to call during an emergency, and so on. Infrequent treatment patients should also meet with the business manager if either party has any questions regarding insurance coverage or the payment arrangement.

Recurrent treatment patients should meet with the business manager, who should answer any questions regarding insurance coverage; discuss payment and copayment arrangements, deductibles, and so on; and review all appropriate practice policies. The business manager should also negotiate a payment schedule, if appropriate. All of these arrangements should then be written into the method of payment form, which the patient should sign. The method of payment form then becomes a contract between the practice and the patient. It also gives the patient a written document to refer to regarding expectations and financial commitments.

The final part of the patient education process involves communicating the fee or likely fee to the patient and discussing how it may be distributed between personal payment and insurance coverage. A small fee can be directly presented to the patient by the doctor. The doctor can easily handle this by writing the fee on a charge slip and instructing the patient to present it to the receptionist at the front desk. In one variation on this theme, the doctor uses a superbill, which lists frequently occurring procedures and their associated fees. The doctor checks the appropriate procedures and tells the patient to present the superbill to the receptionist. In either case, the patient should be directed to discuss any insurance coverage questions with the collections administrator.

The doctor should discuss a large fee with the patient before the start of treatment. However, if this turns into a negotiation, the doctor should turn it over to the collections administrator, and orchestrate it from behind the scenes. If the doctor feels uncomfortable discussing the fee, he or she should discuss the clinical aspects of the treatment and then direct the patient to the collections administrator, who will discuss the financial arrangements. If the procedure involves a standard fee, the collections administrator will be able to handle this as a routine matter. If the fee is not standard, the doctor can explain the contingency issues to the collections administrator, who will then make payment arrangements with the patient. This approach has the added advantage that the collections administrator, who is knowledgeable about insurance matters and the patient's coverage, will handle all of the financial arrangements.

TYPES OF PROBLEM ACCOUNT PATIENTS

Sometimes it is helpful to understand the reasons for delinquency when formulating a strategy to collect on an account. Patients don't pay bills for an almost infinite number of specific reasons. Almost all, however, are variations on four themes:

1. economic hardships or misfortune
2. perceptions of inequity
3. irresponsibility
4. extreme irresponsibility possibly resulting from a personality disorder

Economic Hardship

Unexpected economic misfortune can befall anyone. Unfortunately, you are probably not the patient's only creditor. Imagine that there is a line of creditors forming. If you get too far toward the end of that line, you may not recover your fee. One objective, therefore, when dealing with economic hardship cases is to

Exhibit 10-3 Method of Payment Form

Frederick Flair, M.D.
5555 Greenwood Road, Suite 6
Hampton Roads, VA 23462

STATEMENT OF FEE AND METHOD OF PAYMENT

This form is utilized to establish a clear understanding regarding the details of your financial account with this practice. Please read it, and do not hesitate to ask any questions. Your signature is an acknowledgment of your understanding and agreement with the provisions of this agreement.

Name of Patient: _____ Date: _____

Name of Responsible Party: _____ SS no. : _____

Relationship to Patient: _____

I, _____, agree to be responsible for payment in full of the charges for pro-
   Responsible Party
fessional services that have been rendered to the above mentioned patient by Frederick Flair, M.D. I also understand and agree to the following provisions regarding the fee and method of payment:

1. Frederick Flair, M.D., will file primary insurance claims on behalf of the patient for rendered services. Insurance payment shall be made directly to the practice. Should any payment be made to the Responsible Party or any other individual, the Responsible Party agrees to promptly forward payment to the practice.

2. The patient or Responsible Party will supply the practice with any insurance forms that may be necessary to expedite the insurance-filing process.

3. The Responsible Party shall pay a copayment at the time of service. This amount is *estimated* to be the portion of the fee that is uncovered by insurance.

4. The Responsible Party shall pay any outstanding balance that is not covered by insurance, such as deductibles, copayments, denied claims, unfiled claims, etc., irrespective of who is responsible for the denied claims. The patient or Responsible Party may receive a statement whenever there is an outstanding balance. *The Responsible Party, not the insurance company, is ultimately responsible for the payment for the rendered services.*

5. It is understood that the usual and customary collection procedures may be initiated should the account become delinquent. It is also understood that any collection fees, including any reasonable court costs, legal fees, attorney fees, etc., will be payable by the Responsible Party.

6. If for any reason the account becomes 90 days past due, the Responsible Party will be billed and expected to bring the account current. Please remember that the practice files insurance as a courtesy to its patients and that any insurance contract is between the Responsible Party and the Responsible Party's insurance company. The practice considers, therefore, payment to be the obligation of the Responsible Party if a delay occurs from the insurance company. *Any balance not paid by the insurance company is the obligation of the Responsible Party.*

7. A fee of $15.00 will be charged for any returned checks.

8. The Responsible Party will be charged if an appointment is missed or cancelled with less than 24 hours notice. Insurance will not cover this charge.

9. I hereby authorize Frederick Flair, M.D., to provide my insurance company with any clinical or financial information the company may require.

Exhibit 10-3 continued

10. Additional details or considerations regarding the terms of payment may be outlined below:

_____

_____

_____

_____

_____

Signature of Responsible Party	Date
Signature of Business Manager	Date

move yourself as far toward the front of the line as possible. You can do this in a number of ways:

1. *Be assertive.* The squeaky wheel does tend to get greased first. If you are visible, either through letters, telephone calls, collection procedures, and so on, you will be paid before the creditor who blends into the background.

2. *Give the patient a solution.* Remind the patient that he or she can use a credit card. Suggest that the patient get a part-time job or obtain a loan. Ask the patient about assets that could be converted into cash, such as an IRA account. Have the patient complete a financial information form. This may disclose some assets as well as help you to develop a payment plan. Consider a plan that will pay off the debt over a short period of time. If the amount is small, try to get the patient to make a payment *now* and close the account with a second payment. The patient may not follow through with the plan, but you may collect some of the debt. (Your suggestions may not be in the patient's best financial interests. This is, however, an adversarial situation, and solutions here are intended merely to maximize your revenue collection. You should assess these solutions in light of your views as to what is ethical or socially responsible.)

3. *Consider giving the patient a deal.* For example, assume a patient has a $500 balance. Tell her that it will be turned over for collection on Friday, at which time legal fees of $250 will be added to the balance. If, however, she pays $400 by Thursday, the account will be closed, thereby saving her $350. Once Friday arrives, the matter will be "out of your hands." You might want to calculate the "discount" that you will offer by determining your legal fee if you place the account in collection and subtracting a portion of this from the patient balance.

4. *Don't be intimidated by threats of bankruptcy.* Bankruptcy protects the creditor as well as the debtor. In addition, it is unlikely that asserting your debt will be the final act that pushes the patient into bankruptcy.

5. *Accept known financial hardship cases with open eyes.* Intake procedures may identify potential financial hardship cases. For example, patients without insurance or without a job are likely to be hardship cases. You can then decide whether to take potential hardship cases that are likely to require ongoing treatment. If you do, be certain that the payment terms are agreed to in writing. If you feel that you have an obligation to take house cases or treat some patients at reduced fees, be certain that you closely monitor the proportion of these patients in your practice. You also have an obligation to your employees, your other patients, and your family to stay in business.

Perceptions of Inequity

Some patients don't pay because they feel that a fee is unreasonable given the quality or quantity of service. Equity problems can be reduced, although not eliminated, by providing sufficient information to patients. Be certain that patients understand that fees are for service rendered and are *not contingent upon the success of treatment.* Educating patients concerning your fees, their insurance coverage, likely clinical outcomes, and so on, will allow them to make informed decisions regarding whether to seek your services. Generally, a patient is less likely to feel a fee is unfairly high when all of the facts are known and the patient seeks treatment fully apprised of the clinical and financial implications.

Irresponsibility

Some people are ineffective at managing their lives and their responsibilities. Generally, these people's lives are characterized by unorganized and inappropriately directed activity. Obligations are not responded to based on their objective importance. A major debt, such as a $300 gynecology fee, has no greater importance than a minor luxury, such as going out to dinner. Irresponsible patients fail to pay for a number of reasons, including these:

- *Paying is inconvenient.* The inconvenience, however, may be perceived as trivial by most people. Watching a basketball game on television, for example, may be more important than paying two months of back bills.
- *Irresponsible patients are often disorganized.* Bills are lost, misplaced, or never opened. Payments may sit on a desk for weeks because there are no stamps or envelopes in the house.

- *They often don't plan ahead.* The end of the month may well reveal debts in excess of available cash. In addition, these patients are usually responsible for a disproportionate number of cancellations.
- *They impulse buy.* A patient with a $300 balance buys a "cute, irresistible" puppy for $500, even though your bill remains unpaid.
- *They devise reasons why they can't pay now.* Excuses such as "Doctors are rich anyway," "I'll pay after my next paycheck," and "It's inconvenient to draw money out of savings" provide sufficient justification in the mind of the irresponsible patient.
- *They tend to deny the significance of their debts.* Irresponsible patients often feel that their obligations will disappear if they can postpone them long enough. Unfortunately, this belief is grounded in reality. Some creditors do in fact go away, either out of exhaustion or as a result of disorganized or inefficient collection methods.

The irresponsible patient often responds to personal impulse and to the most immediate or salient force in the environment. Therefore, the primary objective when dealing with an irresponsible patient is to provide structure and consistency. When the irresponsible patient does address financial commitments, you want to be the first creditor to come to mind. Providing constant reminders is an effective strategy with the irresponsible patient. Monthly statements and telephone calls will make you an imposing presence. It is also essential to provide structure by enforcing cancellation fees, late payment charges, and, ultimately, termination of treatment for failure to meet financial obligations.

Personality Disorders

People with personality disorders possess basic personality flaws. Patients with personality disorders may at first simply appear to be irresponsible. Unfortunately, there is no clear indicator that will differentiate irresponsible patients who have personality disorders from those who do not. The distinction is one of degree, with the depth, persistence, and creativeness of the irresponsible behavior being an indicator.

There are several types of personality disorders, but all of them are characterized by a high degree of self-centeredness and limitless ability to deny personal obligations. Patients with personality disorders either have no conscience or only a minimally developed conscience. Some are incapable of feeling guilt, obligation, or remorse and tend to view the world as existing solely to meet their needs. If lying or deception are necessary in order to satisfy a personal need, then that is what will be done.

Another characteristic of people with personality disorders is that they have an uncanny ability to involve others in their disputes. They are adept at "triangling," or passing on their responsibility to another party For example, the patient who manages to get your business manager to agree to charge her "estranged" husband for your services has adeptly removed herself from the collection process. The husband may or may not be estranged, and he may or may not have any legal obligations in the matter.

Case Example 1

Mrs. Phlegmatic brought her youngest child to Dr. Phillips for treatment of allergies. She was poor, but she had insurance, and she told Dr. Phillips's business manager that Social Services had agreed to cover the copayment and deductible. After several visits and no sign of payment from Social Services, the business manager contacted the agency and was informed that Mrs. Phlegmatic had already exhausted her benefits.

At her next visit Mrs. Phlegmatic was told that she would have to make payments on the account. She made payments for two weeks, at which time they stopped and the business manager received a call from Reverend Mooney. He told the business manager that Dr. Phillips was inhumane, uncaring, and trying to take advantage of this poor woman. Reverend Mooney then stated that he would try to obtain the money for Mrs. Phlegmatic. Several weeks passed, and the business manager had additional discussions with Reverend Mooney regarding the account. During this time, Mrs. Phlegmatic's child continued treatment, and the personal balance approached $1,000. The contacts between the practice and Reverend Mooney became increasingly strained and adversarial. On several occasions the business manager delayed calling Reverend Mooney because the conversations had become so unpleasant. Finally, Reverend Mooney informed the business manager that he would not be able to obtain the funds. The practice then looked to Mrs. Phlegmatic for payment, who responded, "I've paid enough, and I'm not going to pay anymore. I'm leaving, and I'm not coming back!"

Mrs. Phlegmatic was very successful at triangling the business manager. She was also no fool. She chose well when she selected Reverend Mooney to champion her cause. She deflected her responsibility to Reverend Mooney, who was more than happy to adopt her cause and confound it with his own agenda—trying to get doctors to behave in a more socially responsible way. Unfortunately, the business manager took the bait and focused his attention on Reverend Mooney instead of Mrs. Phlegmatic. The net result was that Dr. Phillips was not paid, Reverend Mooney had more fuel for his indignation, and Mrs. Phlegmatic had taught her child another valuable lesson regarding how easy it is to manipulate others and evade personal responsibility.

Logic, rationality, equity, and guilt are useless when trying to collect from a patient with a personality disorder. Success will depend on power. Sanctions, legal procedures, and collection agents are the only alternatives when such a patient does not want to pay.

Often the personality disorder patient will threaten to file a malpractice suit if the doctor attempts to collect on the account. If this happens, the doctor must make a judgment that balances the outstanding fee and the principle of resisting what amounts to blackmail against the time and effort that could be expended in a legal defense.

Case Example 2

Rose was a medical secretary for Dr. Jonathan, a general surgeon. When she needed surgery, Dr. Jonathan recommended her to Dr. Apple, who performed a septal rhinoplasty and billed Rose's commercial insurance carrier for $1,800. The carrier directly reimbursed Rose $1,000, but Rose never forwarded the payment to Dr. Apple. After several months, Dr. Apple sent her a collection letter. At that point, Rose forwarded Dr. Apple two bad checks for the insurance amount of $1,000. Finally, after a call from Dr. Apple's business manager, Rose forwarded a good check. Dr. Apple's office then attempted to collect the personal balance. After several fruitless phone calls and collection letters, the office obtained a warrant in debt on Rose, and she was served with papers by a uniformed sheriff at work. Rose immediately responded by calling Dr. Apple's office. She stated that Dr. Apple had not taken good care of her, that she had a poor clinical result, and that she was thinking about filing a malpractice suit. In addition, she conveyed this information using abusive and defamatory language. Dr. Apple decided to write off the account. Rose was obviously a "loose cannon," and her threat to file a malpractice suit was sufficient to intimidate him.

PREVENTING PATIENT PAYMENT PROBLEMS

One tactic essential for successful revenue collection is to collect personal fees at the time of service. Front office staff must be trained to respond appropriately to the typical payment excuses presented by patients. This training should be provided by the collections administrator or business manager. Appropriate responses include suggesting credit cards when checkbooks and cash are "forgotten" and giving the patient an addressed envelope with instructions to mail the payment today. In addition, the receptionist should approach the patient with the *expectation* of payment, not offer the patient excuses for failure to pay, and direct any patient who will be missing a second consecutive payment to the business manager. Examination of the reward contingencies for those with cash collection responsibilities is also important.

Patients who repeatedly fail to make payments should meet with the business manager. Some patients test how far they can go before there will be consequences. Other patients may truly not have the funds. In either case, the business manager needs to ascertain the reasons for the delinquency and either reiterate and enforce the agreement as stated in the method of payment form or patient pamphlet; negotiate new terms, taking into account any change in the patient's financial circumstances; or recommend suspension of the patient's treatment. Patients with personal balances should be billed on a regular cycle, which is usually every month.

COLLECTING OVERDUE BALANCES

Success in collecting overdue balances depends on consistency and timeliness. Consistency means that you have a plan and that you follow through with it in an automatic, mechanical manner. The collection process should progress step by predetermined step with clockwork regularity. There should be *no* exceptions. Timeliness is important, because you are less likely to collect from older accounts. This is true for a number of reasons, including these:

- Patients move and thereby become difficult to locate. If a patient moves far away, the collection mechanics become more difficult and expensive.
- As a debt becomes older, you will move further toward the back of the line in the mind of the patient. The longer you wait, the more time the patient will have to go even further into debt. In addition, other creditors will have time to collect, thereby depleting the patient's assets and decreasing your chances of collecting.
- Patients are more likely to consider older debts to be "ancient history." The anxiety, fear, or pain you alleviated will become less salient with time, and thus the patient's feeling of guilt and associated motivation to pay the debt will be reduced.

When patients don't pay, their overdue balances will appear on an aging analysis. Whenever this happens, the practice must immediately contact the patient. Perhaps the simplest initial step—and the most appropriate when the failure to pay is truly an oversight—is to send another bill. The amount overdue, however, should be clearly indicated by labeling it as overdue. Computerized billing software normally ages balances, so that old debt is printed on the statement in an overdue or aged category, such as "60 Days Overdue." Alternatively, you can begin to send a series of collection letters. Generally, the first collection letter should be sent when the account passes into the 60 days past current category.

Some doctors attach a special mystique to collection letters. They assume that if they could only assemble the right combination of words, they would be able to convince even the most irresponsible patients to settle their accounts. This attitude is naive, especially when you consider that an irresponsible patient is probably well aware of the debt and has *chosen* not to pay. Unfortunately, there is no magic available to write collection letters. They will be more effective, however, if their contents are governed by logic:

1. A collection letter should be short. This will focus the patient's attention on the overdue balance.
2. Don't dissipate your strength by giving the patient excuses or alternatives to payment.
3. The initial contact should assume that the patient is not malevolent. The overdue balance could be due to lost mail or to an oversight. Don't give excuses to the patient, but don't preclude them either. If the patient wants to save face while at the same time paying the bill, that shouldn't make any difference to you.
4. Command the patient to action. Clearly state that the patient *must do something*, either pay the bill or contact the office *by a stated date*.
5. Always enclose a statement of the account with the first collection letter.

Exhibit 10-4 contains a sample first collection letter.

Exhibit 10-4 First Collection Letter

(Date)

(Guarantor Name)   Acct. #: (Account Number)
(Billing Address)   (Patient Name)
(Billing Address)

Dear (Guarantor):

   A recent audit of your account indicates that you have an outstanding personal balance of $ (balance), which is long overdue. I ask that you pay this amount before (enter date ten days from date of letter).

   We have provided services in good faith, and we rely on the good faith of our patients to promptly pay their bills. If you have any questions regarding your account, please contact me at (phone number). Thank you for your attention to this matter.

Sincerely,

(Name of Business Manager)
Business Manager

If the first letter is unsuccessful, it should be followed by a second and final letter. The second letter should state that if the bill is not paid within seven days, either the account "will be turned over for collection" or "legal action will be taken." Exhibit 10-5 contains a sample final collection letter. The second letter should also command the patient by telling the patient what to do as well as by providing a reason why the patient should act. The time interval between the two letters should be short. The fact that the letters are sent and that they provide specific dates of action is far more important than their specific wording. Do not waste your time, energy, and resources by sending more than two letters. If a patient does not respond at this point, the account should either be written off or given to a collection agent.

If the patient or guarantor is in the military, send a copy of the second collection letter to the commanding officer. The military is very concerned about the credit reputation of its personnel, and commanding officers will apply considerable pressure on personnel to settle their debts. Your patient intake form should request that all military personnel provide their base or ship, and the name of their commanding officer. If you don't have this information, a telephone call to the patient's residence or to the base's officer of the day often can be a means of getting the name of the commanding officer. Finally, the government maintains a

Exhibit 10-5 Second Collection Letter

(Date)

(Guarantor Name)   Acct. #: (Account Number)
(Billing Address)   (Patient Name)
(Billing Address)

Dear (Guarantor):

   This is your final notification that you have an outstanding personal balance of $ (balance). As you will recall, you signed an agreement with this practice to pay for our services. We have provided services in good faith, and assumed good faith on your part that you would live up to your responsibility to pay for these services.

   If complete payment is not received by (date), your account will be turned over to our attorney for legal action, which can include a hearing in general district court, garnishment of wages, and attachment of bank funds. This will result in additional costs to you, since collection fees, attorney's fees, court costs, and finance charges will be added to your balance. Once an account is turned over to our attorney for collection, we cannot call it back, and you will be assessed these additional charges.

Sincerely,

(Name of Business Manager)
Business Manager

personnel locator service. The charge is $3.50, and you must supply a full name and social security number. The request must be made in writing to: Worldwide Locator, U.S. Treasury, NMPCN 0216, Washington, D.C. 20370.

There are other techniques that should be used in addition to collection letters. The first and most obvious is to suspend services. This tactic is most effective when the patient is receiving continuing treatment, since it creates immediate consequences for the patient. Naturally, termination must be done in a medically and legally appropriate manner to avoid a malpractice charge of abandonment (see Chapter 9). Doctors with high proportions of continuing patients, such as psychiatrists, gynecologists, family physicians, and allergists should systematically apply this tactic using established rules. These rules should be communicated to patients through patient pamphlets or method of payment forms. For example, failure to make two payments or failure to pay two consecutive mailed statements will automatically result in the suspension of treatment. At a minimum, suspending services will put a cap on the outstanding balance.

The telephone is a very effective collection tool, because it is both intrusive and selective. The telephone places you in the patient's office, living room, bedroom, or kitchen. (Consult your attorney regarding state laws governing collection methods. Often state law precludes collection calls outside of certain hours.) When the telephone rings, people stop whatever they are doing to answer it. Letters may be lost or be opened and discarded by the wrong person. You may never know for certain if a patient ever receives your letter. With the telephone, however, you can be sure you have reached the correct person.

Practices often delay using the telephone, either out of fear of a direct confrontation with the patient or due to a feeling that it is inappropriate to make such a personal intrusion except as a last resort. Instead, the telephone should be used *early* in the collection process, because the telephone allows you to evaluate why the patient is delinquent. If the patient has a grievance, this can be determined and the business manager can begin to resolve the problem. If there is an economic hardship, then it becomes possible to arrange a payment schedule or some other commitment. If the patient is irresponsible, then some structure can be applied in order to direct and motivate payment. If the patient's behavior suggests a personality disorder or simple intransigence, then aggressive collection strategies can be implemented more quickly than normally would be the case.

Here are guidelines to follow when using the telephone:

1. *First, identify the answering party and only talk to the patient (or whoever is responsible for the debt).* If Mr. Smith is the guarantor of the account, then you are wasting your time discussing the matter with Mrs. Smith. In addition, talking to the wrong person may breach confidentiality.
2. *Try to determine the patient's "state of mind" regarding the debt.* You need to determine whether you are confronting someone, for example, who

accepts this as a legitimate debt, who will be aggressive, or who will seek sympathy. One tactic for determining this is to identify yourself, state the nature of the debt, and then listen. Listen for both *what* the patient says and the *way* in which it is said.

3. *Control the conversation by offering the patient alternatives that meet your objectives.* Phrases such as "How large a payment can you make?" "When will you make your next payment?" or "What would be a good time for you . . . ? convey weakness. Determine what *you* need. Make a proposal and let the patient accept it or make a counterproposal. You can then accept or reject the counterproposal. The questions above could be replaced with "I need a payment of $200.00" (determine a level that will be satisfactory and propose it), "I expect to receive your final payment by Friday, February 18" (let the patient tell you what is not possible), and "Let's meet this Friday at 10:00 AM" (you can always state an alternative if the patient objects).

4. *Get to the point.* Brief conversations allow your business manager more time to contact more patients. Brief, no-nonsense contacts also communicate the serious business nature of the discussion.

5. *Obtain specific commitments from the patient.* Do this by getting specific agreements regarding amounts and time. "I'll send you a substantial payment in a few days" is virtually worthless. In addition, always restate the agreement to the patient and tell him that you are making a note in the financial record. For example, "You agree, then, that you will mail a check for $200.00 so that I will receive it by Monday, March 23, and I am noting this in your financial record." Whenever a payment arrangement is negotiated over the phone, it should also be put into a letter and mailed to the patient.

6. *Be persistent and follow through with your promises.* If a patient does not meet a commitment, immediately contact the patient. This tells the patient that you will not go away, and it also provides validity to future promises. For example, consider the following statement: "Mr. Johnson, I did not receive your payment for $200.00. If I don't receive it by Wednesday, I will turn your case over to our lawyer for collection on Thursday." Is Mr. Johnson more likely to respond to this message if it is communicated on the day that the $200.00 had been due or if it is communicated three weeks later? The telephone offers you the ability to provide immediate follow through on broken promises.

PLACING AN ACCOUNT "IN COLLECTION"

Some patients will not respond to your statements, collection letters, or telephone calls. When this happens you will need to implement collection proceedings. The first step is to write off any account that will cost more to collect than it will generate in cash. The automatic write-off criterion for your practice should be determined by looking at the time, effort, and cost likely to be expended by your staff. Next, you must decide whether the practice will institute the legal process or whether you want to turn the account over to a collection agent.

If you are not faced with large numbers of accounts that must be placed in collection, you may want to consider undertaking collection in small claims court. The advantages of pursuing this course are as follows:

1. You will retain control over your cases.
2. You will collect your money more quickly from some of your patients. Generally, patients who are employed and for whom you have good addresses are good bets. In about 75 percent of these cases, obtaining a warrant in debt will result in a quick settling of the account.
3. You will save legal fees, which can consume 50 percent or more of the balance due.

The small claims process varies from state to state, but generally it proceeds in the following manner. The practice obtains a warrant in debt against the patient. Some jurisdictions will let a practice obtain a warrant by mail, whereas others require that this be done at the courthouse. The warrant specifies the delinquent amount and sets a court date. The cost is nominal ($10–$20), and it generally can be added to the patient's account. The patient is then served with a copy of the warrant by the sheriff and/or through the mail.

At this point, most patients contact the office and arrange to make payment. It is amazing how a legal notice delivered by a uniformed sheriff will get a patient's attention! When the patient contacts the office, negotiate payment arrangements that will close the account *before* the court date. This will leave you with the option to pursue legal action if the patient breaks the agreement.

If the patient does not arrange to make payment, the business manager will have to appear in court and present evidence that the services were provided and that the patient's account is still unpaid. The court will grant a judgment against the patient. If the patient still refuses to pay, you will then be faced with the challenge of collecting on the judgment. Once again, your options will be restricted by state law, but the normal choices involve garnisheeing wages and attaching assets, such as bank accounts, cars, and so on.

Medical practices should not routinely use small claims court. You "win" in those cases that pay off the account as a result of the warrant in debt, since you will obtain payment with relatively little expenditure of time, effort, or money. The other cases, however, will require considerable collection effort.

Some patients will contest the case in court. Many patients, however, will simply fail to appear, and in essence they will challenge you to collect on the judgment. Most of these cases will be hard-core collection veterans. It will be difficult to locate their bank accounts and employers, and they may well have falsified some of the information on the intake form with the objective of misleading you. Finally, these people can be abusive and vindictive. Your personnel are not trained to collect from these types of people, nor do they have the time or the resources available to track them down and force them to pay. As a result, the small claims procedure should only be considered for those cases in which there is a very high probability that the patient will pay as a result of receiving the warrant in debt. The business manager will have to make an educated guess based on the type of patient (hardship, equity, irresponsible, personality disorder) and the patient's response to the initial collection attempts.

The alternative to small claims court is to utilize a collection agent, which can be a collection agency or an attorney who performs this type of work. In either case, you should select a collection agent based on (1) cost, (2) recovery rate, and (3) methods employed.

Cost and recovery rate are interrelated. An agent with a recovery rate of 70 percent and a fee of 50 percent returns 35 percent of the account to the practice. An agent with a recovery rate of 50 percent and a fee of 40 percent only returns 20 percent of the account to the practice. Obviously, you must simultaneously consider both the fee and the recovery rate when selecting a collection agent.

Using a collection agent can be very cost-effective if the agent can assign the collection fees to the patient. This is a matter of state law. For example, Exhibit 10-6 illustrates a collection arrangement used by an attorney in Virginia. The attorney assigns a 50 percent fee to the patient. The physician then pays the attorney 50 percent of the total collection. If the attorney collects the full amount, then the physician will receive 75 percent of the outstanding fee. In this case, the $125 collection fee paid by the physician will certainly be worth the time, effort, and stress that is transferred from the physician's office to the attorney's office.

Exhibit 10-6 Analysis of a Collection Using an Attorney

Outstanding Account Balance	$500.00	
Attorney's Assigned Fee (50% of Account Balance)	$250.00	
Total Balance Due		$750.00
Total Collected by Attorney	$750.00	
Attorney's Fee (50% of $750.00)	$375.00	
Total Received by Physician		$375.00

Seventy-Five Percent ($375/$500) of Outstanding Balance Received by Physician

Note: Court costs are passed on to the patient.

The methods employed by the agent are also a legitimate concern. To some extent, the agent will be representing your practice to the community. Particularly inappropriate, inhumane, or disproportionate collection methods can damage your reputation. It is important, therefore, to contact several professional references when evaluating a collection agent. Question the references about customer or patient complaints, the actual level of collection experienced, and the time that it takes to collect on accounts. Also inquire about how cooperative and responsive the agent's staff is in responding to questions from clients.

Once you have retained a collection agent, it is important to monitor the agent's results. Does the agent successfully collect on your accounts or have the accounts simply been moved into another black hole? If patients complain about collection methods, it is important to discuss this with the agent. Most likely, the patients will be objecting to legitimate, appropriate, successful tactics. It is important, however, for you to protect your reputation and to feel comfortable with the methods used by your agent.

Another element to successfully using an agent is to forward your delinquent accounts in a timely manner. If your final collection letter says that the account will be placed in collection if the balance isn't paid in a specific number of days, then be certain to turn the account over to the agent on the day after the due date. Some agents will give you better terms for younger accounts, and there are good reasons for this. As we have seen, old accounts are more difficult to collect.

Finally, once an account has been placed with a collection agent, never take the account back from the agent or accept a payment from the patient. Some patients will contact the practice in an attempt to avoid collection fees or attorney's fees after the agent has applied pressure. If you take the account back, you may be responsible for these fees. In addition, the patient will invariably renege on promises made to you. If you accept a payment from a patient, it may not cover the collection fee or interest charges. The agent may look to you for payment if you interfere with the collection process.

COLLECTING FROM INSURANCE COMPANIES

The most favorable payment arrangement for the doctor is to collect fees at the time of service, with patients receiving payment from their insurance companies. Competition for patients and patient expectations make this type of arrangement infeasible for many doctors. In fact, insurance collection probably will be the single largest revenue source for your practice, and anything that affects the insurance collection process will have a magnified effect on practice receipts. Ensuring the validity and consistency of the insurance collection process is essential, therefore, to financial survival.

A particularly dangerous aspect of insurance collection is the long period between the time that a claim is generated and the receipt of a payment or denial. This delay in feedback makes it possible for a significant problem to arise before it is perceived by the practice. Using efficient insurance billing procedures, monitoring insurance billing results, and identifying and correcting problems as early as possible are essential to protect the practice's revenue stream and its financial viability.

Effective insurance collection begins with effective insurance billing procedures. The object should be to bill as often as possible, with daily insurance claim filing being the ultimate goal. Filing insurance daily or as frequently as feasible is analogous to dividing up a ship into compartments. A catastrophe in any one compartment can be localized and will not threaten the existence of the ship. Individual events, such as the post office losing a bundle of mail, billing software developing a bug, the power going off during an insurance-billing run, an insurance check being lost, a hardware failure, or incompetence on the part of a particular claims agent, will then only affect a small and limited part of your revenue. If you file insurance claims on a weekly or monthly basis, then the same events might affect a week's or month's worth of revenues.

Some insurance companies are capable of processing electronically submitted claims. Electronic submission has a number of advantages, including faster payment, quicker error detection, reduced postage and mailing costs, and reduced clerical labor. Some electronic claims systems immediately indicate whether the claim will be paid or denied, which provides greater integrity to the billing process. You should, however, evaluate the total cost of electronic submission, including the cost of additional equipment and access fees. Generally, electronic submission is only financially justifiable in offices with a very high volume. Some doctors, however, have concluded that immediate problem detection and reduced paperwork in the front office are worth the extra cost.

The next important consideration is to file your claims correctly and comply with any authorization procedures. Normally, there will be a "provider support" office to help practices deal with denied claims and comply with claim-filing procedures. It is sometimes possible to have major carriers send a training representative to your office to train your staff in correct filing procedures. Many Blue Cross companies provide this service. This training can be particularly useful if you are just going into practice or if your office has had turnover in critical billing positions.

Insurance companies are very large bureaucracies. One characteristic of a bureaucracy is that it solves problems by applying standards and rules. If you find that you are not getting your problems resolved, you have to get the ear of a person who is high enough in the bureaucracy to make exceptions to the standards and rules. The way to do this is to speak with a supervisor. If you don't get resolution to your problem, ask, "If you agreed with my position, would you be able to . . . ?" If the answer is no, then you need to ask for *that* employee's supervisor. If the answer is yes, then you must determine whether continuing up the corporate ladder is worth the time and effort. Generally, ascending two levels of supervision above the normal claims representative will place you in middle or top management.

Some companies appear to go out of their way to make the billing process difficult. They require the use of company-specific forms or they create their own procedure codes instead of using the standard CPT codes. Unfortunately, there is not much that you can do about this other than refusing to participate with these companies and not accepting assignment of payment. Methods for dealing with nonstandard filing requirements include selecting flexible computer hardware and software, training employees to deal with requirements, and developing special office procedures. Unusual codes and forms will result in higher claim error rates. By segregating these claims and working on them as a separate batch, employees can pay particular attention to the different codes and filing procedures required by these companies.

Some companies are very unresponsive to claim inquiries or take an unreasonably long time to process a claim or forward a payment. If a company is particularly unresponsive, you may want to consider filing a complaint with your state's insurance commission. Each state has an insurance commission or an agency that regulates insurance company operations. The power of the commission or agency—and therefore the degree to which insurance companies will be responsive to complaints filed with it—will vary from state to state. If you feel that a claim has been unreasonably denied or has not been responded to in a reasonable amount of time *and* you have exhausted all internal remedies, you have little to lose by writing a letter to your state's insurance commission.

The result of filing an insurance claim has more significance than simply receiving no response, a denial, or a payment. An outstanding claim or a denial *may* indicate that something has malfunctioned in your billing system. Further, the problem, if there is one, will probably continue until someone identifies and corrects it.

The doctor should routinely review practice aging analyses and other management reports that relate to insurance collection. Other reports useful for understanding the collection situation include these:

- number of procedures per month
- revenue generated per month
- revenue by insurance company per month
- insurance receipts by company per month
- aging analysis by insurance company

- gross receipts per month
- write-offs and adjustments per month

Weekly or daily reports can also be useful. Generally, most practices find that monthly reports reveal significant trends while being less subject to the random variations that make reports over shorter time periods difficult to interpret.

All too often, the doctor will avoid the responsibility of looking at aging analyses, using the rationalization that it is really the business manager's job to identify and resolve billing problems. The doctor's objective, however, is different from the business manager's. The business manager reviews aging analyses to determine which accounts need immediate action. The doctor reviews aging analyses to determine whether the business manager is doing his or her job and to evaluate the overall collection success of the practice.

On occasion, a business manager may not want the doctor to regularly review aging analyses and other management reports. The business manager may pander to the doctor's ego and imply that this task is beneath the doctor. Reviewing these reports is critical, however, to the doctor's ultimate responsibility, which is to ensure the financial soundness of the practice. A good business manager will be proud of his or her achievements, and these achievements ultimately appear in the collection and financial reports. Whenever a business manager in any way suggests that the doctor should not routinely review collection and financial reports, the doctor should immediately become suspicious.

The significance of an unpaid claim is the most difficult to interpret, because there is no overt message indicating that something is wrong. Unpaid claims are typically identified when money begins to move into older categories, such as 60 or 90 days past current. In order to discover this, the business manager must regularly run aging analyses, examine them, and then act upon the results.

Dealing with a rejected claim is arguably the business manager's *highest* priority. First, a rejected claim means that the money represented by the denied claim will not be paid unless action is taken, and it is therefore a higher priority than current claims, which may be paid. Second, the denial may be symptomatic of a larger billing problem. This may mean that many other claims for this patient and for other patients may be destined for denial. This circumstance can, if left unattended, threaten the financial soundness of the practice.

Any rejected claim must be immediately examined by the business manager to determine the cause of the problem. The business manager must always be thinking of the implications of a denied claim for other outstanding claims. If there are implications for other claims, the business manager must immediately address them. Often, the first indication of a software or a filing procedure problem will be a denied claim. If the symptom is not immediately detected, many additional claims will be denied. This not only delays the receipt of cash, but it also requires the refiling of more denied claims, which can add up to a substantial amount of additional work.

Case Example 1

MCCC, a large midwestern insurance company, is the carrier for about 10 percent of Dr. Feldstone's patients. It requires the use of its own procedure codes as well as patient information that Dr. Feldstone does not normally provide on claims filed with Blue Cross and other commercial carriers.

In August, Dr. Feldstone replaced his business manager. At about that time, MCCC supposedly mailed Dr. Feldstone a new set of procedure codes. The new codes either were never received or were lost as a result of the personnel transition. They were never entered into the practice's computerized billing system, and the practice continued to file claims with the obsolete codes. The new business manager was somewhat overwhelmed with her job, and consequently she did not attach great significance to the returned MCCC claims. They were placed in an in-basket, where they would receive attention when "things calm down."

At about the same time, CCC, the insurance carrier for 40 percent of Dr. Feldstone's patients, changed one procedure code, which was used in about 15 percent of his billings for these patients. CCC had notoriously bad provider services, so it was not clear whether the information was never conveyed to the practice or was simply lost during the personnel transition. Once again, the new procedure code was not entered into the computer, nor were the billing personnel aware of the need for the code modification.

At about the same time, Blue Cross/Blue Shield's processing software began to have an intermittent problem that was limited to only a few practices, including Dr. Feldstone's. Claims would be randomly rejected for failure to have a diagnostic code when one was in fact present. The business manager attached no diagnostic significance to the rejected Blue Cross claims. (This Blue Cross company did not return rejected insurance claims but forwarded a form requesting the additional or missing information.) She simply assumed that the claims had been inappropriately submitted and proceeded to supply Blue Cross with new diagnosis codes. As a result, Blue Cross was unaware that it had a software problem.

MCCC, CCC, and Blue Cross together represented about 70 percent of Dr. Feldstone's monthly revenue. The new business manager did not appreciate the significance of the increasing proportion of rejected claims, and she continued to deal with them on a case-by-case basis. Over a three-month period, the revenues generated remained about the same, receivables in the "current" and "current plus 30 days" categories grew significantly, and cash receipts were down. Cash receipts for the third month were at 69 percent of normal levels.

Dr. Feldstone did not routinely review the practice's financial reports. He had noticed that cash receipts were down, but he attributed this to the new business manager's "learning curve." By the time Dr. Feldstone determined that he had a major collection problem, he was faced with

1. a cash crisis
2. a backlog of MCCC rebilling, which could not begin until the billing personnel were trained in the use of the new procedure codes (average turnaround for this company was about seven weeks)
3. a backlog of CCC rebilling (average turnaround was eight weeks)
4. a delay in Blue Cross cash of about eight weeks
5. greater than normal vulnerability for the next several weeks to any other problem in the collections system, such as a hardware breakdown or software bug

Case Example 2

Field Psychiatric Association was a group psychiatric practice. In addition to providing psychiatric services, it employed several psychologists and clinical social workers who were paid on the basis of monthly collections. Monthly collection figures were obtained from earned receipts reports for each producer. Dr. James, the practice administrator, was responsible for reviewing monthly management reports and attending to the business aspects of the practice.

On March 3, the February earned receipts by producer report indicated a large drop in collections, and as a result the subsequent payroll, which would be due on the tenth of the month, would be roughly 60 percent of normal levels. The drop was uniform across all producers, with the exception of Dr. James, whose receipts were at normal levels. She did not participate with any insurance companies, and all of her patients paid full fee at the time of treatment.

Dr. James was very concerned, because her monthly fixed expenses could not be covered with the practice's share of the gross receipts (see the section on breakeven analysis in Chapter 7). She was also very concerned about the financial well-being of her therapists. Dr. James's first reaction was panic! Where should she look for the cause of the problem? What information was available that could give her a clue regarding what had happened? She then focused her mind on the fact that this problem was not caused by magic or demons. It was solvable, and the answer, or at least some indication of the problem's source, would be found in the practice's financial data. Dr. James began the investigative process to determine the cause of the cash problem. She identified six hypotheses:

1. Cash receipts had been lost or stolen.
2. Insurance claims had not been mailed on a regular basis.
3. There had been a precipitous decline in procedures due to vacations during the holiday season, resulting in reduced receipts several weeks later.

4. Insurance claims had been improperly completed due to software or personnel problems.
5. Insurance receipts had been lost or stolen.
6. One or more insurance companies were having a problem processing claims.

Dr. James first determined that the cash shortage was approximately $15,000 by comparing a report of the practice's gross receipts for the month with the gross receipts for the previous three months. She then noted that the cash collections for February totalled $17,793, whereas the collections for the previous three months averaged $18,396. Since cash collections were stable, this largely eliminated Hypothesis 1. It also suggested that the problem had to be associated in some manner with insurance collections.

Next, she examined Hypothesis 2 by looking at a sample of accounts in the computer. Insurance claims were uniformly sent either on the day of treatment or the following day. In addition, all information relating to the patient computer accounts appeared to be correct. Finally, November through February monthly reports of revenues generated by insurance company did not indicate any substantial monthly variability. These data, in combination, largely eliminated Hypothesis 2. Wealth was being put into the pipeline, and the question was where and when it would come out—or even whether it would.

Revenue reports and reports on the number of sessions for December revealed less than a 10 percent decline in the number of procedures. This eliminated Hypothesis 3.

Hypothesis 4 could be time consuming to fully investigate. The business manager stated that she had not received an unusual number of returned claims. Her word was accepted at face value, although it was recognized that in theory she could be covering up a problem. Examination of a sample of accounts in the computer and a test running of the computer's claims-filing program indicated that the practice was generating payable claims. A very unsettling theory, however, was that the computer was *saying* that it was generating all of the claims when in fact it was only generating a *portion* of the claims. In order to eliminate this hypothesis, it would be necessary to examine a sample of the patient business charts. If copies of claims were missing for dates on which the computer had indicated that a claim had been generated, then this would support Hypothesis 4. Checking this would be a long, tedious task. As a result, Dr. James decided that she would postpone examining this hypothesis until after she had examined the others.

Hypothesis 5 would take time to investigate, although the strategy would be easy to implement. Company X and Company Y paid a large proportion of the practice's insurance claims. If insurance funds amounting to $15,000 were lost or diverted, at least some of the money would have to come from one or both of these carriers. These companies could be questioned by telephone on claims that should have been paid by now. If there were funds that had been diverted or lost, then one or both insurance companies would indicate that they had paid on claims that the practice's computer indicated were still unpaid. Once again, this would be a personnel-intensive process. Dr. James postponed further investigation of this hypothesis until other, more easily researchable alternatives had been eliminated.

Two sources of data would be used to examine the sixth hypothesis. An examination of an aging analysis by insurance company revealed that Company X receivables in 30 days past current were much higher than normal. Reducing the revenue in this category by the approximate write-off and then guessing at the proportion in the category that might be old enough to be payable resulted in an estimate that could account for $15,000. An examination of insurance receipts by insurance company revealed that February Company X receipts were $6,399, whereas they averaged $22,118 for the previous three months. These data directly pointed to a problem with Company X claims.

Dr. James now knew that the source of the problem was associated with Company X, although she still did not know with certainty whether the fault lay in the claims that her practice was sending, whether Company X funds had been lost or diverted, or whether the problem was with Company X's processing of the claims. She decided that she would first test the hypothesis that would create the least difficulty for her. She called Company X's administrator and stated that her 30 days past current claims were very high and that her cash receipts were down. She asked him if there had been a problem in the processing of her claims. The administrator stated that someone would look at the practice's accounts. Later that day a subordinate called back to tell Dr. James that the processing department had gotten behind, temporary and overtime help was being enlisted, and the fault lay with the insurance company. The data that Dr. James had used to confront the insurance company was incontrovertible. Company X knew that if it denied the problem existed, Dr. James would begin inquiring about specific accounts. To its credit, Company X quickly admitted the problem.

Dr. James stated that she and her employees should not have to suffer as a result of the company's problem, and she asked for a $15,000 advance against the outstanding claims. The Company X administrator countered with an offer to pull all of Dr. James's claims and "put them on the top of the stack." Dr. James agreed, and three days later she began to receive payments.

THE COLLECTION PLAN

The collection plan integrates all of the parts of the collection system. Having a plan will help ensure that problem accounts are quickly identified and that revenue collection is pursued with consistency. An example of a collection plan is found in Exhibit 10-7. The plan should provide an outline of the various parts of the collec-

Exhibit 10-7 Sample Collection Plan

Patient Intake Process

1. Each patient will complete an intake form that provides sufficient biographical information to pursue collection should the account become delinquent.
2. The business manager will scan each intake form for obvious signs of financial hardship. If a patient is likely to be a hardship case, the business manager will advise the physician of this possibility so that the physician can make an informed decision should long-term treatment be necessary.
3. The intake form will provide for authorization to bill the patient's insurance company.
4. The intake form will unequivocally state that the patient is ultimately responsible for settlement of the account.
5. New referrals that have been scheduled more than one day in advance will be reconfirmed the day before the scheduled appointment.

Patient Education Process

1. A sign will be posted at the receptionist's window stating that payment is expected at the time of service.
2. When a new referral is taken over the telephone, the receptionist will inform the referral that payment or copayment is expected at the time of service. If the referral has any questions, he or she will be immediately forwarded to the business manager.
3. Each new patient will be provided with a copy of the new patient pamphlet.
4. Any patient who will be undergoing continuing treatment will be scheduled for a brief meeting with the business manager. During this meeting, the business manager will review the patient's insurance coverage and copayment arrangements and answer any financial questions.

Payment Arrangement Process

1. The physician will indicate the procedures performed on a billing slip, which will then be handed to the patient with instructions to present it to the receptionist.
2. When the physician determines that there should be a fee variation for a specific visit, this will be directly communicated to the business manager by the physician.
3. When treatment will result in large fees, the physician will discuss this matter with the patient before the onset of treatment.
4. The physician will apprise the business manager of patients who will be undergoing large fee treatment, and the business manager will negotiate any payment plan, taking into account the patient's insurance coverage and financial circumstances and the needs of the practice.
5. The physician will not negotiate fees or payment plans with patients. The physician will direct any patient who wishes to discuss the fee to the business manager. The business manager will then inform the physician of the patient's circumstances. The physician, with the advice of the business manager, will determine the appropriate patient fee. This and all other fee negotiations will take place between the business manager and the patient.

continues

Exhibit 10-7 continued

Verifications and Preauthorizations

1. Insurance information will be obtained from referrals at the time they schedule the initial office visit. All patients with CHAMPUS, OPTIMA, or any other plans requiring preauthorization will be informed of their preauthorization responsibilities at this time.
2. Any patient with a preauthorization responsibility will be flagged in the appointment book by the receptionist taking the referral.
3. Upon a flagged patient's arrival for the initial office visit, the receptionist will verify that the patient has in fact received preauthorization.
4. If a flagged patient has not received preauthorization, the receptionist will immediately inform the business manager, who will determine the best way to handle the situation.
5. Treatment authorizations will be placed in the patient's clinical chart. The need for additional authorizations will be monitored by the physician. The physician will inform the business manager when an additional authorization is required, and the business manager will be responsible for obtaining the authorization or informing the physician of a denial.

Copayment Collection Procedures

1. The receptionist is responsible for all initial payment, copayment, and deductible collections.
2. The receptionist is responsible for maintaining a current and accurate list of all patients with copayments.
3. The receptionist is responsible for one collection attempt at the time of service. If the attempt is not made, the receptionist is responsible for contacting the patient that day and requesting payment by mail.
4. The business manager is responsible for ensuring that the receptionist is effectively performing his or her collection tasks. The business manager is also responsible for developing collection methods to deal with patients who cannot or will not pay, employee collection training, and guidelines for when to refer patients to the business manager.

Insurance Billing Procedures

1. The business manager is responsible for the accurate collection and transmission of all information necessary to receive insurance payment.
2. All procedures will be entered into the computer each day, and insurance will be generated and mailed at least three times each week. The ultimate goal, however, is daily insurance billing.
3. The business manager will maintain a file of all changes in billing procedures or notices received from insurance companies.

Problem Account Detection

1. Any denied insurance claim will be given the highest priority. The business manager will immediately investigate the denial, resolve the situation, do any rebilling necessary, and correct any problems with practice procedures, software, and so on.
2. The business manager will immediately inform the director whenever there are any insurance-billing problems that are related to computer software or that have larger insurance-billing implications.
3. The business manager will generate both aging and write-off reports each month. These will be forwarded to the director.

continues

Exhibit 10-7 continued

4. The business manager is responsible for maintaining aging balances at acceptable levels, as determined by the director.
5. Any account that has money in 90 days past current will be periodically analyzed by the business manager. The patient will be billed for personal fees. Insurance fees will be pursued with either a tracer or by resubmission of a claim.

Collection Steps and Sequencing

1. Patients under continuing treatment will be informed that a missed copayment must be paid by the time of the next visit.
2. If a patient misses two consecutive copayments, the business manager will inform the physician, and, with the concurrence of the physician, the patient's treatment will be suspended until the fees have been paid.
3. Any patient fee that moves into 90 days past current will generate a series of two collection letters that will be sent with a ten-day interval.
4. The business manager will contact the patient by telephone if there is a need to send the second collection letter.
5. The second collection letter will require a response within five business days.
6. If there is no response to the second collection letter, the business manager will forward the account to the collection agent after informing the physician.

tion process. Particular attention should be given to any of the following items that are appropriate for your practice:

1. specific collection responsibilities associated with each job
2. the patient intake process
3. the patient education process
4. the billing method and payment arrangement process
5. verifications and preauthorizations
6. copayment collection procedures
7. insurance billing procedures
8. problem account detection methods
9. use of financial information (by the business manager for operations and by practice management for control and problem resolution)
10. the collection sequence (including the timing of first and second collection letters, writing off accounts, and referring accounts to the collection agent)

The collections administrator is responsible for developing the daily procedures that operationalize the collection plan. Perhaps the most important single element of the daily operational procedures is a method for determining when to initiate the next collection action. For example, if your business manager has 600 accounts to manage and 75 are in some stage of delinquency, how does he know that Fred Kringle should have responded to his second collection letter by today or that Anne Blert promised to get her payment in by yesterday?

The simplest solution to this problem is to use a daily calendar. Whenever an action that has a deadline is taken, a note is made of what should happen by the deadline date. If Fred Kringle was given until November 14 to respond to a second collection letter, an entry to that effect is made for November 14. On November 14, the business manager will check the status of the account, and if Fred has not responded adequately, the business manager will *immediately* initiate the next collection step.

The same objective can be achieved by creating a collections database in a computer. This approach has the added advantage of allowing you to determine quickly the status of any account in the database and easily track each account's history. An example of a screen from a collections database is found in Figure 10-1. Cases can be selected and sorted by any variable, so it is easy, for example, to call up all accounts requiring action on or before February 5 that are being evaluated by a particular collections person, and then sort them by last name and producer.

CONCLUSION

You should now be able to evaluate whether your practice has an effective, comprehensive collection plan. If it does not, you should be able to give your

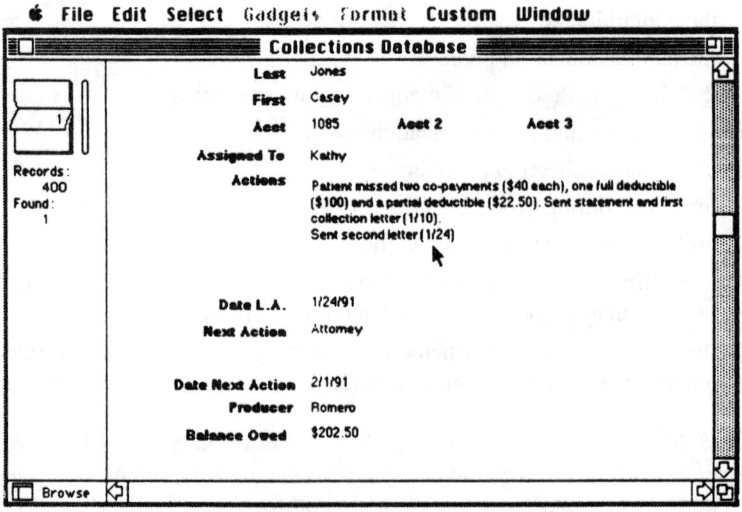

Figure 10-1 Screen from a Collection Database

collections administrator or business manager guidance regarding the development of a collection plan and also be able to assess the results of his or her efforts. You should now be familiar with the reasons why patients don't pay their bills and be able to implement procedures that reduce collection problems before they occur. In addition, you should now appreciate the diagnostic significance of insurance receivables and be able to formulate a collections plan that will compartmentalize insurance collection problems.

Finally, this chapter should have clarified your role in the collection process. As a doctor, you will not be involved with the daily collection of fees. Your collection role, however, is crucial to your practice's financial security. Your ultimate responsibility for revenue collection is too important to delegate to a salaried employee. By reviewing financial reports and involving yourself in the design of your practice's collection plan, you will be able to ensure the collection effectiveness of your practice.

NOTES

1. G. Belden, *Strategies for the Harassed Bill Payer: The Bill Collector and How to Cope with Him* (New York: Grosset and Dunlap, 1974), 120–22.
2. A study that this author conducted in one practice documented a claims loss rate of 8% with one insurance company. This rate dropped to almost zero when the claims were hand delivered and signed for.

Chapter 11

Using Computers

CHAPTER OBJECTIVES

This chapter is primarily directed at doctors who are entering private practice or who currently do not use a computer in their practices. These doctors need to understand the business applications of computers so that they can use computer technology effectively in the management of their practices. They also must understand how to evaluate software and hardware so that they can make suitable purchases. Doctors who currently use computers will be able to use this chapter to assess how effectively they are utilizing their computer equipment.

This chapter covers the following topics:

1. medical office management software
2. uses of generic software, accounting software, word processors, spreadsheets, telecommunications, local area networks, and databases
3. selecting IBM-compatible or Macintosh equipment
4. considerations when selecting software and hardware
5. sources of software and hardware information
6. using computer consultants
7. where to buy software and hardware
8. daily operational considerations
9. backing up data

INTRODUCTION

Computer technology is as essential to performing the business tasks of a medical practice efficiently as a secretary or a business manager. Notice that the comparison made was to people, not machines. Computer hardware and software

371

should be thought of as employees, not office equipment. Computers do not replace other pieces of office equipment; they replace personnel. Computers cost less than human employees because you don't pay them salaries or provide them with benefits, such as vacation time, FICA, retirement, workers' compensation, and sick leave. Although hardware sometimes breaks and software may develop bugs, they do so less often than human employees become sick, quit, or have to be fired. Most practices will find that annual computer repair and replacement costs will be less than employee turnover costs or the cost of benefits. A computer will never cheat or steal from you, and although on a rare occasion it may give you false information resulting from data entry errors, this will not have the malicious character of a human lie. Finally, computers will not consciously attempt to cause internal conflict or dissension within your practice. In short, the most cost-effective and least troublesome employees you will ever have will be your computer software and hardware.

It is important to have reasonable expectations for what a computer can do to improve business operations in a medical office. A computer can help your office to operate more efficiently and make fewer mistakes. You should be able to collect fees faster, pursue delinquent accounts more efficiently, generate more useful management reports, and market more effectively. On the other hand, a computer will not create order out of chaos. It will not compensate for a disorganized office or one that is staffed by incompetent or unmotivated employees. In fact, computerizing an office will bring preexisting problems into sharper focus and magnify their effects. This will occur because computerizing operations always creates stress. Employees are asked to learn new ways of doing things, and they will have to perform important functions while still feeling less than completely confident.

Using a computer gives employees the power to do many routine tasks more quickly and with fewer mistakes. There is a hidden danger, however, to this power. The knowledge required to use a computer effectively gives power to those who possess this knowledge. Employees who have critical know-how can hold you hostage. It can be frightening to face the prospect of disciplining or firing an employee who is the only person who really understands how to generate your insurance claims or post insurance payments to accounts. It is absolutely essential, therefore, that employees (including you perhaps) be cross-trained to operate *critical* software so that your office will still function if any single employee leaves or becomes unable to work. It is also essential for your practice to have a plan for training new employees. If an employee with critical software knowledge leaves, you must be able to train the replacement personally or use a cross-trained employee or an outside trainer.

Using computers creates a dependence upon the operation of the hardware and software. It is easy to say that you should have backup procedures available to operate your office if the computer system goes down. The reality, however, is that when the system does go down, the functions it performs for the most part also go down. Practices that have been computerized for a while will often have additional hardware that can be pressed into emergency service. For example, a computer that is currently being used for word processing may be temporarily used to handle patient accounts. Software problems, however, are more difficult to compensate for. If your insurance billing program begins to malfunction and reloading the program does not solve the problem, there is usually no alternative except to revert to a manual system until you can get a solution from the software publisher. (Problems of this severity are exceedingly rare with quality software. To put the issue in perspective, a manual insurance billing system becomes totally inoperative whenever the insurance clerk is absent.)

Computer systems, or combinations of specific software and hardware, should be designed around the required office tasks. Medical practices can generally benefit from using a computer for patient account management, accounting, word processing, and database management. These various areas of use are called *applications*, and the programs used to perform work in these areas are called *applications software*.

Selecting applications software and the other components of a computer system should be done in the following manner. First, identify the tasks that will be performed with the computer. Next, identify software that will perform those tasks. Which software to choose will depend on a number of issues, including cost, required training, technical support, and software capabilities. Finally, select the hardware that can best operate the software. Considerations when selecting hardware include cost, the compatibility of the software and the hardware, the reliability of the manufacturer and vendor, and the physical size of the equipment.

All of these decisions should only be made after considerable research into and thought concerning the available choices. The necessary research and decision making are certainly well within the ability of any doctor. Those doctors who view the selection process as an intellectual challenge or as an opportunity for demonstrating their hands-on style of management will probably want to become very involved in the decision making. They have the options of personally undertaking the required tasks or working closely with a consultant.

Other doctors might feel no more excitement than they would feel selecting a copier. They don't have the personal desire to obtain the necessary information, nor are the choices particularly meaningful to them. A doctor who is uninterested in becoming involved should hire decision-making expertise in the form of an external consultant. The doctor should not delegate the selection process to the business manager or any other nonowner, because employees generally will not have

- current knowledge of the available software and hardware
- the personal skills to deal with computer salespeople, who will have objectives that are not necessarily compatible with the best interests of the practice

- a vision of the practice's future direction (which lack prevents them from making purchase recommendations with that future in mind)

Finally, employees may favor software and hardware based solely on current familiarity. Purchasing systems that they have previously used will be less frightening and will give them immediate power. These are inappropriate reasons for purchasing decisions, because avoiding a one-time learning curve is not worth the reduced performance incurred over the life of the software and hardware.

APPLICATIONS

Managing Patient Accounts

Patient accounts will be managed with medical office management software (MOMS). The MOMS program you choose will be the centerpiece of your practice's computer system. Exhibit 11-1 contains a checklist of the capabilities that your MOMS should possess. Practice personnel should be able to set up a new patient account quickly; record daily activity, such as procedures, adjustments, and write-offs; and generate standard production data, patient bills, insurance claims, and management reports easily. In addition, your MOMS should allow you to develop your own customized reports. For example, you may wonder whether your patients' diagnoses are related to their zip codes or insurance plans, or perhaps you want to give other employees in your office access to patient biographical information. Your MOMS program should have the ability to export the appropriate data into a program that will allow you to answer questions about the relationship between variables or create separate databases.

Speed is an important consideration when selecting MOMS. A slow computer system can be very frustrating to employees and patients and can also waste valuable personnel time. When evaluating the speed of various MOMS, you should consider the following:

1. How fast does the overall system operate with a large patient account database? Demonstrations given by MOMS sales representatives are often on very small databases. The system may behave very differently when it has to deal with 1,500 accounts.
2. How rapidly can an account with many transactions be accessed and worked? Once again, the software may handle an account with 15 transactions very differently than an account with 500 transactions. This consideration will be more important to doctors who see many patients over a long period of time or for many procedures.
3. How rapidly does the software respond when it is being simultaneously accessed by more than one work station? (This is important if multiple

Exhibit 11-1 Characteristics of Medical Office Management Software (MOMS)

MOMS should be able to record the following types of information:
1. Patient procedures
2. Financial transactions, including patient payments, insurance payments, write-offs, adjustments, and discounts
3. Patient, guarantor, and spouse biographical information, such as address, telephone number, and date of birth
4. Insurance information, including plan, policy number, primary or secondary designation, and signature on file
5. Medications, including date of prescription, dose, and frequency

It should be able to generate the following:
1. Practice daily activity reports
   - Daily activity by producer, including fees and procedures
   - Daily receipts and adjustments
2. Billing reports
   - Individual patient statements
   - Batch printing of statements, with or without finance charges and for a selected range of dates
   - Statements that break out personal balances from insurance balances
3. Insurance reports
   - Individual patient claims
   - Batch insurance claims for a selected range of dates
   - Secondary insurance claims automatically when a primary claim is posted to an account
   - Aged insurance by patient
   - Aged insurance by plan
   - List of families by insurance plan
   - Insurance receipts by selected time period
   - Batch insurance tracers by insurance plan
4. Management reports
   - Gross receipts for selected time periods
   - Earned receipts associated with specific procedures and producers for selected time periods
   - Uncollectible write-offs by selected time period
   - Practice aging analysis for accounts above a minimum balance
   - Sales tax collections
   - Overpaid families
   - Patients by producer
   - Last visit on or before a selected date
   - Marketing reports of various types, such as patients by procedure or diagnosis, patients by birthdate, and professional courtesy
5. Database reports
   - Selected family information and merge capability into word processing, spreadsheet, or database program for further analysis
   - Management reports exported into word processing, spreadsheet, or database program for further analysis
   - Selected transaction information and merge capability into word processing, spreadsheet, or database program for further analysis

work stations will be accessing the MOMS.) In addition, does the system have a way of preventing simultaneous writing to the same file at the same time by different work stations? If a program does not have this protection, it can result in major problems.

Your office will become highly reliant on this software and the personnel who operate it. You should be very concerned, therefore, about both the complexity of the operations required to use this software and the training time necessary to become proficient in its use. Since your MOMS will be the cornerstone of your practice's business operations, you can easily become dependent on the personnel who operate it. This dependence will be directly proportional to the software's operational complexity and the amount of training time necessary to develop proficiency in its use.

Finally, you should ascertain who will provide MOMS consulting support and what the likely support response time will be. Because of the specialized nature of this software, it is essential that consultants be very knowledgeable and readily accessible. Generally, MOMS publishers will provide a toll-free telephone number for software support. Software support is usually contracted for on an annual basis or a fee is charged for consultation time. Response time should be on the order of two to four hours. Validate whatever you are told by contacting current customers.

Since your MOMS will be so critical to the operation of your practice, selecting it will be your most important computer-related decision. There are many acceptable choices in all other software categories. Your strategy, therefore, should be to (1) find the MOMS that will best meet your practice's requirements and (2) satisfy other practice needs with software and hardware that complement your MOMS.

Accounting Software

A theme expressed throughout Chapter 7 is that an important part of the doctor's management role is to be a consumer of accounting information. Consistent with this theme, you should not try to replace your accountant with accounting software. Instead, you should look for accounting software that can provide you with accounting information useful in the daily operation and management of your practice. Appropriate uses for accounting software include

- reporting accurate accounting data to your accountant in a timely manner
- producing management accounting information that can be used in management decision making
- managing daily practice finances, such as checking account balances and payroll calculations, including appropriate withholdings and deductions, and making timely and accurate payroll tax deposits

There are a number of factors to weigh when deciding whether to use accounting software. Since many of the tasks performed by the software are bookkeeping functions, they could be contracted out to a bookkeeper or an accountant. This would also provide an extra measure of financial control, since an independent party would be examining the practice finances. Practices that are thinly staffed may find that it is more feasible to contract out the work, even though they may occasionally have to wait a few days for a report.

Case Example

Harold Lint, C.P.A., did Dr. Tillery's practice accounting. Dr. Tillery's business manager handled the practice's checkbook and did the check reconciliation by hand. After Dr. Tillery turned over the "books" to Lint for preparation of his 1990 taxes, Lint told Dr. Tillery that he would have to spend two days, at $75 per hour, resolving inconsistencies in the payroll and the checking account. In addition, Dr. Tillery noted that he had experienced several problems making timely and accurate 941 federal withholding payments during the past year. Dr. Tillery asked Lint what to do. Lint suggested two alternatives:

1. Lint would handle all of the bookkeeping. Dr. Tillery would turn over his cancelled checks and checkbook memos to Lint at the end of each month. Lint would reconcile the checkbook and produce monthly income statements and balance sheets as well as compile payroll records. Lint would charge Tillery $250 per month. Since all of the accounts would be proofed each month by Lint, tax preparation costs at the end of the year would be reduced to about $400 from its current level of about $2,000.
2. Dr. Tillery could purchase accounting software and turn over higher quality data to Lint at the end of the year. Lint had determined that the methods currently used by the business manager did not provide enough structure and error detection. Lint would still have to perform quality checks on the data at the end of the year, but the accounting software should largely eliminate many of the problems that had plagued Dr. Tillery's bookkeeping.

Dr. Tillery investigated various software programs that were compatible with his computer. He found that he could purchase a general accounting and payroll program for about $375 and that training for his business manager would cost an additional $400. Dr. Tillery decided to combine the two approaches by having the business manager use software to manage the accounts and then forward the cancelled checks and the bank statements to the accountant for reconciliation. Lint reduced his charge to $100 per month, since the data were largely "clean" and in a form easy to enter into his computer system. Dr. Tillery had the security of having the reconciliation performed by an independent agent.

If you determine that some accounting tasks should be performed within your practice, you will need to obtain accounting software. It is very important to consult your accountant when selecting accounting software, since the accountant may have strong preferences regarding how information should be reported and which program features you need. You should not, however, delegate the software selection process to your accountant. The software characteristics that a professional accountant might look for could be very different from those that would work best in your office. In addition, the accountant may be biased due to familiarity with his or her own software. Remember, the software will be used by a clerical worker, not a CPA. Capabilities that an accountant might personally use and find desirable might also make the program very intimidating and difficult for a clerical worker to learn and use.

The tasks performed by accounting software fall into the following categories:

1. general ledger
2. accounts receivable
3. accounts payable
4. payroll

Any accounting software that you select should have integrated modules. This means that when you post an entry, the information is automatically forwarded to the appropriate general ledger, accounts receivable, accounts payable, and payroll modules. Generally, your accounts receivable will be handled through your MOMS, since your receivables will be largely composed of patient fees. As we have seen, your MOMS should provide you with considerable accounts receivable information and capabilities, including the ability to generate reports, age receivables, assess interest charges, and produce patient statements. Accounts receivable should not be a major factor, therefore, in selecting accounting software.

The simplest type of accounting software is a "one-write" program. One-write programs provide general ledger, accounts receivable, and accounts payable capabilities, although they are less sophisticated than general accounting programs. One-write programs are analogous to manual one-write check systems, which produce carbon copies when you write checks and make deposits. With computer-based one-write systems, you can post cash disbursements into accounts, balance bank statements, and run reports such as balance sheets, income statements, and cash receipt and disbursement journals.

One-write systems are simpler to operate and much less expensive than general accounting programs. They require less training time than general accounting programs and will be less intimidating to your personnel. One-write programs typically do not provide a payroll function. If payroll is important to you, however, that function can be performed by a stand-alone payroll program.

General accounting programs provide more features than one-write systems. Additional features typically include an integrated payroll function, the ability to produce additional reports, forecasting, inventory reporting, a more extensive budgeting capability, ratio analysis, the ability to handle more bank accounts, and generally greater flexibility and customizability. Some general accounting programs also have multiuser capability. This can be an important feature if your practice operates two or more offices.

Databases

A database is a large amount of stored information on a particular subject. Table 11-1 is an example of a simple biographical information database. A database is composed of records and variables. Each record contains values for each variable. In Table 11-1, each person is represented as a record or row in the database, and each record (person) has a value for each variable or column in the database. Using hindsight, you should be able to see that a MOMS program is really just a very specialized program for managing a patient account database. An accounting software program is a specialized database program for managing a financial database.

You may find that you wish to maintain additional databases in your practice. For example, it may be helpful to establish a "New Referrals" database. (MOMS software often lets you store referral information. Generally, however, the amount of information that can be stored on a referral and the data analysis capabilities are limited.) Exhibit 11-2 contains a list of referral variables used by one medical practice. Data for each new referral are entered into this database. It is then used to answer marketing questions such as these:

- Where are referrals coming from?
- Which physicians are generating the most referrals?
- Which practice physicians are generating referrals for other physicians in the practice?
- How many referrals are coming from specific referral sources, such as the Yellow Pages?
- What is the relationship between insurance plans and referral sources?
- What is the relationship between "lag" and "show/no show" status?

Database programs let you easily manipulate large numbers of records by permitting you to find records with certain variable values and by sorting records. For example, you can select the records of patients between ages 20 and 30 who also have Blue Cross insurance plans, and you can then examine the referral sources

Table 11-1 Biographical Database

Last Name	First Name	Age	Race	Sex	Marital Status
Smith	Robert	37	W	M	S
Allison	Frederick	14	W	M	S
Bellview	Melinda	29	B	F	M
Lewis	Allen	29	H	M	D
Johnson	Lisa	38	B	F	M
Boston	Nelson	missing	W	M	M

for these patients. In addition, most database programs can calculate statistics, such as means, medians, modes, counts, standard deviations, and correlations between groups of selected records. These functions can be used, for example, to determine whether different referral sources generate patients with different "no show" rates. These finding, sorting, and statistical functions give you the power necessary to draw conclusions from the information in the database.

Database programs come in two varieties. Flat file database programs treat each database as a distinct entity. Relational databases allow you to link together databases with common variables. If Fred Smith's age appears in three different databases, changing his age in any one database will also change it in the other two databases. Generally, relational databases take more time to learn, are more com-

Exhibit 11-2 Variables in a New Referrals Database

1. Last Name
2. First Name
3. Age
4. Sex
5. Zip Code
6. Date of Referral
7. Physician Assigned
8. Physician Generating Referral
9. Referral Source (narrative entry)
10. Referral Source Type (select appropriate category, such as Yellow Pages, physician, other professional, CHAMPUS, etc.)
11. Show/No Show
12. Diagnosis
13. Insurance Coverage
14. IOV Date (initial office visit)
15. Lag (calculated variable defined as the number of days between date of referral and IOV date)

plex to operate, and are more expensive to purchase than flat file databases. Most doctors will find that flat file databases are adequate for their database needs.

Database programs provide data analysis capabilities that MOMS programs typically do not possess. It is important, therefore, for your MOMS program to be able to communicate easily with your database program. This communication is achieved by exporting data from the MOMS program into the database. Once the data are in the database, you can select, sort, and analyze them so as to obtain a greater understanding of clinical, business, and marketing issues. Ease of communication between the MOMS program and the database program should be an important consideration when selecting database software.

Word Processing

The practice should select and use only one word processing program. This should be a sophisticated program that has many time-saving features such as the following:

- *Mail Merging.* The ability to merge a list of names and addresses into a form letter.
- *Spell Checking.* The program should be able to quickly check spelling and offer corrections.
- *Dictionary.* The program should be able to find uncommon words. In addition, a medical dictionary can be helpful.
- *Glossaries.* These are passages of boilerplate text that can be entered into a document with a single keystroke or command.
- *WYSIWYG.* The acronym for "what you see is what you get." A program that displays text on the screen as it will appear on the printed page will let secretaries produce better documents in less time.
- *Tables.* The program should have the ability to produce tables and sort their contents.
- *Style Sheets.* A style is a set of formatting instructions for a particular type of document, such as a letter, medical evaluation, or court report. By storing a combination of tabs, fonts, indents, margins, and so on, as a style, the secretary can easily create consistent documents.

Another important consideration when selecting word processing software is whether it has the ability to communicate with other software. For example, a word processing program will be much more useful if it can easily receive names and addresses directly from the MOMS program. It is also important for the word processing program to be able to communicate with the database program. For example, suppose that you want to send a form letter to all patients with a particular diagnosis code. If the MOMS, word processing, and database programs can communicate, the procedure would be as follows:

1. MOMS exports a list of all patient names, addresses, and diagnosis codes to the database program. (If the MOMS program has some database capabilities, such as selecting and sorting, it would be possible to go directly from MOMS to the word processing program.)
2. Those cases with the desired diagnosis code are selected in the database program, sorted into alphabetical order, and exported to the word processing program. (It is always desirable to put long lists into some logical order. For example, if letters have to be paired with address labels, it is much easier to ascertain they are properly matched when both the labels and letters are printed in alphabetical order.)
3. A standard form letter is written in the word processing program and merged with the mailing addresses imported from the database program. The word processing program then prints the individualized form letters.
4. Alphabetized address labels are printed using either the database or word processing program.

Spreadsheets

A spreadsheet is composed of rows and columns that resemble an accountant's ledger pad. Exhibit 11-3 contains a spreadsheet. One useful spreadsheet feature is the ability to define a cell as a function of other cells. For example, cell B6 can be defined as the mean of cells B2 through B5. If any changes are made to cells B2 through B5, the spreadsheet will automatically recalculate the value of cell B6.

Spreadsheet programs are useful for displaying data, for testing what will happen if you change the values of interrelated variables, and for making projections. For example, individual aging analyses generated by a practice's MOMS program were entered into a spreadsheet to produce Table 7-8. The relationships between fixed and variable costs can be entered into a spreadsheet and projections can be calculated for various revenue levels, such as in Table 7-13. Spreadsheet programs also provide graphing capabilities. Figure 7-2 contains a graph generated from the data in Table 7-13.

Although a spreadsheet looks like an accounting ledger, spreadsheet programs should not be used in place of accounting software. It is possible to use a spreadsheet to create accounts receivable, accounts payable, and general ledgers, but unless you are very skilled at programming a very sophisticated spreadsheet, you will not be able to build in the logic checks and other error detection features that accounting software normally possesses.

Exhibit 11-3 Sample Spreadsheet

	A	B	C	D	E	F
1	NAME	AGE				
2	Smith	18				
3	Jones	19				
4	Lawson	25				
5	Franklin	21				
6	MEAN	20.75				
7						
8						
9						
10						
11						
12						
13						
14						
15						
16						
17						
18						

The spreadsheet program should be able to communicate easily with your other programs. For example, producing documents with tables and graphs can best be accomplished by constructing the tables and graphs in a spreadsheet, then exporting them into the word processing program. All of the tables and graphs in this book were constructed with *Excel* spreadsheets, which were then exported into the word processing program *Word 4.0*.

Telecommunications

A telecommunications capability that some doctors might find desirable is electronic insurance claims (E-claims) submission. This topic was discussed in Chapter 10. The issue boils down to the costs associated with E-claim submission versus the potential savings in supplies and postage, faster problem claim resolution, and a reduced clerical workload. E-claims require a modem and software that will allow your computer to communicate with the insurance company's computer.

Generally, insurance companies that support E-claims have their own proprietary software that you must purchase or rent. These programs generally are compatible with only some computer brands. If you anticipate using E-claims with a particular carrier, you should contact that company before making your computer hardware and software selections. Keep in mind, however, that insurance companies have been notorious for changing paper-claim-filing requirements with little or no notice. This fickleness may well begin to characterize E-claims hardware requirements.

Telecommunications can also be used to conduct on-line literature searches. By linking a private practice's computer by modem and communications software with comprehensive medical databases, such as MEDLINE, HEALTHLINE, and BIOETHICSLINE, the doctor can quickly research a subject. In addition, some journals are now available on computer, so that if an article is located, it may not be necessary to go to the library to obtain the text.

Other Uses

Computers can be used to schedule appointments and utilize practice resources more efficiently in large practices. Scheduling software can schedule across several locations, coordinate the use of facilities and equipment, generate patient and chart-pull lists, and keep patient waiting time to a minimum. Smaller practices, however, may find the familiar appointment book to be advantageous. If the scheduling is put on a computer, then constant access to the scheduling system is essential. One computer or terminal must be devoted at all times to scheduling. Small practices may find that funnelling all scheduling and scheduling changes through one computer may become a choke point, and result in a slow, frustrating process.

Electronic transfer of mail (E-mail) allows the transfer of letters, reports, data, and so on, from one computer to another. E-mail may have increasing application to private practice doctors as databases develop for medical diagnosis and decision making. Currently, most sophisticated diagnostic and decision-making databases are located at medical schools and hospitals. It is inevitable that these databases will become available to private practices by modem in a manner similar to current bibliographic databases.

LOCAL AREA NETWORKS AND MULTIUSER SYSTEMS

Local area network (LAN) software is used to link several computers together. A LAN could be useful, for example, if several employees must have simultaneous access to MOMS. A LAN could also be useful if you have two or more waiting rooms and want to enter patient payments immediately from both locations. Computers networked into a LAN can still operate independently if the network goes down.

A LAN will add considerable complexity and cost to your computer system. The cost of a LAN version of a MOMS program is often one and a half to two and a half times more expensive than the single user version. Many LAN networks require the use of a separate computer that is totally dedicated to functioning as a "file server" or "network server." In addition, all of the locations will have to be wired together. LAN versions of MOMS and generic software often operate more slowly than the single user version, and on occasion one station can tie up the system so that other stations cannot obtain information. Finally, LANs are particularly susceptible to software bugs and interaction problems between stations. Unless you are a "hacker" or have a very good relationship with a systems analyst, you should avoid LANs in their current state of development.

In a multiuser system, all of the software and data are stored in a central computer. Users operate "dumb" terminals, which have no processing capability without the central computer. If the central processor goes down, all of the terminals go down. Multiuser systems usually cost significantly more than LANs. Since multiuser systems are designed for business use, they usually have well-integrated software and hardware. In addition, the software can be of very high quality, since multiuser manufacturers tend to concentrate on particular vertical markets, such as medicine, accounting, and engineering.

The problems that LANs and multiuser systems are designed to address can often be solved using simpler means. Before implementing a LAN or purchasing a multiuser system, you should evaluate the real *necessity* for multiple employees to simultaneously have access to the most current information or be able to enter changes to a database. For example, suppose that the MOMS is based in a back office with the business manager and that a front office receptionist only needs to consult the MOMS for patient addresses and telephone numbers. These data can be easily copied and placed on the receptionist's computer as a separate database. If necessary, the copy can be updated daily by simply carrying a floppy disk from one computer to the other. Most questions directed to a receptionist regarding patient accounts can be easily answered by using a day-old copy of the MOMS. The rare question that requires more recent information can be handled by the business manager, or the patient can be asked to wait for a few minutes while the receptionist consults the business manager's computer.

In summary, LANs and multiuser systems add considerable cost and complexity to a practice's computer system. Before seriously considering either alternative, you should be certain that there is a real need for the features that each one provides.

SELECTING COMPUTER SOFTWARE AND HARDWARE

Most computer consultants will tell you to perform a "needs analysis" to determine whether you really need a computer. The position taken in this book is that virtually all medical practices will be better off managing their patient accounts on a computer. Unless your practice is exceedingly small, you will find that the accuracy and management power that a good MOMS can provide is reason enough to computerize your office. Once the initial decision is made, the training and financial costs associated with acquiring additional software will seem relatively inconsequential.

Some small practices with two or more clerical workers may find that managing patient accounts essentially consumes all of the available time on one computer. Thus, there will not be enough time available on the "MOMS computer" for word processing and other functions. Under these circumstances, a needs analysis may be appropriate to determine whether the volume of other work can justify the purchase of an additional computer versus a dedicated word processor or typewriter. When making this decision, the doctor should consider that the purchase of additional computer equipment will provide backup hardware should the MOMS computer develop a problem.

At this point we come to a major fork in the road. You must decide whether to select software that is compatible with IBM formatted computers or with Apple Macintosh computers. A specific applications program, such as the word processing program Wordperfect, utilizes the computer's *operating system* to communicate with the computer. The operating system acts as an interface between the applications program and the computer hardware. IBM adopted an operating system called MS-DOS, which is an acronym for Microsoft-Disk Operating System. Various hardware manufacturers, including IBM, subsequently modified MS-DOS to suit their own needs, and as a result programs vary in their compatibility across IBM and IBM-clone computers.[1] Collectively these variations of MS-DOS will be referred to as DOS. IBM's newest machines use an entirely different operating system called OS/2. OS/2-based machines will operate DOS software, but DOS machines will not operate OS/2 software. Finally, all programs that run on MS-DOS or OS/2 are incompatible with programs designed to run on the Apple Macintosh's operating system. Some software, such as Wordperfect, is published in DOS, OS/2, and Macintosh versions. However, programs that are very successful in one operating system may not be as effective in another. For example, DBASE IV is a very successful DOS database management program that has had very little success in its Macintosh version. Similarly, Excel is the predominant Macintosh spreadsheet, but it has been much less successful in obtaining DOS or OS/2 market share.

Your first impression may be that deciding between the IBM and Apple Macintosh worlds will be easy. After all, IBM has set the standard for small business computing, and most small businesses use IBM formatted software and hardware. However, the fundamental differences between the two companies' approaches to computing have significant implications for the user, and you should make your decision only after examining the operation of software on both types of computers. The difference between operating DOS and Macintosh software lies in the demands that they place on the computer user. DOS formatted applications are *command* driven. For example, if you wish to delete a letter called Myletter, you would have to type

DEL MYLETT.TXT

To copy a document named File 1 from a disk in disk drive A to a file named Harry1.QAL on hard disk C, you would have to type

COPY A:\FILE1 C:\HARRY1.QAL

Although these tasks may sound simple, you must remember large numbers of commands to effectively use DOS programs. Proficiency in some DOS programs can require considerable training, continual reference to software manuals, and extensive experience. In summary, the learning curve can be steep.

Another difficulty in using DOS software is that there can be considerable diversity in the way that different programs interact with the user. For example, pressing the CONTROL and \ keys may save text in one program, whereas the same command may delete text in another program. Needless to say, this lack of consistency can be very frustrating for a clerical worker who is trying to use several different programs!

To some extent software publishers have tried to reduce the learning curve and the inconsistencies between programs through the use of "shell" programs. Shell programs present the user with more easily used menus and a higher degree of consistency across software. In addition, Microsoft offers a program called *Windows* that emulates to some degree the graphic environment of the Macintosh, which will be described below.

Macintosh applications are *graphics* driven. To delete a document called Myletter, you simply point to a small picture of the document, which is called an icon. You do this with a hand manipulated control device called a "mouse." You move the Myletter icon into an icon of a trash can. In effect, you simply throw it out, just as you would a paper letter. There are no commands to learn. To move a document from one disk drive to another, you point to the document's icon and "drag" it across the computer screen to the icon of the other disk drive. Once again, there are no commands to learn, and the operation of the computer is largely intuitive. A typical Macintosh screen with icons on it is presented in Figure 11-1.

The Macintosh's user interface is a model of consistency across programs. Virtually all Macintosh programs use the same screens and menus. As a result, there is considerable transfer of learning from any Macintosh program to all others, and the time necessary to train employees is considerably shorter with Macintosh software. Most Macintosh software programs communicate information very easily with each other, even when the programs are from different publishers. For example, data can be easily transferred from Healthcare Communications' MediMac MOMS software to Claris' Filemaker II database manager for analysis,

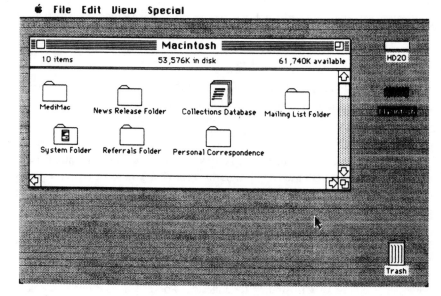

Figure 11-1 Apple Macintosh Screen. *Source:* Icons courtesy of Apple Computer Co, Inc., Cupertino, CA.

then subsequently transferred to Microsoft's Word 4.0 for inclusion in word processing documents. In addition, it is possible to *simultaneously* operate MOMS, word processing, and other programs. Finally, the intuitive nature of the software means that employees learn faster and consult training manuals far less often than with DOS software.

IBM has tried to compensate for some of these Macintosh advantages with their new OS/2 operating system. Software that uses OS/2 has been slow to obtain market share because of the large investment that users have in DOS hardware. In addition, there currently are few programs written for OS/2. It is clear, however, that OS/2 will be the future standard of the IBM world and that the days of DOS are numbered.

You should not underestimate the advantages of intuitive software operation and shorter employee training time. Since your employees will become more proficient sooner with Macintosh software, your practice will experience a smaller productivity decline when there is employee turnover. In addition, you will be less likely to become a hostage to an employee's unique software knowledge, and as a result you will have more flexibility when dealing with problem employees. Finally, you may find that the learning curve is sufficiently flat that you yourself can master some aspects of your MOMS. It is always advantageous for the owner of a small business to be able to personally inspect all aspects of the business whenever he or she chooses.

There are, however, two disadvantages to using a Macintosh:

1. *There are fewer software choices.* This can be a consideration when selecting MOMS. But if you find a program that meets your needs, it is irrelevant whether there are five or twenty other viable alternatives, since you will only be using one MOMS program. Availability is not a problem in the other applications areas, where there are many good Macintosh choices.

2. *Macintosh hardware is generally more expensive than IBM-clone equipment.* Nonetheless, it is often no more expensive than IBM equipment and the equipment of other high-end manufacturers, such as Hewlett-Packard and Compaq. Purchasing inexpensive IBM-clone equipment is risky. These brands come and go, and the original savings in price will seem trivial if you cannot obtain service or parts.

In summary, you must make a choice between Apple Macintosh and IBM DOS or OS/2 software. Once you go down one of these roads, your investment will be such that it will be very expensive financially and in training and practice efficiency to go back. Since your MOMS software will be the cornerstone of your practice's business operations, you should only make this choice after carefully examining MOMS programs run in each of the three operating systems. OS/2 represents the future of IBM compatible computing, and you should probably reject DOS-based MOMS unless you already have a considerable investment in DOS equipment. The additional cost associated with Macintosh equipment is minor when amortized over the life of the hardware. If you find a Macintosh-based MOMS that is compatible with your needs, then Macintosh should be your equipment of choice.

Evaluating Software and Hardware

Selecting your practice's hardware and software will be a major business decision. It will both involve a considerable investment of money and have a major effect on the productivity of your business office. It is essential, therefore, to only make the decision after obtaining sufficient information about the available software and hardware and how they function as a working system. You can obtain this information from a number of sources, including

- colleagues
- consultants
- medical conference presentations and demonstrations
- MOMS sales representatives
- medically oriented computer publications

- general computer publications
- users groups

Consulting colleagues in the same specialty is a very important strategy. Usually, computer users will be very happy to talk about their experiences, preferences, likes, and dislikes regarding software and hardware. By talking to experienced colleagues, you will be able to learn about the subtle strengths and weaknesses of a program, which only become apparent after using it for a considerable period of time.

It is important, however, to be wary of "dissonance reducers." Dissonance reducers cognitively distort their degree of satisfaction to justify their decisions. Dissonance reducers inflate the strengths of a system and minimize its weaknesses so that they can rationalize having selected it. Much of this dissonance reduction will occur at a semiconscious or unconscious level. Dissonance reducers are not lying; they are using a cognitive mechanism to make rational sense out of their behavior. It is important to understand this so that you can get the most out of consulting with your colleagues. The object of your consultations should be to obtain a description of how their systems operate. You should be much less concerned about eliciting conclusions regarding a system's adequacy and should focus on the mechanics and uses of the system. For example, you should find out about data entry procedures, training requirements, available reports, consistency with office routine, response time, and so on. You should then determine how well this system would work in your practice and make comparisons with the other available systems.

Since MOMS software is highly specialized, you will have to do a good deal of investigation to obtain a thorough understanding of what is available. Displays and demonstrations at medical conferences allow you to examine a lot of software in a short period of time. In addition, software companies usually send well-trained personnel to medical conferences so you will get knowledgeable answers to your questions. Many medical conferences are now offering paper sessions and workshops on computer issues. These can be useful for learning about generic office automation issues as well as the latest developments in applications and hardware.

Journals such as *Physicians and Computers* and *M.D. Computing* offer evaluative articles, reviews of MOMS, and descriptions of how to use generic software in medical practices.[2] Reviewers often subject the software to demanding tests, such as very high patient counts or large batches of insurance claims. As a result, you may get an indication of how the software might behave a few years from now. Since MOMS publishers are competing for a narrow market, they are likely to advertise in medically oriented computer journals, which are consequently good sources of information about the newest software.

General computer publications are usually not good sources of MOMS information because of the very specialized nature of this software. They can be excellent sources, however, of current information about generic software, such as spreadsheets, databases, word processing programs, and accounting packages. In addition, routinely reading these magazines will keep you abreast of the latest hardware, software, and computing issues. Generally, your business manager will not have the motivation or the skills to think creatively about potential uses of computer systems. This is a task that belongs to top management, and if you don't take the time and the effort to learn about new possibilities, this proactive planning function will probably remain unrealized.

Some users groups can be of great assistance. For example, there is a medical-dental interest group in the Boston Computer Society. Members of local users groups can be helpful with general computing issues and generic software, and they may assist you in finding local physicians with automated offices.

Finally, consultants can be an excellent source of computer information. Consultants go by a number of titles, including *systems analyst*, *systems consultant*, *systems integrator*, and *vertical specialist*. No matter what the titles, it is important to make a distinction between *medical* consultants and *computer* consultants. Medical consultants may not be particularly knowledgeable about the latest computer software. This is because they have an orientation toward medical practice issues in general, not just office automation issues. Therefore, a medical consultant who recommends a "pet" software program may be meeting his or her needs more than the client's needs. The software may work, as it did three years ago, but whether it is the best available today for a given price is another question. On the other hand, a medical consultant who is current on the latest software and hardware can be a very cost-efficient source of information.

Computer consultants often work with a wide range of businesses and may not immediately appreciate the unique software needs of a medical practice. If, for example, a computer consultant does not understand the advantage of being able to link payments with procedures when printing a complete account summary, he or she will not include this characteristic among the software selection criteria. The consultant may be able to elicit the importance of this characteristic from your business manager, but then again he or she may not.

In short, you must be an informed consumer of consultants. You must critically interview each medical consultant to determine whether computers really make his or her eyes dazzle. If they don't, then you may be getting outdated or uninformed advice. Similarly, you want to be certain that each computer-oriented consultant either currently appreciates or is able to appreciate the intricacies of insurance billing, remit posting, and account auditing.

A consultant can supply you with a number of services. The consultant can assess your practice's software and hardware needs, research the compatibility of various software and hardware combinations, and make purchase recommendations. In addition, the consultant can purchase the equipment for you and provide employee training and software and hardware consultations. If you use a consultant to purchase equipment, it is particularly important to be aware of the quality of the equipment. The consultant may be keeping overall costs down by recommending inferior clone equipment. This will allow the consultant to charge his or her fee while keeping the overall cost of the contract at competitive levels. The true cost may not be discovered until service problems arise and you find that the equipment manufacturer is no longer in business or the distributor no longer stocks parts.

Where to Buy Software and Hardware

Because of the very specialized nature of MOMS, you will find that this software is almost always sold through a single area distributor. As a result, your ability to negotiate price on MOMS may be very limited, unless the seller is also a source for other software and hardware.

There will almost certainly be a number of competing vendors selling generic software and hardware, however. It is important to remember that price is not the only significant consideration when selecting vendors. Effective training, knowledgeable consultation, and timely equipment repair should be of more concern than a few hundred dollars reduction in the initial sales price.

There are a number of different kinds of software and hardware vendors. *Retail stores*, such as Computerland, Businessland, and Sears Business Centers, are high-visibility storefront outlets. Retail stores market to the general public as well as to small businesses. Generally, these vendors will have high prices, and their main goal is to sell equipment, not provide service and training.

Value-added vendors tend to specialize more in business sales and vertical markets. A vertical market is a specialized field, such as medicine, law, architecture, and professional accounting. Vertical markets are characterized by complex software and very specific hardware requirements. Value-added vendors employ systems analysts with experience in developing software and hardware solutions for a particular type of business. Remember that, unlike an independent consultant, a systems analyst who works for a value-added vendor will have a vested interest in solving your computer problems with the vendor's products. Value-added vendors' prices will usually be the same or somewhat below those of retail stores. By purchasing a complete package of MOMS, generic software, hardware, and employee training, you may be able to negotiate some additional savings.

Mail order vendors offer the lowest prices. Do not purchase MOMS by mail order, since the vendor will not be able to provide training. Obtaining services can be a problem with mail order–purchased computers and printers. Shipping a dead computer or printer back to the mail order vendor is a time-consuming nuisance. The costs of downtime and the inconvenience associated with one repair will not be worth the savings in initial sales price. Printers have mechanical parts, and they will need occasional adjustment. Taking a mail order–purchased computer or printer to a local repair shop will result in one of two frustrating outcomes: (1) The shop will refuse to service your equipment, even if it is a local "authorized" repair shop; (2) Your equipment will sit on the bench so long that you will not bring it back again. Only consider buying computers and printers by mail if a local repair shop will sell you a service contract.[3] Realize, however, that the repair shop may still be less responsive to your needs than to the needs of a client who also purchased equipment there.

Mail order vendors can be used to buy some hardware and software. Self-contained and simple hardware devices, such as external disk drives and modems, are reasonably safe mail order purchases. These items either work or don't work. When they don't work, they are usually replaced instead of repaired. Generally, the local repair shop will send a damaged disk drive back to the manufacturer anyway, so you actually may save time by doing this yourself.

Mail order software purchases should be limited to (1) software that requires minimal training, (2) software for which a local consultant can provide training, or (3) software that your employees do not have to master immediately. For example, a year from now you may decide to purchase a page layout program to publish your own newsletter. By then you may be a "hacker" and want to self-train in the program at your leisure. Another candidate for mail order purchase might be a backup program that several magazines have reviewed favorably. (A backup program is used to make a copy of your software and data to protect against damage or theft.) Finally, you may want to convert your office to a new database program. You locate a consultant who can provide the training, and you purchase the program by mail order for $100 less than the price in the local computer store.

The mail order industry has had its share of bankruptcies and disreputable operators. It is safest to order from major advertisers in the larger computer magazines. Full-color, multipage ads that run for several months provide some indication that a mail order house is reputable and financially viable. Mail order vendors will often ship software by overnight air freight at a minimal cost. If you identify a product that can improve your productivity, you can have it in place by the next day. However, you should ascertain that the product is in stock before ordering it.

"Warehouse" outlets, such as the Price Club, and office supply superstores, such as Office Warehouse, are good places to purchase computer supplies such as floppy disks, paper, printer ribbons, and laser printer toner. Do not buy hardware from these outlets, since it will probably be of an obsolescent design or from a defunct manufacturer.

The Selection Process

Irrespective of who supplies you with software and hardware, you should have a clear written statement describing what will be purchased, who will supply training and support, and what the availability of support and repair services will be. The recommended course of action is as follows:

1. Hire a consultant to evaluate your office needs and recommend software and hardware. You should only consider doing this yourself if you are truly knowledgeable about computers, have had several years of computing experience, *and* are willing to take the time to thoroughly research the alternatives.

2. Even if you do use a consultant, develop your personal knowledge of computers by asking for software demonstrations from MOMS sales representatives, attending demonstrations at medical conferences, reading medically oriented computer journals, meeting frequently with the consultant, and so on. This step is not essential, but it is consistent with the philosophy adopted in this book—that you are your own best advocate.

3. Validate the consultant's report by getting a demonstration of the proposed system and at least one other demonstration for comparison. Consider having another consultant comment on the report. If you have done the research yourself, consider validating your conclusions by discussing them with a consultant.

4. Contract separately with a consultant to obtain purchase bids for MOMS software, hardware, training, and so on. (This consultant needn't be the same one who assisted in the software and hardware evaluation process.) You also have the option of obtaining purchase bids yourself based on the vendors identified in the consultant's report or through your own research.

5. Evaluate lease and purchase alternatives using the present value concepts discussed in Chapter 7.

6. Have all contracts, including agreements with consultants and vendors, reviewed by your attorney.

COMPUTER OPERATING CONSIDERATIONS

The success of your computer system will to some extent be a function of some very mundane but nevertheless important considerations. The personnel who will train your employees and set up your equipment should make certain that the recommendations given below are followed:

1. All equipment should be on surge suppressors. This is not the place to cut corners. Buy good surge suppressors that protect all poles (positive, negative, and ground).

2. Take into account the work flow and the floor plan of your office when locating computer equipment. Placing a printer next to a telephone, for example, can create an annoying distraction. Consider relocating furniture to create a better work flow.

3. Consider the ergonomics of operating a computer. Are chairs and desks at a comfortable height? Are desks large enough to fit a computer and still have usable writing and working areas? You may have to purchase or relocate suitable office furniture.

4. Evaluate the security of the computer equipment location. The more deterrents that you place between thieves and their objectives, the more likely they are to go someplace else to steal. Ideally, rooms with computer equipment should have deadbolt locks, solid core doors, and steel frames. Consider installing an office security system. If possible, place computers so that they are not within eyesight of patients who are in the waiting room or are scheduling appointments or paying fees at the receptionist's window.

5. Whenever an employee terminates, always change access codes for password protected programs and the office security system.

6. Create standards and procedures for computer operations, such as powering up and down, deleting files, naming files, and backing up files.

7. Be certain that employees receive education on how computer equipment works. This can prevent problems, such as placing documents over ventilation holes and frying the equipment or placing disks next to a telephone and having them become corrupted by electromagnetic interference.

In summary, the setting up should involve more than simply unpacking the equipment and plugging it into the wall. The installation should take into account how your office operates as well as introduce standard operational procedures that will result in effective and efficient computer operations.

Backing Up Data

The object of backing up data is to make a copy and put it in a remote location so that you will have a recent, usable record in the event that (1) the equipment is physically stolen; (2) the equipment is physically damaged, such as by fire, water, or dropping; or (3) the data become corrupted for any reason, including a personnel error, a software bug, a computer virus, or sabotage.

Backing up your data is an absolutely essential task that must be performed every day without exception. Many people view backing up records as a necessary evil intrinsic to an automated office. This is an inappropriate way to view this task. Instead, it should be realized that manual offices continually face much more exposure to the loss of information because it is so difficult and time consuming to back up manual records. Computerized offices can provide greater security for financial and patient information, and you should take advantage of this added security on a daily basis.

Data are copied, using a backup program, onto other storage media, such as floppy disks, tapes, or other hard disks. If you don't have a lot of data to back up, floppy disks are an inexpensive and easily used storage medium. Unfortunately, each floppy disk holds a relatively small amount of information, so if there are a lot of data to back up, you will have to use many disks. If you find that a secretary is feeding disks to the computer for more than a few minutes, you should consider purchasing a tape system or an extra hard disk drive. Tape backup systems have much more storage capacity and do not need any clerical attention during the backup process. An extra hard drive has the same advantages as a tape system, but it has the added advantage of giving you a backup piece of hardware. If the hard drive with the original data becomes inoperable, you can substitute the backup hard drive.[4] The disadvantage of using a backup hard drive is that the backup is tied to the equipment. You can only have one duplicate copy, whereas with a tape or floppy disk backup system you can make multiple duplicate copies.

It is important to implement a thorough backup procedure that will ensure the integrity of your data under any conceivable circumstances, *including failure of the backup media*. Disks, tapes, and drives are extremely reliable, but why tempt fate when the costs are so minimal? Exhibit 11-4 outlines a backup routine that will protect against virtually any plausible set of mishaps.

Alternating the backup disks or tapes on a daily basis achieves two purposes. First, it protects against a catastrophe, such as a sprinkler releasing, a fire, or a computer "crash," that strikes *during* a backup. Second, it provides extra security by putting very recent data in two remote locations. It is important that personnel store the alternate daily backups in separate rooms.

Weekly backups provide security against a catastrophe that engulfs your whole office, such as the theft of all of your equipment and furniture or a serious fire. Alternating weekly backups provides you with additional time to identify corrupted data. For example, if an employee damages your data just before a weekly backup and you then back up that data over your old backup, you will have no

Exhibit 11-4 Daily and Weekly Backup Routines

Daily Backup Routine

Two sets of backup floppy disks or tapes marked A and B.

Monday, Wednesday	Use Set A
Tuesday, Thursday	Use Set B

Store set A and Set B in separate rooms under lock and key.

Weekly Backup Routine

Two sets of backup floppy disks or tapes marked A and B. The sets are used on alternating weeks and are stored in separate rooms at a practice owner's residence. A backup is made every Friday.

---

good copy of the data. Alternating weekly backups will give you a week to determine that something is in error before the normal weekly backup corrupts the second weekly backup.

Weekly backups should be stored outside of the practice, and they should be under the control of a practice owner. Ideally, the weekly backup should be made by a practice owner, although this arrangement is often tempered by the labor relations climate or the length of time necessary to perform a backup.

Finally, be certain that normal office procedures generate enough of a paper record to reconstruct past work and payments for a period of time. Daysheets, copies of superbills, appointment books, and other documentation should be retained for several months so that there is enough time for any data losses or corruptions to become evident.

CONCLUSION

You should now have an understanding of the uses of medical office management, accounting, spreadsheet, database, word processing, and telecommunications software. You should know why it is important to make an informed choice regarding whether to use DOS, OS/2, or Macintosh software. You should be familiar with several sources of software and hardware information and know where and how to purchase software and hardware. Finally, you should understand that some thought must be given to integrating the computer system you choose into your office. Daily procedures, work flows, and standards must be developed, and your practice must have thorough and consistently used backup procedures.

NOTES

1. The term *IBM clone* refers to computers not manufactured by IBM that are supposed to operate like an IBM computer and use software designed for IBM equipment. Clones can vary in their degree of "cloneness," and it is not unusual to find IBM compatible software that will not run easily or at all on some IBM clones. IBM clone equipment is generally less expensive than IBM equipment.

2. *Physicians and Computers*, 233 Waukegan Road, Suite S-280, Brannockburn, IL 60015, tel. (708) 940-8333; *M.D. Computing*, Springer-Verlag, Inc., 175 Fifth Avenue, New York, NY 10010, tel. (212) 460-1500.

3. Computerland, G.E., and Honeywell are three national companies that currently offer service contracts on equipment they did not sell.

4. A backup hard drive does not need to be an unused piece of equipment. For example, it might be used during the day in another room but have sufficient excess storage capacity. It is important, however, that during the night the backup hard drive be secured in a locked location remote from the original data to reduce the chances of theft.

Chapter 12

Strategic Management

CHAPTER OBJECTIVES

This chapter explains why doctors who are going into private practice or are currently in practice should develop a practice strategy and use it to guide operational decisions. You will learn

1. how to develop a practice strategy
2. how to evaluate your strategy based on market competition and internal practice considerations
3. generic practice strategies and when they may be useful
4. why operational decisions that are inconsistent with your strategy may jeopardize your personal happiness and your practice's existence

INTRODUCTION

Strategic management is the process of examining and evaluating options for the future of your practice. Strategic management and the resulting strategic plan can be contrasted with operational plans, which focus on immediate or near-term objectives instead of long-term goals. Strategic plans and operational plans should be consistent with each other. Strategic planning addresses questions such as these:

- What do I want this practice to be like in a few years?
- What changes are occurring in medicine, the community, my patients, my competitors, and so on, that may affect the way I practice in the future?
- What things must I begin to do now or in the near future to ensure that my practice will have the characteristics I desire and will be competitive in the medical environment a few years hence?

The concept of strategic planning was introduced in Chapter 8. It was emphasized that marketing decisions should be based on a thorough evaluation of your practice's strengths and weaknesses and the environment's opportunities and threats. You were also asked to consider your long-range vision of the practice. This *strategic* thinking was then to be translated into a marketing plan—an *operational* plan describing immediate and near-term tactical goals and courses of action. Developing your marketing plan as suggested in Chapter 8 is an example of strategic planning.

Strategic management, as well as thinking in strategic terms, is applicable beyond specific functions such as marketing. An awareness of strategic issues should characterize your approach to managing your practice. You need to develop an awareness of the long-term implications of daily events or emerging trends. There are tools and techniques, discussed in this chapter, that you can use to help identify issues of strategic importance and evaluate your strategic plans.

Managing your practice's strategy should be an ongoing process. Changes in your practice's circumstances, your personal goals, local demographics, insurance, regulations, or the competitive environment should all generate strategic thought. Strategically managing a practice is characterized by a *state of mind* in which management is continually evaluating events in terms of their long-range implications.

Some doctors will conduct a strategic analysis before entering private practice with the object of creating practices that are competitive and that meet their personal needs. Many doctors, however, will not reevaluate their strategic options once their practices are operating. It is important to go beyond the initial strategic thinking that occurs at the inception of a practice. The world in which your practice operates is not static. The important strategic considerations of several years ago may have been replaced by other considerations. As a result, doctors should make strategic planning an ongoing practice process. Doctors who do not do this risk the following:

- They may develop a practice that is unsatisfying in some fundamental aspect, such as the relations among colleagues, the kinds of patients, or the quality of the doctor-patient relationship.
- They may find that profitability is eroding due to new forms of competition, changes in revenue-expense relationships, and so on.
- They may discover that some of their skills have become obsolete due to new medical technology they neglected to anticipate or pursue.

Some organizations choose to make strategic evaluation an annual event. This can be useful, because it ensures that strategic reevaluations will occur. However, relying on a "strategic planning time" may not be responsive enough to changes encountered by your practice. Strategic *thinking*—interpreting events as they occur in light of their strategic implications—is an important supplement to examining your practice's strategy on a regular basis. A doctor who wants to remain competitive must constantly monitor the medical environment for changes and try to anticipate them. Since changes in medicine often imply significant capital expenditures and extensive training, it is essential to plan for these changes and to integrate them in an orderly manner into your practice's operational plans.

The following discussion will provide you with a framework and some tools for undertaking formal strategic management. By becoming familiar with this approach to management, you should also become more sensitive to those daily occurrences that have strategic implications. As a result, you will be able to act more responsively to strategically significant events.

STRATEGIC MANAGEMENT: TOOLS AND TECHNIQUES

Strategic management is a mindset. It is a way of thinking about events in the larger context. In order to think strategically, it is important to separate yourself emotionally and psychologically from present circumstances. You need to break from the present and be able to look at events unaffected by the compulsions of the moment. Figure 12-1 presents some tasks that can help you to think in strategic terms. They are separated into planning tasks and action tasks. The planning tasks involve defining the mission of your practice, translating that mission into long-

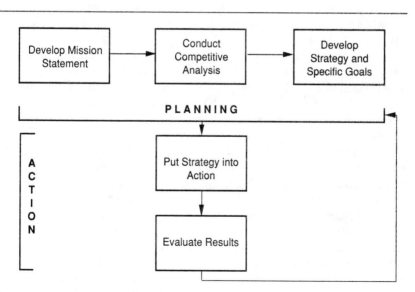

Figure 12-1 A Plan for Strategic Management

and short-term objectives, and developing a strategy for achieving those objectives. Once you develop the strategy, put it into action and then evaluate the results. The evaluation will be helpful in future planning.

The planning process begins with defining the mission of your business. This may seem like a trivial task, since its mission is defined, to some degree, by the content of your medical training. The object, however, is to define the mission of your *business*, not to simply restate the training that you received in medical school. Providing medical services is one aspect of the mission of your business. Other aspects could include

- personal financial security
- self-fulfillment and personal satisfaction
- developing collegial relationships
- income
- working with state-of-the-art techniques
- fulfilling various social responsibilities

Defining your practice's mission is important because it will provide you with guidance when responding to daily events. Exhibit 12-1 contains a sample mission statement for a psychiatric practice. The process of defining the practice's mission should not take untold days or weeks of introspection, long meetings with partners, or hours of exploration with a consultant. Be honest with yourself. If you have partners, be sincere with each other. What are *all* of the reasons you are practicing medicine? What are you trying to achieve both professionally and personally? By answering these questions, you can define the essence of your mission.

The mission statement will help you to deal with daily operational problems. For example, should you overlook a colleague's superiority attitude vis-à-vis the front office staff? Should you take a big financial risk to develop a managed care contract with a large local employer? Your mission statement will provide you with a touchstone to evaluate the options. A practice with the mission statement found in Exhibit 12-1 would have some guidance in resolving these questions.

Don't view a mission statement as an inflexible constraint. Instead, it should be a constant reminder of what you are about and why your practice exists. Operational policies that are inconsistent with this mission should be examined very carefully. A practice that routinely violates its mission statement runs the risk of becoming fragmented and uncoordinated in its actions. It may go off in several different, perhaps inconsistent, directions, thereby decreasing the chance that the ultimate objectives of the practice owners will be achieved.

Next, translate the mission statement into a strategic plan. This plan will contain specific short- and long-term goals for the practice and will specify how the practice will achieve these goals. A practice that has clear performance objectives, determines how it will reach these objectives, and then aggressively pursues them

Exhibit 12-1 Mission Statement for a Psychiatric Practice

Our Mission

Our mission is to provide *personalized* service to our patients and to do so in a manner that ensures the financial security of the practice, the satisfaction and development of our employees, and financially rewarding careers for our physicians.

Our Patients

Personalized service means that our patients will recognize that their health is important to us. We will do whatever is necessary to ensure that our patients understand this. Our commitment to personalized service will be reflected in all aspects of this practice, including treatment modalities, business arrangements, practice design, and the amount of time allocated to individual treatment.

Practice Finances

The practice will grow in an orderly manner so that its survival is never dependent upon the success of any single new program, idea, provider, or treatment modality. It will be managed in a fiscally conservative manner, with strong management controls, which will ensure its survival irrespective of changes in the business cycle, insurance considerations, and other external factors.

Our Employees

Our employees will be treated in an honest, respectful manner and will receive compensation that is consistent with community standards.

Our Services

We will provide the services needed by our patients, including both medical and psychotherapeutic services. We will provide inpatient psychiatric services at the leading area hospitals.

Financial Rewards

We will operate this practice so that we will receive financial rewards consistent with our education and work level. This will be reflected in our patient business policies, our compensation and retirement plans, and our fundamental financial decisions.

---

will generally outperform a practice that is managed on the basis of the momentary needs of its members or the immediate pressures of the marketplace. In order to identify specific short- and long-term goals and develop a strategy for attaining them, it is necessary to perform a competitive analysis.

A Competitive Analysis

The purpose of a competitive analysis is to identify those features of your practice's internal and external environment that will govern the feasibility of attaining goals and adopting strategies for achieving them. Figure 12-2 presents a competitive analysis model. You can use this model to examine both market competitive issues and your practice's specific circumstances. The resulting data will then allow you to evaluate strategy options and to select a specific strategic plan. You should consider the following:

The Economic Characteristics of Your Market

1. Is your market growing?
2. How many rivals do you have?
3. What is the pace of technological change?
4. What is the geographical range of your competition—local, regional, or national?

The Driving Forces

1. Are there changes in who is buying your services? (HMOs, PPOs, and employee assistance programs may represent changing sources of patients.)
2. How are advances in technology or medical knowledge affecting the type and price of services you provide?[1]

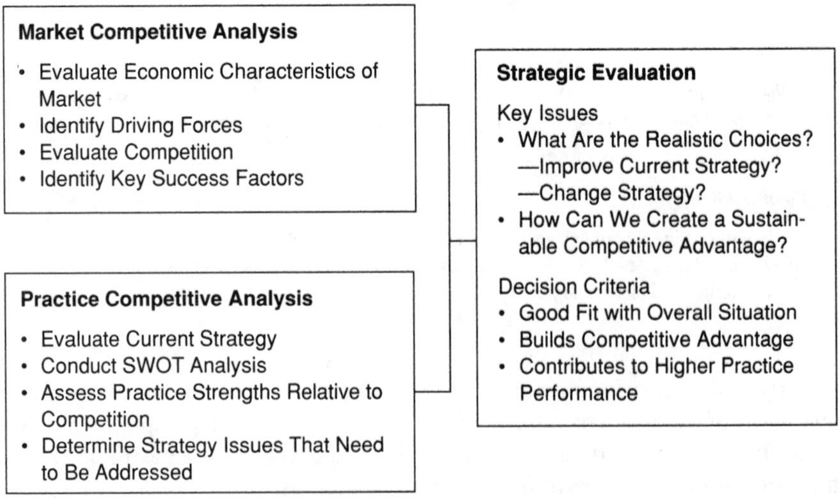

Market Competitive Analysis

- Evaluate Economic Characteristics of Market
- Identify Driving Forces
- Evaluate Competition
- Identify Key Success Factors

Practice Competitive Analysis

- Evaluate Current Strategy
- Conduct SWOT Analysis
- Assess Practice Strengths Relative to Competition
- Determine Strategy Issues That Need to Be Addressed

Strategic Evaluation

Key Issues
- What Are the Realistic Choices?
  —Improve Current Strategy?
  —Change Strategy?
- How Can We Create a Sustainable Competitive Advantage?

Decision Criteria
- Good Fit with Overall Situation
- Builds Competitive Advantage
- Contributes to Higher Practice Performance

Figure 12-2 A Competitive Analysis Model. *Source:* Adapted from *Strategic Management: Concepts and Cases*, ed. 5, by A.A. Thompson and A.J. Strickland, p. 58, with permission of Richard D. Irwin, Inc., © 1990.

3. How are innovations in marketing, such as promotional methods and changing standards, affecting the practice of medicine?
4. Are there changes occurring in cost and efficiency?
5. Are there regulatory and governmental changes that may affect your practice?
6. Is society changing its attitudes toward your services?

The Competition

1. Who are your rivals and what things can you do to gain a competitive edge?[2]
2. What is the potential for new competition?
3. What is the potential for alternative health care fields to provide substitute services?
4. How much power do buyers have? Will individual consumers, PPOs, HMOs, and employee assistance programs affect the pricing in your market?
5. What market strategies are used by your competition?

Key Success Factors

Key success factors are those things that a practice must do well in order to succeed. The key success factors may change with time, so it is important to be aware of changes in the preferences of patients and clients (PPOs, HMOs, referring physicians, and so on). Key success factors may include

- professional image
- location
- cost-effectiveness
- superior or unique medical skills
- marketing skills
- reputation for innovation

The second part of a competitive analysis consists of a review of your practice's specific situation. You can analyze your own competitive situation by examining the following:

Your Current Strategy

Your current strategy can be evaluated using a number of criteria, including income relative to competitors, financial reserves for future growth, ratio of time spent in clinical practice to time spent in management, and professional reputation.

1. Are there parts of your strategy that aren't working?
2. Are there parts of your strategy that are particularly effective?
3. If you don't have a formal strategy, identify the strategy that has evolved.

SWOT Analysis

SWOT is an acronym for strengths, weaknesses, opportunities, and threats. A strength is something that your practice is good at doing. A weakness is something your practice lacks or something that puts it at a disadvantage. An opportunity is an opening in the market that your practice can take advantage of. (Not all practices will be in a position to take advantage of a given opportunity.) Threats are environmental issues that may affect all medical practices, some medical practices, or only your own. Exhibit 12-2 lists some considerations to look for when performing a SWOT analysis. An effective strategy will do some or all of the following:

1. It will build upon practice strengths.
2. It will compensate for weaknesses.
3. It will take advantage of opportunities.[3]
4. It will provide defenses against threats.[4]

Your Practice's Strength Relative to Competitors

How does your practice compare with competitors on key success factors? Sometimes it is useful to rate your competitors. Table 12-1 contains a sample competitive strength assessment. Don't become overly fixated, however, on the numbers.[5] Instead, focus on the *reasons* you are stronger or weaker than other practices.

Strategic Issues That Need to Be Addressed

Review the market competitive analysis and the practice competitive analysis. At this point most of the major issues should be clear, and your objective should be to identify major strategy alternatives. Issues to consider include these:

- Is your present strategy likely to succeed given the information at hand?
- How well does your present strategy fit with projected future key success factors?
- How well will your present strategy fare against future external threats and internal weaknesses?

Exhibit 12-2 SWOT Analysis—What to Look For

Potential Strengths
1. A distinctive competence
2. Adequate financial resources
3. Good competitive skills
4. Well thought of by patients
5. Well respected by peers
6. Access to economies of scale
7. Insulated from competitive pressures
8. Proprietary technology or skills
9. Cost advantages
10. Effective marketing
11. Proven management
12. Superior skills
13. Strong referrals from other physicians
14. Other

Potential Weaknesses
1. No clear strategic direction
2. Obsolete facilities
3. Sub par profitability because . . .
4. Lack of managerial depth or talent
5. Missing key skill or competence
6. Internal operating problems
7. Very narrow scope of services
8. Weak market image
9. Poor location
10. Below average marketing skills
11. Limited financial resources
12. High costs relative to competitors
13. Other

Potential Opportunities
1. Serve additional customer groups
2. Enter new markets or segments
3. Broaden services to meet more patient needs
4. Diversify into related services
5. Move into new geographic markets
6. Complacency among rivals
7. Fast market growth
8. Other

Potential Threats
1. Entry of more competitors
2. Entry of alternative health care providers (chiropractors, nurse practitioners, psychologists, etc.)
3. Slow market growth
4. Costly regulatory or licensing requirements
5. Vulnerability to recession, business cycle, changes by major employers, etc.
6. Growth of consumerism
7. Changing patient tastes and needs
8. Adverse demographic changes
9. Other

Source: Adapted from *Strategic Management: Concepts and Cases*, ed. 5, by A.A. Thompson and A.J. Strickland, p. 91, with permission of Richard D. Irwin, Inc., © 1990.

- How vulnerable is your practice to external attack?
- What aggressive moves could be made to take advantage of opportunities, make the practice more competitive, reduce costs, and deter or block threats?

Next, evaluate your strategic situation. *Realistically* examine the choices that are available to you. Is it possible to improve on your current strategy? Modifying a current strategy will generally be less disruptive and risky than going off in a totally new direction. What things, if any, can you do to create a sustainable competitive advantage? When answering these questions, use these evaluation criteria:

Table 12-1 Competitive Strength Assessment

Key Success Factors	You	A	B	C
Professional Competence	9	9	7	5
Effective Marketing	5	6	2	8
Location	7	9	5	5
Access to Patient Referral Groups	2	5	5	8
Management Skills	7	3	?	?
Mean	6	6.4	4.75	6.5

Rating Scale: 10 = strongest; 1 = weakest; ? = no information available.

1. the fit between the strategy and internal and external findings
2. the degree to which a strategy will create a competitive advantage
3. the extent to which changes will result in increased performance, greater productivity, better patient care, and so on

Strategic Options

A successful strategy will be consistent with both the external and internal findings of your competitive analysis. Table 12-2 outlines some generic strategies and summarizes some of the internal and external issues to consider when evaluating strategies. When you are evaluating strategy alternatives, it is important to keep the following considerations in mind:

1. Do not set as an objective the attainment of a competitive advantage that is impractical to achieve.
2. Realistically evaluate whether practice personnel have the skills, time, and motivation to follow through on a strategy. An overly ambitious plan may create internal problems and put strains on your resources and personnel. In addition, a strategic change may not be consistent with the personal objectives of all employees or partners. As noted earlier in the discussion of motivation, people work to achieve their own objectives. A change in strategy may result in turnover, hostility, and perhaps sabotage if it is perceived as inconsistent with an individual employee's objectives. This should not deter you from pursuing strategic change, but you should take into account potential resistance to change (see Chapter 6).
3. A strategy that is a radical departure from your current course can be very risky. Such a strategy should only be undertaken after considerable analysis and thought.

Table 12-2 Generic Strategic Options

Medical Environments	Practice Positions	Situational Considerations	Market Share Options	Strategy Options
Rapid growth	Dominant leader	External	Grow and build	Competitive Approach
Consolidating to a	Leader	Driving forces	Capture bigger market	Low cost
smaller group of	Aggressive	Competitive pressures	share and grow faster than	Differentiated services,
competitors	challenger	Anticipated moves of	competitors	location, hours, skills,
Mature/slow growth	Content follower	key rivals	Invest heavily	technology
Aging/declining	Weak/distressed	Key success factors	Fortify and defend	Offensive initiatives
Fragmented	candidate for	Internal	Protect market share	Attack, end run, guerrilla
Rapid change,	turnaround/exit	Current performance	Grow as fast as medical	warfare
increasing high	No clear strategy or	Strengths/weaknesses	market	Defensive initiatives
technology	market image	Threats/opportunities	Retrench and retreat	Fortify/protect
		Cost position	Surrender weakly held	Retaliatory
		Competitive strength	positions when forced	Harvest
		Strategic issues and	Fight hard for core markets	Turnaround
		problems	Maximize short-term cash	Revamp strategy
			flow	Operational changes—
			Minimize reinvestment of	reduce cost, increase
			capital	revenues, sell assets,
			Overhaul and reposition	etc.
			Try to turn around	
			Abandon/liquidate	
			Sell out	
			Close down	

Source: Adapted from *Strategic Management: Concepts and Cases,* ed. 5, by A.A. Thompson and A.J. Strickland, p. 158, with permission of Richard D. Irwin, Inc., © 1990.

4. Avoid a strategy that can work only if everything goes smoothly. There will always be surprises, and few things in life go exactly as planned.

5. Prepare for the responses of your competitors. If the strategy works, how will your competitors react? Are there any defensive strategies that you might implement along the way so that you can retain your competitive advantage?

Specific strategies only make sense given the particular details of your situation. Here are some generic strategies to consider. They are intended to stimulate your thinking.

The Low-Cost Producer. This strategy may be relevant when trying to attract groups of patients from a large employer, group of employers, or managed health care system or when targeting certain types of patients.[6] The strategy is to offer lower prices and thereby gain market share and make a profit on volume. Another option is to offer services at going rates, treat a lower volume of patients, and obtain a higher profit margin by controlling costs. Offering low prices relative to competitors means that the practice must be cost conscious in every aspect of business. Tight budgeting, elimination of waste, frugal design of office space, and thin personnel staffing are intrinsic to this strategy.

Differentiation. A differentiation strategy is based on identifying patients with different sets of needs. One or more of these needs form the basis for a practice strategy. Practices that can successfully differentiate their services may be able to command premium fees. Medical services can be differentiated on several bases, including technical superiority, image quality, and location. For example, a physician who is the sole provider of a service in an area has achieved differentiation. Structuring a practice around a unique service can generate many referrals at premium fees. Differentiation can also be based on providing superior quality services or more complete services. For example, the orthopedic surgeon who can offer hip replacement patients a complete inhouse package of x-ray examination, surgery, and physical therapy may have a competitive advantage.

Differentiation can have its disadvantages. If patients do not *perceive* the differentiated product as truly beneficial, then there will be no competitive advantage. If the differentiated service is successful, it may well generate imitators. True differentiation only occurs when you can generate an advantage that is not easily imitated. Differentiation can also fail in the following situations.

- The differentiation is based on something that doesn't really lower the price or isn't perceived as really increasing the patient's well-being.
- The price is set too high.
- The value is not perceived by patients even though it is real.[7]

Attacking. Generally, it is not acceptable in medicine to *directly* attack your competitors. You can, however, attack your competitors' strengths and weak-

nesses. Opening satellite practices, using image advertising, and using price reductions to obtain managed cost contracts are all legitimate forms of attack.

End Run. An end run attack achieves market share by changing the rules of the
game. Opening a satellite practice in a new area and introducing a technological
innovation are both end run strategies. Recently, a Richmond surgeon became the
first in Virginia to use laser surgery for gallbladder removal. By effectively promoting the advantages of this technique throughout the state, he greatly expanded
his market, took the "high ground," and put all other competitors in the *state*
market in the position of having to catch up.

Guerrilla Warfare. Guerrilla warfare is characterized by attacks directed at the
weak points of carefully selected competitors. It can be a very effective strategy
for small practices in a market with mature, larger, well-entrenched competitors.
This strategy also can be useful for new practitioners in a saturated market. Guerrilla attacks must focus on weakly defended or over extended services or patient
groups. For example, if you know that an employer has been unhappy with the
services provided by a practice, you can attack by going after that employer's
contract. Similarly, doctors in markets where little advertising has occurred may
be particularly vulnerable to effective marketing of services through the media.

Fortifying and Protecting. This is a defensive strategy designed to block the
advances of adversaries. Generally, service businesses use a fortifying and defending strategy to protect referral sources. Written contracts, wining and dining,
acknowledging referrals, and providing quality service make it difficult for chal-
lengers to divert referrals.

Harvesting. Harvesting is a strategy for orderly withdrawal from a market
while at the same time collecting a harvest of cash.[8] Harvesting is accomplished
by cutting budgets to a minimum, reducing advertising expenses, reducing quality
in those areas where it will not show, eliminating nonessential services, reducing
or eliminating equipment maintenance, subletting or selling excess office space,
and so on.

Harvesting is appropriate when a practice is in an undesirable position and the
doctor wishes to totally restructure the practice or kill it off. Harvesting can create
the capital necessary to finance a turnaround or it can precede liquidation. In any
event, it is a strategy that can buy time for a final decision. Consider the following
case example:

> Ralph Early did not enjoy his solo private practice. He found the experi-
> ence to be lonely, he did not enjoy cultivating referral sources, and he
> did not find managing the day-to-day affairs of a small practice to be
> rewarding. His lease expired in six months, and he decided that he
> would prefer working for a large hospital doing clinical, educational,
> and administrative work. While negotiating an agreement to work for a
> hospital, he began a harvesting strategy. He eliminated a part-time cleri-

cal position, a nursing position, and a telephone line and reduced his supply inventory to a minimum. He also accelerated into his remaining months of private practice any personal expenses that he thought his future employer might not compensate him for. Finally, he limited the time each day that his business manager would take patient calls so that she could work back accounts and maximize collections.

Turnaround. A turnaround strategy is appropriate when a practice is in crisis, it is worth saving, but the current strategy has led to very serious financial or management problems. The first task in a turnaround strategy is diagnosis. A misdiagnosis can be fatal, since the practice by definition is already in a weakened state. It is essential at this point to determine whether the crisis has been caused by poor implementation or an ineffective strategy. Common problems that can precipitate the need for a turnaround strategy include

- buying market share with low fees while underestimating the actual cost of delivering the services (this can be a real danger of fixed fee, HMO, and PPO arrangements)
- excessive fixed costs associated with underutilized office space, equipment, or personnel
- never gaining or even losing market share as a result of competitors' actions
- overreliance on a new procedure or technological innovation that does not generate the expected revenues

Attempting a turnaround can be very risky. Hall studied 64 companies that had attempted a turnaround; none of them succeeded.[9] The turnaround attempts failed because the firms either waited too long to begin or had insufficient cash or managerial talent to recover in slow growth industries. Following are five generic approaches to undertaking a turnaround:[10]

1. *Revamp the existing strategy.* If the cause of the problem is strategic as opposed to operational, then this approach is appropriate. Strategic problems are essentially flaws in the approach to the market. Operational problems usually result from incompetent execution of the strategy. Revamping can be undertaken with any of the strategies noted above.
2. *Increase revenues.* This approach is necessary when there is no way to cut expenses. The strategy for approaching the market remains the same. However, operational changes are made to increase revenues. Revenues can be increased by hiring additional physicians or allied health care professionals, offering additional services, adding office hours, and so on. If demand is inelastic and you are a nonparticipating physician, you can raise your

fees. If demand is elastic, raising your fees may result in driving patients to your competition, thereby reducing your revenues.

3. *Reduce costs.* Once again, the strategy for approaching the market remains the same. However, operational plans stress cost reductions in all aspects of the practice. Reducing costs will only work if the items associated with the costs do not generate revenue or if their associated costs can be reduced at a greater rate than their associated revenues. In order to use this tactic, cost inefficiencies must be identifiable and the cost-revenue relationship must be understood. Costs can be reduced by eliminating unneeded or underemployed positions, eliminating underutilized services (e.g., E-claims), increasing the use of budgets, and undertaking a general belt tightening.

4. *Sell assets.* Big ticket capital items (e.g., x-ray equipment, computers, lab equipment) that are not being efficiently utilized can be sold. The cash generated can then be used to finance other revenue-generating programs and services.

5. *Use a combination of approaches.* A turnaround need not be elegant. Use any and all of the approaches that seem relevant. A change of strategy can be coupled with the other approaches, or these approaches can be used with the current strategy. Generally, the more serious the problem, the more likely it is that you will have to consider a broad, rapid attack on the problem.

IMPLEMENTING THE STRATEGY

After identifying a strategy, the next step is to implement it. The object is to achieve the tightest possible fit between the strategy and how your practice operates in each of the functional areas covered in this book. Everything this book may have taught you regarding staffing, performance evaluation, leadership, motivation, organizational structure, budgeting, marketing, revenue collection, and computers must be applied *in the context of your strategy.*

Both professional and nonprofessional employees must have the qualifications, skills, and motivation to achieve your objectives in the way specified by your strategy. To the extent that the necessary skills are difficult or costly to acquire through training, the practice must acquire them through employee or partner selection.

Employee rewards must act as a link between employees' perceptions of their own personal objectives and the implementation of the strategy. As noted in Chapter 5, people don't work for you, they work for themselves. If you properly structure the situation, people will work *with* you to achieve your goals because of the mutually desirable consequences. Rewards must be based on results, and the results rewarded must be consistent with the practice strategy.

Your budgets must provide the financial means for implementing the strategy. They must also ensure that resources are used efficiently so that you will have sufficient funds for the most critical parts of your strategy. Your marketing plan will be your blueprint for approaching the market, and it must be in harmony with your overall practice strategy. Some marketing people would maintain that your marketing strategy *is* your practice strategy. Computer hardware and software, as well as all other capital equipment, must be selected based on their ability to contribute to achieving your objectives by way of the specified strategy.

Supporting all of this should be shared values, shared ethical standards, and a productive work environment. If employees or partners don't truly believe in the practice's mission and the means of achieving that mission, then they will not have the commitment to follow through in difficult times. In addition, they won't have a *theory* instructing them how to behave in those circumstances where there is no clear policy or procedure.

Finally, the doctor's role in this process is to orchestrate the implementation of the strategy. Possible leadership styles range from the directive to the delegative, and the doctor may choose to pursue strategic imperatives quickly or slowly. The decisions regarding leadership style and pace must be based on the immediate circumstances. A doctor who is already in practice and who is modifying a previously developed strategy (or one that simply evolved) can adapt his or her leadership style to the demands of the situation. If things are going along well and the desired changes will be relatively minor or subtle, then a consultative approach and a longer period of implementation may be suitable. As pointed out in Chapter 5, consultation with others spreads the ownership of an idea, thereby creating motivation on the part of others to make the idea work. If, on the other hand, the practice's existence is being threatened, it may be necessary to use a more directive approach and to put the changes into place sooner.

A doctor who is entering private practice has the opportunity to define a strategy before creating his or her practice's structure. However, the doctor can easily be faced with too many strategic decisions and not enough time or information. There are no easy solutions to this problem. Perhaps the best tactic is to approach strategy implementation with some degree of humility. Admitting that you don't know and asking for opinions and advice is a far better tactic than acting with bravado on the basis of rudimentary information. Consulting with peers and colleagues and judiciously using consultants can give you a perspective on how best to put your strategic plan into effect.

Case Example

Dr. Fred Stanley was the founder of a group psychiatric practice. He had been dissatisfied working for other physicians, so he decided to develop his own practice. He envisioned a practice composed of two or three other owners that would provide a very high standard of care in a well-appointed, upscale office suite. He was looking for a relaxed team atmosphere in which he could work with respected, cooperative colleagues. Consistent with this strategy, he rented an office suite in a "class A" office building and proceeded to decorate the waiting room with Chippendale reproductions and his own office with art deco furnishings highlighted by a large black marble desk. He had five other treatment offices, and by the time that he opened his doors he had hired three other providers.

During the practice's first year, Dr. Stanley hired George Michael, Ph.D., to fill one of the two open offices. Dr. Michael had a full caseload, but his patients required considerable front office attention. They tended to be more remiss in paying their copayments and generally had less desirable insurance coverage. In addition, Dr. Michael was very demanding of the office staff. He was abrupt, often interrupted conversations between the office staff and others, and was almost always running too late to be courteous. In addition, he required far more typing, transcription, and scheduling support than any other provider. All of this created tension within the practice. Nevertheless, Dr. Michael generated substantial revenue for the practice, so Dr. Stanley tolerated and to some degree tried to manage his behavior. Dr. Stanley discussed these problems on several occasions with Dr. Michael, and on more than one occasion the discussion degenerated into a confrontation.

Toward the end of the practice's first year, the building owners contacted Dr. Stanley regarding his first right of refusal on the unrented office space adjoining his suite. An attorney had offered to rent the space, so Dr. Stanley either had to rent the space now or be precluded from expanding during the four remaining years on his lease. A month before Dr. Stanley had been notified about the office space, Lionel Filbert, M.D., had contacted him about joining his practice. Dr. Stanley at first rejected the idea, although he did not immediately communicate this to Dr. Filbert. Dr. Filbert's caseload was almost entirely composed of chemically dependent families and adolescents. Because of the nature of their problems, these patients tended to be irresponsible. They often cancelled or did not show for appointments, avoided their financial responsibilities, and came up with many creative ways of not paying their bills. In addition, Dr. Filbert had a reputation for being demanding of office staff, having unrealistic expectations, and responding emotionally to everyday problems. On the other hand, Dr. Filbert treated in excess of 45 patients each week, plus hospital rounds, and his reputation with this patient population was excellent.

In light of the office space option, Dr. Stanley reconsidered his decision regarding Dr. Filbert. Using a break-even analysis, Dr. Stanley calculated that Dr. Filbert's contribution margin would just about cover the additional monthly rental. The added office space could provide room for five additional providers.

Dr. Stanley calculated that if he could fill several of the other offices, he would have a very profitable practice. Balanced against this was the knowledge that his present office suite was still not filled and that, in the event he was not able to recruit additional providers, he could have a serious financial problem if Dr. Filbert ever decided to leave. In addition, he anticipated that it would be difficult to work with Dr. Filbert.

Dr. Stanley, tempted by the opportunity to have a larger practice, retained Dr. Filbert with a partnership option and leased the additional office space. The next year and a half were very difficult for him. He had numerous problems with Dr. Filbert's patients, hired three secretaries for Dr. Filbert (none of whom Dr. Filbert considered to be adequate), and received a fairly steady stream of "emergency" calls from him on weekends and evenings regarding "office problems." In addition, Dr. Filbert and Dr. Michael formed an "alliance of misery." Staff meetings were largely consumed with responding to their complaints, and from Dr. Stanley's perspective they never had anything positive to say or to contribute to the practice atmosphere. Finally, other producers were becoming dissatisfied because the "squeaky wheels" in the practice did get oiled. The secretaries and the business manager attended first to the needs of Drs. Filbert and Michael.

During this period of time, Dr. Stanley was able to hire two additional producers. The office morale, however, was very low. Dr. Stanley became concerned that two other producers, whom he eventually wanted to become partners, would become so dissatisfied that they would leave. In addition, Dr. Stanley was becoming very frustrated with his practice, as indicated by these comments:

> In hindsight I can see what happened. I lost sight of what was really important to me and where I wanted to go. Dr. Filbert didn't fit with the practice strategy. Unfortunately, I wasn't thinking *strategy* when I hired him. I knew what it would be like to work with him, but I only saw that as a daily inconvenience. I didn't understand that in combination with Dr. Michael, I would be inadvertently changing the fundamental philosophy and reason for being of this practice. We went from a low-volume, high-quality, calm practice to a high-volume, frantic crisis center. Our location, our rent, our furnishings, our marketing are all based on my original mission statement. These are all wasted on our current clientele. I could just as easily attract them in a strip shopping center office space with crate furniture at 50 percent less rent. In addition, the office chaos and animosity has given us a reputation as a bad place to work. I now find it very difficult to attract additional producers.

> Dr. Filbert and Dr. Michael are not bad people. They simply don't belong here. To make them belong here, I would have to adjust our mission—to include their approach to practice. It's not a question of right or

wrong, good or bad. It's simply an issue of fit. Right now we don't have a fit, and life is difficult for everyone.

Beyond the satisfaction issues, Dr. Stanley anticipated some additional long-term consequences due to the lack of fit. Dr. Michael would probably leave in six months when his contract expired. Dr. Filbert might well leave when his contract expired in eight months, simply because he was always dissatisfied about everything! In addition, the continuing presence of both Drs. Michael and Filbert for the next several months might drive away Dr. Stanley's other producers. Dr. Stanley saw the prospect of having a large office suite to himself in eight months. Dr. Stanley stated,

> I have to go back to my initial strategy. This will be very difficult and dangerous. I could choose to continue going in the direction in which my practice has evolved, but I can see now that it would mean developing a very different practice, and I don't *want* to do that. I will have to terminate both Dr. Michael and Dr. Filbert. In addition, I must do it soon so that the others will see that I intend to change the direction of this practice.

> A break-even analysis shows that we should be able to scrape by if we are really careful about costs, sublet the added office space, and cut our nonessential spending to the bone. Hopefully, over time, the reputation of the practice will improve so that I will be able to recruit other producers and fill my original office space.

CONCLUSION

Having a clear practice strategy will help you to make operational decisions that are consistent with practice objectives. In the absence of a strategy, decisions are often made that have very significant unintended consequences. This chapter should have made you aware of why you should think in strategic terms and encouraged you to undertake strategic planning at the inception of a practice and on a routine basis.

There are a number of tools that can help you organize your strategic thinking. There are also a number of generic strategies that you can use as points of departure when evaluating your practice's strategic options. Discussion of these tools and options, as well as case examples of doctors who had to contend with the consequences of implicit and explicit strategic choices, should provide you with the means and the motivation to evaluate your strategic choices and put your strategy into effect.

NOTES

1. For example, there appears to be a trend in general internal medicine toward providing more care at the office and less in the hospital. In addition, the nature of office care seems to be changing, with an increased emphasis on preventive care and health maintenance. As a result, internists now devote more of their time to talking to and educating their patients. These trends may have implications for office staffing and design. See S. Wartman, "Internal Medicine," *JAMA* 263 (1990): 2649–51.

2. You can answer this question by examining the local market as well as national trends. For example, a report by the AMA's Council on Long Range Planning and Development stated that the primary source of competition for internists in coming years will be subspecialty internists and that some subspecialties may expand their range of services to obtain a larger and more secure patient base. See "The Future of General Internal Medicine," *JAMA* 262 (1989): 2097–100.

3. For example, the American Academy of Family Physicians found that only 40 percent of its members provided some level of obstetric care and that an additional 40 percent had discontinued obstetric services. The risk of malpractice litigation was cited as the reason for this trend. At the same time, the decrease in the availability of obstetric services may create an opportunity for less faint-hearted family practice physicians. See R. Bredfledt, J. Colliver, and R. Wesley, "Present Status of Obstetrics in Family Practice and the Effects of Malpractice Issues," *Journal of Family Practice* 28 (1989): 294–97.

4. The Clinical Laboratory Improvement Amendments of 1988 will soon require the accreditation of office laboratories, and the accreditation process will include proficiency testing. For some physicians, compliance testing and federal paper work may be a threat to their ability to provide in-house laboratory testing. Anticipating this threat by developing a strategy for compliance would constitute a defense. See M. Goldsmith, "Federal Proficiency Testing Requirements Set to Start for Physician Office Laboratories," *JAMA* 263 (1990): 2355–56.

5. An alternative rating scheme would be to weight each of the key success factors and use the weights to adjust the practice ratings. This approach, however, places an emphasis on numbers instead of the reasons for the underlying strengths and weaknesses.

6. For an example in which low cost was an inherent part of a practice strategy, see J. Norman, "Can a Practice Serving the Poor Avoid Financial Quicksand?" *Medical Economics*, February 5, 1990, 79–87.

7. A.A. Thompson and A.J. Strickland, *Strategic Management: Concepts and Cases*, 5th ed. (Homewood, IL: BPI/Irwin, 1990), 114.

8. P. Kotler, "Harvesting Strategies for Weak Products," *Business Horizons* 21, no. 5 (1978): 17–18; P. Kotler and R. Clarke, *Marketing for Health Care Organizations* (Englewood Cliffs, N.J.: Prentice-Hall, 1987), 98, 342; F. Paine and C. Anderson, *Strategic Management* (Hinsdale, Ill.: Dryden Press, 1983), 246–47.

9. W.K. Hall, "Survival Strategies in a Hostile Environment," *Harvard Business Review* 58, no. 5 (1980): 75–85.

10. C.W. Hofer, "Turnaround Strategies," *Journal of Business Strategy* 1 (Summer 1980): 19–31; Thompson and Strictland, *Strategic Management*, 155.

Chapter 13

Great Expectations: The Personal and Emotional Aspects of Private Practice

In life, what usually creates the most pain, hurt, disappointment, and difficulty for us are our own great expectations—or, better stated, our own unrealistic expectations of ourselves and others. What happens when expectations are unrealistic? They play havoc with our emotions, thereby interfering with our interpersonal relationships, with our feelings about ourselves, and with our ability to act in a rational, problem-centered manner. Fear, anger, and anxiety begin to control us, and we act in ways that are ineffective and self-defeating.

Many doctors initially have unrealistic expectations concerning the demands of running a business. For some, reality causes them to adjust their expectations to more realistic levels. Other physicians, however, begin with unrealistic expectations and never give them up. They continue to assume that their expectations are correct and that the world simply isn't cooperating! In fact, their experiences are typical of what people encounter when they run a business, but their expectations are unrealistic.

Understanding and mastering the personal and emotional aspects of private practice is essential to success. The purpose of this chapter is to help doctors anticipate some of the personal and emotional effects of running a practice. This is important for three reasons:

1. You may be able to react more quickly to and work more effectively with personal and emotional issues if you are aware that they are real and that they can affect your practice.
2. If you believe your difficulties are unique, you may begin to feel helpless and hopeless. By understanding that they are not unique and that others have undergone similar ordeals, you may be less frightened or troubled during times of great stress.
3. Understanding what underlies your personal reactions to a situation may give you a more positive mindset. This may help you to deal more effec-

tively with employees, patients, and business issues and get more enjoyment out of running your own practice.

What, then, are typical expectations concerning the operation of a private practice? They basically fit into three categories. The first category includes expectations of others, including employees and associates. The second category includes expectations of oneself. The third category includes expectations regarding how the business world operates.

EXPECTATIONS OF EMPLOYEES AND ASSOCIATES

Starting a practice is a very exciting process. It is easy for you to become caught up in the excitement of opening your own business. It is also easy to fall into the trap of expecting others, especially employees, to have similar feelings and degrees of commitment. Others may initially be enthusiastic, but their enthusiasm usually fades. No one will care as much about "your baby" as you do, and no one will be as willing as yourself to sacrifice and struggle when times are difficult. This can also be a problem with other partners, who perhaps don't have as large a financial stake or who simply don't have the same degree of psychological investment in the practice.

Others' lack of caring may manifest itself in a number of ways. For example, your receptionist might walk through the waiting room and fail to pick up a candy wrapper that is lying on the floor. On a more serious plane, one of your partners might promise to review the practice aging analysis on Saturday but spend the entire weekend on a camping trip. These incidents have two levels of significance. First, you should be concerned because someone did not perform a task you felt should have been performed. At another level, you may be exasperated because the events are symbolic of an uncaring, irresponsible attitude. They may indicate that people whom you trusted really don't *care*. You then begin to wonder, "What other things are they doing where they also don't care about the results?"

When this happens, you are likely to be surprised. Then you might have an emotional reaction—probably disappointment, anger, or some combination of the two. How appropriate are such reactions? And should you have them? The answers to these questions depend on the degree of investment in the practice that the other person should have. It is unrealistic to expect that employees who have no ownership should have a degree of commitment beyond what their immediate jobs call for. To expect more than this is simply setting yourself up for disappointment. To expect, for example, that employees will routinely provide you with overtime or weekend hours or will frequently change their schedules to meet practice needs is unrealistic. You can *demand* these things, and you may be able to obtain them, but don't expect that employees will cooperate because they feel a commitment to the success of your practice.

Employees work for the goals that are important to them. Expectancy theory, discussed in Chapter 5, suggests that you should not expect employees to work as though they were owners when they will not in fact enjoy the rewards or benefits of ownership. Nonexempt employees, especially, will perceive demands beyond the ordinary duties of their jobs as inequitable. Generally, employees who perceive inequity will regain equity indirectly, for example, by being cold or uncaring toward a patient or by not picking up a candy wrapper in the waiting room. It is important, therefore, that you look at the situation from the employees' perspective so that you don't have unrealistic expectations of your employees. Unrealistic expectations on your part will result in disappointment, doubts about your own management ability, and employee turnover (if I was a good manager, he never would have . . .). Should you comment about the wrapper to the secretary? You probably should, and the secretary may pick up the next wrapper that she sees. Don't expect, however, that the secretary will translate this into the concept of a duty and then apply it to the next equivalent but different event.

When a partner behaves in ways that you perceive as unfair or irresponsible, then feelings of disappointment, anger, and even betrayal are appropriate. What should you do about the situation? You don't have many choices. You must immediately discuss the matter with your partner. Discuss the problem at both the factual *and* the emotional level. Tell the partner about your expectations and how her actions made you *feel*. If you were disappointed or angry, let your partner know. This will be helpful to you, because you will reduce your frustration by "getting it off your chest." It also tells the partner how her behavior has affected you, and the discussion process may help to clarify any misperceptions regarding mutual expectations. Pretending that nothing has happened will only allow time for your resentment to grow and will create the opportunity for similar occurrences.

Usually, directly addressing the circumstances will result in both parties adjusting their behaviors and expectations. However, suppose your partner continues to behave in ways that you perceive as inequitable. Assuming you have tried to clarify your expectations, you may then conclude that the transgressions were the result of conscious decisions. Your partner simply doesn't care about your feelings or what you need. In effect, your partner is not functioning as a partner and is probably focusing more on her own personal needs. When circumstances reach this point, you may need to consider getting a "divorce." This is the time to look out for your own interests and to weigh the financial and personal value of continuing the partnership against the frustration, inconvenience, and financial costs associated with dissolving the business relationship. Once again, the underlying theme is that people work for themselves. If a partnership is such that one party will tolerate a disproportionate share of the burden, then the other party will invariably take advantage of this situation. Conducting civil war to regain equity will almost certainly lead to a practice that is dysfunctional. If you and your partner cannot work together without one or both of you feeling unfairly treated, then you may be best off to recognize this reality and end the relationship.

PERSONAL EXPECTATIONS

Doctors are intelligent, well-trained, high-achieving professionals who expect to reach their goals. They have to be this way in order to survive the selection and educational processes required to become doctors. Most doctors receive no formal business training. In addition, many doctors, especially those who are going into practice for the first time, have had relatively little experience dealing with people other than health care professionals and patients. As a result, doctors often have unreasonable expectations regarding the amount of control that they will have over their practices.

In many ways, this is analogous to the situation of first-time parents. First-time parents often have a vision of parenthood that is an amalgam of their recollections of childhood and their present needs as adults. They are certain that if they can only plan well enough and work hard enough, their child will develop in the way they desire. Intellectually, they may understand that the child will be a distinct human being and have his or her own set of desires, needs, and abilities, but they never fully accept this vulnerability to uncontrollable forces.

You may have similar hopes and aspirations for your practice, along with similar expectations that you will be able to realize them by controlling events. You may have a vision of an office staff that will be dedicated to helping you attain your personal goals. You may also imagine that if you can work hard enough, you will achieve success and be able to maintain control over your business. Some doctors envision a practice that effortlessly (perhaps magically) takes care of all those things that are necessary to support their clinical needs. They seldom anticipate having to deal with the messy details of running a business because there is nothing in their background to prepare them for the reality. This is about as realistic as the image of a crying, wet baby in which the crying and the wetting don't have any disagreeable qualities.

The expectation that you will be truly in control and that you can force events to occur the way that you wish is a fallacy. You can influence events to varying degrees, but you cannot control your practice as if it were an extension of yourself. As soon as you hire your first employee or obtain your first patient, you lose this degree of control. The larger your practice becomes, the more it takes on a life of its own which to some extent meets the competing needs of your employees, partners, patients, the community and to some degree yourself. You cannot be everywhere all of the time, and when and where you are absent, partners, employees, and patients may make decisions based on their needs, decisions that are not always in your best interest.

Someone once said that running a business is like being in a war. You are going to have casualties, and the casualties may be your needs and desires. The goal is to take *acceptable* casualties in relation to the objectives you achieve. No secretary will be perfect. Some fees will not be collected and some telephone messages will be lost. Occasionally charts will be misfiled, and employees, partners, and patients will not live up to their promises. The list of daily failures can appear endless *if you choose to log them*. If you are of a mind to, you can create an inexhaustible list of events over which to become upset. What you must keep in mind, however, is whether, in spite of these failures, you are achieving the objectives stated in your practice's mission statement (see Chapter 12). This is not to say that you should be unconcerned about setting high performance standards, since if you don't set them, no one will. Instead, this is a call for *balance* and *realism* in the enforcement of those standards. If a secretary is getting 90 percent of the job right and the 10 percent that is not right is also not critical, think long and hard before trying to get that last 10 percent. Ask yourself whether that last 10 percent will show up significantly in either better patient care or on the financial bottom line, and then ask yourself what price you may have to pay in order to get it. Experienced managers know when to push. They push when it makes a difference and they back off when it doesn't.

It is vitally important that you examine your own need for perfection. A perfectionistic attitude can result in pushing for perfection at the wrong times or in the wrong places. Virtually every element of a doctor's development and training encourages perfectionism. Perfectionism is adaptive in the practice of clinical medicine, since inattention to detail can significantly affect the well-being of patients. Medicine attracts people who are intellectually oriented toward facts and details and who enjoy pursuing cause-and-effect relationships, and the demands of medical education tend to eliminate people who are not concerned with nuances. Finally, the doctor-patient relationship is an unequal one. The patient is in a dependent position, which tends to reinforce the doctor's expectation that his or her demands will be followed unquestioningly.

Unbridled perfectionism can result in striving for that last 10 percent when it really doesn't matter. If you don't choose when to be demanding, you will waste a lot of energy fighting battles of no great consequence and you will create a tense, confrontational work environment within your practice.

BUSINESS EXPECTATIONS

It is important to have realistic expectations of the way that others will act in business relationships. In many ways, business relationships are like the criminal justice system. In the criminal justice system, each side advocates its strongest possible position. The competition of ideas and facts, as filtered by the law, reveals the truth, which is determined by a judge or jury. In the business world, each business seeks to maximize its own gain by presenting its most competitive product or service. Business law, business ethics, standards of practice, and community standards serve as the law in this competition, and the marketplace, which is both jury and judge, will determine the value of the competing services. Your gain is generally a competitor's loss, and vice versa.[1] In addition, everyone in your business environment is trying to survive, and someone else's survival might be at your expense. Every time that you turn around, someone will be trying to take money out of your pocket. Employees expect pay raises, cities increase taxes on revenues and personal property, suppliers raise their prices, insurance companies increase their premiums while simultaneously tightening their claims payment criteria, some patients will not pay for services, equipment will break—the list is endless.

This sounds like the Law of the Jungle, and it is. For many doctors, however, these business realities are masked by a very forgiving jungle in which there is a plentiful supply of patients. Tigers can become fat and complacent when the food supply is abundant. Businesses, including medical practices, may begin to expect that revenues will always flow in irrespective of the competition and the changing market conditions. For some doctors in some specialties, this may always be the case. Others, however, may enter a market in which increasing competition or declining patient demand will mean that at some point the doctor will be confronted with the need to run a leaner, more effective business.

A realistic business expectation is that others will act so as to increase their chance of immediate financial gain. Any other consideration will only be important to the extent that it increases their chance of future financial gain. It is important to understand this, because it may help you discover openings that will maximize your own financial gain, as well as avoid being taken advantage of in an increasingly rough world.

Case Example

Dr. Jones, a general surgeon, leased office space from Johnson Realty Associates. Her lease contained a cost-of-living adjustment clause. After the first year of the lease, Johnson Realty did not assess a rental increase. After the second year of the lease, Johnson Realty assessed an increase for both the first and second years, stating that an employee, who had subsequently been fired, had neglected to assess the first year's increase. Dr. Jones, after clarifying with her attorney that she did owe the first year's assessment, met with Johnson officials. She informed them that she was very upset about their failure to notify her of the assessment after the first year. As a result, she had assumed that there would be no assessment the first year and had therefore not budgeted for it. The Johnson Realty officials were very apologetic and offered to let Dr. Jones spread the payments over six months. They stated that they wanted to keep Dr. Jones content because they wanted her to renew her lease after it expired in two years.

Johnson Realty did not offer to mitigate Dr. Jones's immediate financial problem out of altruism or a sense of fairness. They did not feel sorry or in any way ethically burdened because of the bungled first year's assessment. Instead, they offered Dr. Jones a payment plan because they were afraid that she might be upset enough over the incident to leave in two years. Their ultimate concern was the added cost of having to rent the office space to another tenant, plus the risk that it would sit idle for several months. Dr. Jones, being an astute listener, learned for the first time how Johnson Realty perceived *their* business vulnerabilities. Dr. Jones, seeing an opportunity to maximize her gain, offered the Johnson Realty officials an alternative. She told them that if they reduced the increase by 50 percent in compensation for her inconvenience, she would pay them immediately and not allow the incident to influence her decision in two years. Johnson Realty countered by saying they would agree to these terms if Dr. Jones would immediately extend the lease for an additional year. Dr. Jones stated that she would not extend her lease now and that if Johnson Realty did not agree to her terms, she definitely would allow the incident to affect her decision two years hence. Johnson Realty agreed to Dr. Jones's proposal.

This case illustrates that actions are driven by their financial consequences. In this adversarial climate, the practice that does not operate by these rules is working at a disadvantage. Was it unfair or unethical for Dr. Jones to press for a "take back" that Johnson Realty was not obligated to give her under the terms of the lease? It should be remembered that Dr. Jones was truthful and that the subject of the negotiation was the *degree* of reparations that Johnson Realty should pay for the inconvenience they had caused Dr. Jones. Dr. Jones took an aggressive approach. Johnson Realty was willing to pay for some good will, since it might affect the negotiations in two years. The eventual outcome was fair to both parties, since each side made a choice based on what was of value to it at the time. The underlying philosophy presented here is one that has been stated many times in this book: *You are the only person who will look out for your own interests. If you will not represent the best interests of your practice, who will?*

Sometimes it will be in your interest to forgo a short-term gain in order to achieve a long-term objective, as Johnson Realty did. Releasing a patient from a financial obligation, providing community services or seminars at cost, or taking employees' personal needs into consideration can all be done for ethical reasons. If, however, these actions come into conflict with immediate organizational goals, you should test them against your long-term objectives. If they are inconsistent with your long-term objectives, then you have a choice of satisfying the competing needs or the needs of your business. If you make such decisions only after careful consideration, then you may be able to avoid situations in which you compromise your interests to a degree that threatens your survival in the jungle.

THE JOYS OF THE BUSINESS ASPECTS OF PRIVATE PRACTICE

Attending to the business aspects of your practice can be exciting and enriching. You have an opportunity to create something new, to breathe life into something that was formerly just a dream. The character of your practice can be an expression of your personality and your professionalism. The decisions you will make regarding strategy, personnel relations, marketing, revenue collections and so on, are *your* decisions. You can, if you wish, shape your practice so that it contributes substantially to your ability to provide quality clinical services. Most people work their whole lives for other masters. Making the decisions and accepting and meeting the challenges and responsibilities of running your own business can give you the sense of freedom that many strive for in our society but few ever experience.

The business aspects of your practice can provide you with an opportunity for personal growth. Many doctors have to learn new skills and, perhaps more importantly, new ways of thinking about problems. Obtaining new knowledge and skills while simultaneously treating patients and running a business may require you to stretch yourself. The business aspects of your practice will challenge your values and priorities and your ability to cope with stress. Nevertheless, as you overcome these new challenges, you will feel a sense of pride and accomplishment that will complement the satisfaction you experience from your clinical successes.

The business aspects can also provide you with the kind of excitement that is a natural concomitant of creative, risk-taking endeavors. There are few real adventures in modern life; opening a small business is one of them. Doctors are generally well prepared intellectually for this challenge. The business world, however, is a great equalizer, and it will throw challenges at you from every direction. Each day can present you with new problems and new opportunities. Solving the problems and taking advantage of the opportunities can give you a kind of satisfaction that those who have never been entrepreneurs will never know. For many doctors, taking the chance regardless of the outcome will be worth the effort. For these doctors, trying and failing—or determining that private practice is not satisfying, as some doctors do—is far better than growing old filled with regrets and wondering, "What would have happened if I had tried?"

Finally, a private practice can provide you with an opportunity to experience the pleasure of finding and working with other professionals who are of like mind. There is satisfaction and security in being able to rely on well-chosen peers and in the realization that together you have created an organization that is better than each could have created alone. Once again, you must look to your own values and what you want to achieve. A solo practice will allow you to be a composer and a performer, whereas a group practice will allow you to be an orchestrator and a conductor. Both alternatives can be fulfilling.

Your education and hard work have given you the chance to create an independent, satisfying life in which you will have more control over your own fate than most people in our society. By successfully managing the business aspects of your practice, you will be able to ensure that you have the necessary support for providing the clinical services that you were trained to provide. Finally, meeting the challenges that arise will give a sense of personal growth and achievement and deep satisfaction.

NOTE

1. This is not true in the case of a high-growth market, where it is possible for all competitors to grow without taking market share from each other. Realistically, even in high-growth markets practices will be trying to take market share from competitors, and in fact market share will typically shift between practices.

Point System of Job Evaluation

KNOWLEDGE

Knowledge is the result of education and experience. Education provides knowledge through formal schooling, whereas experience provides knowledge through training and working on the job. (See Table A-1.)

NONSUPERVISORY RESPONSIBILITY

This factor concerns the degree of analytical ability, judgment, discretion, and timeliness involved in making decisions. It also concerns how education and experience are applied to the job, but it does not cover responsibility for personnel administration, which is covered elsewhere. (See Table A-2.)

Consider the following when evaluating the vertical scale of the chart:

1. What decisions are made?
2. What are the most difficult decisions and actions?
3. Is independent judgment required or are decisions based on precedent?
4. How frequently are decisions made?
5. Consider all of the responsibilities for the position even if some of them are delegated to a subordinate. For example, an office manager may be responsible for revenue collection even if some specific collection tasks are delegated to a billing clerk.
7. Remember, making decisions is more important than making recommendations.

Table A-1 Factor: Knowledge

Experience (in years)

Education	Under 1	1–2	2–3	3–4	4–5	5–6	More Than 6
High school degree	110	120	135	150	170	195	230
High school plus some specialized courses	135	145	160	175	195	220	255
High school plus many additional courses up to the equivalent of one year of college	160	170	185	200	220	245	300
Extensive courses beyond high school, one or two years of college, business school, or technical training	210	220	235	250	270	295	350
Courses equivalent to two or three years of college	265	275	290	305	325	350	405
Bachelor's degree	325	335	350	365	385	410	465
Master's degree or equivalent graduate degree	385	395	410	425	445	470	525
Master's degree or equivalent, plus other graduate degree or certification	445	455	470	485	505	530	585
Doctorate	510	520	535	550	570	595	650

Table A-2 Factor: Nonsupervisory Responsibility

This factor measures the degree to which making decisions and taking action are important to the job. It is composed of the degree of complexity of analytical ability, judgment, etc., when making decisions or taking actions, the degree of review provided, and the inconvenience and cost associated with inadequate performance.

Column A = Decisions/actions reviewed regularly. Limited effect on operations.

Column B = Decisions/actions reviewed regularly. Inadequacies would only result in minor problems.

Column C = Decisions/actions usually reviewed. Inadequacies could cause moderate inconvenience or expense.

Column D = Decisions/actions occasionally reviewed. Inadequacies could cause considerable problems or expense and could affect patient health.

Column E = Decisions/actions occasionally reviewed. Inadequacies could cause extensive inconvenience or expense and could affect patient health.

Column F = Decisions/actions rarely reviewed. Inadequacies could cause extensive inconvenience or expense and could affect patient health.

Column G = Decisions/actions rarely reviewed. Inadequacies may affect long-range practice plans and strategies and could affect patient health.

Column H = Decisions/actions usually final. Inadequacies may affect long-range practice plans and strategies and could affect patient health.

Column I = Decisions/actions usually final and may seriously affect long-range plans or patient health.

Column J = Decisions/actions are final and would seriously affect long-range plans or patient health.

continues

Table A-2 continued

	A	B	C	D	E	F	G	H	I	J
1. Operating procedures are well defined and independent activity is limited.	120	140	165	195	245	315	415	560	765	1060
2. Operating procedures are generally covered by clear rules, regulations, instructions, etc. Decisions/actions required are not complex.	140	160	185	215	265	335	435	580	785	1080
3. Makes operating decisions and takes some actions of importance. Occasional decisions of considerable complexity.	165	185	210	240	290	360	460	605	810	1105
4. Makes operating decisions and takes actions of moderate difficulty. Occasional actions/decisions of considerable complexity.	195	215	240	270	320	390	490	635	840	1135
5. Makes frequent operating decisions and takes actions of considerable difficulty. Assists in the formulation of recommendations on difficult and important issues.	245	265	290	320	370	440	540	685	890	1185
6. Assists in the formulation of and, on occasion, independently formulates recommendations on difficult and important matters.	315	335	360	390	440	510	610	755	960	1255
7. In addition to the above, sometimes makes independent decisions and takes independent action on important matters.	415	435	460	490	540	610	710	855	1060	1355
8. Frequently makes independent decisions and takes independent action on important operating matters.	560	580	605	635	685	755	855	1000	1205	1500
9. Continually makes independent decisions and takes independent action on very important operating matters.	765	785	810	840	890	960	1060	1205	1410	1705
10. Continually makes independent decisions and takes independent action on operating matters of the greatest importance.	1060	1080	1105	1135	1185	1255	1355	1500	1705	2000

Consider the following when evaluating the horizontal scale of the chart:

1. What is the extent to which decisions are reviewed by superiors?
2. What is the potential cost or seriousness of errors? How often are decisions required that could have serious costs or consequences?
3. How much time could elapse before an error is detected?
4. Evaluate the job under normal day-to-day conditions. Don't place disproportionate weight on unusual or unlikely circumstances.

For both the horizontal and vertical scales, if a subordinate position merits more points than the position being evaluated, assign the number of points associated with the subordinate position.

INGENUITY

This factor concerns the creativeness and resourcefulness required by the position. For example, would the incumbent be responsible for creative thinking, developing new ideas, or devising plans? Evaluate the position based on how much ingenuity is normally required, not how much might be required in unusual circumstances. The key issue is whether the job requires ingenuity, not whether a particular incumbent happens to be personally creative. (See Table A-3.)

PERSONNEL MANAGEMENT RESPONSIBILITY

This factor concerns the amount of organizing, leading, coordinating, training, and controlling of employees that is required. It assesses both line and functional responsibilities. *Line responsibilities* are defined as organizing, selecting, training, promoting, dismissing, setting performance objectives, evaluating, and directing the actions of others. As an example of a line relationship, consider a business manager who directly controls the actions of a subordinate secretary.

Functional responsibilities are concerned with implementing programs and policies through employees, however, the position does not have direct line authority over the other positions. As an example of a functional relationship, consider a business manager who must use secretaries for revenue collection, but the secretaries report on a line basis to the office manager. (See Table A-4.)

The following should be considered when evaluating jobs on this factor:

1. Only consider responsibilities for managing employees.
2. It is important to determine whether the position has line responsibilities, functional responsibilities, or both.

Table A-3 Factor: Ingenuity

	A	B	C
1. Requires little original or independent thinking.	100	115	130
2. Requires occasional ingenuity in the refinement of ideas originated by others.	150	170	195
3. Ingenuity is definitely required, but it usually involves the refinement of established ideas, procedures, methods, etc.	225	260	300
4. Some original and independent thinking in originating and developing new or improved ideas.	350	400	475
5. Frequent application of a high degree of original and independent thinking in developing complex ideas in new, undefined areas.	550	625	700
6. Continuous application of a high degree of creativeness, resourcefulness, and inventiveness. Originates very complex creative ideas in new and undefined areas. Creativity has major effect on the practice.	800	900	1000

Note: The B point values should be used when the definition closely matches the job. The A or C columns can be used for jobs that are somewhat above or below the definition but not to a significant enough extent to select a higher or lower degree definition.

3. When evaluating line responsibilities, consider the diversity of supervisory activities involved, the type of employees being supervised, and any extenuating or complicating issues.
4. When evaluating functional responsibilities, consider the diversity of activities, the types of employees with whom the incumbent must work, and any extenuating or complicating issues.
5. It is often more difficult to get things done through employees in a functional relationship than in a line relationship.
6. If a subordinate position merits more points than the position being evaluated, assign the number of points associated with the subordinate position.

OUTSIDE RELATIONSHIPS

This factor concerns the extent to which the incumbent must interact with others outside of the practice, including insurance companies, patients, physicians,

Table A-4 Factor: Personnel Management Responsibility

	Number of Line Subordinates Supervised				
	None	1–5	6–10	11–15	16 or More
1. Little or no line or functional responsibility.	120	130	140	155	170
2. Line responsibilities are primarily simple and routine *or* functional responsibilities are limited to advice or guidance, with no responsibility for control or follow-up.	130	140	150	165	180
3. Line responsibilities are generally routine and involve the same or similar activities *or* some functional advice and guidance, usually without responsibility for control or follow-up.	145	155	165	180	195
4. Line responsibilities are somewhat complex and occasionally difficult but involve the same or similar activities *or* frequent functional advice and guidance, usually without responsibility for control or follow-up.	160	170	180	195	210
5. Line responsibilities are moderately complex and occasionally difficult and involve varied activities or work groups *or* frequent functional advice and guidance, with some control responsibilities, of limited complexity, for upholding standards.	180	190	200	215	230
6. Line responsibilities are generally complex and difficult and involve varied moderately complex activities or work groups *or* moderately complex functional control responsibilities for upholding standards.	205	215	225	240	255
7. Line responsibilities are complex and difficult, somewhat diversified, and involve complex activities or work groups *or* complex functional control responsibilities for upholding standards.	235	245	255	270	285
8. Line responsibilities are highly complex and diversified and involve highly complex activities or work groups *or* highly complex functional control responsibilities for upholding standards.	275	285	295	310	325
9. Line responsibilities are of extreme complexity and involve activities and work groups of extreme complexity *or* functional control responsibilities of extreme complexity.	420	430	440	455	470
10. Line responsibilities are of maximum complexity *or* functional control responsibilities of maximum complexity.	790	800	810	830	860

and so on. It is important to determine whether these outside contracts involve simply exchanging information or whether something more significant occurs, such as influencing the decisions of others. Consider the level of people being contacted, the frequency of contact, and whether the nature of the communication is to elicit or provide information. (See Table A-5.)

Table A-5 Factor: Outside Relationships

	A	B	C
1. Outside contacts are limited to the exchange of information with employees in other organizations who do not make decisions. Little tact or negotiating skills required. Contacts are fairly infrequent.	50	65	80
2. Outside contacts are required that involve some tact and diplomacy; on occasion they may influence decisions *or* contacts may occur frequently but only involve the exchange of information.	100	120	150
3. Outside contacts are inherent in the position and they require tact and diplomacy and frequently influence decisions of moderate importance. They could involve discussions with management at relatively high levels.	190	240	300
4. Outside contacts are a major job responsibility. They involve important decisions, require negotiation and tactical skills, and occur at high organizational levels.	360	430	500

Note: The *B* point values should be used when the definition closely matches the job. The *A* or *C* columns can be used for jobs that are somewhat above or below the definition but not to a significant enough extent to select a higher or lower degree definition.

Index

About the Author

Robert J. Solomon, Ph.D., is associate professor of business administration at the Graduate School of Business, College Of William And Mary, in Williamsburg, Virginia. He received his doctorate in industrial and organizational psychology from the University of Rochester, and he received his B.A. from Case Western Reserve University. Dr. Solomon has consulted with many organizations, including private practices, on such topics as employee and office management, marketing, hiring methods, and collection of receivables. He has published over 25 professional papers on such topics as marketing, employment methods, practice management, and practice decision making. He is also vice-president of a private group practice that offers psychological and psychiatric services.

DATE DUE			
NOV 02 '92			
AUG 30 '93			
OCT 27 1992			